Study Guide for

INTRODUCTION TO HUMAN ANATOMY AND PHYSIOLOGY

■ ■ ■

Third Edition

Eldra Pearl Solomon, PhD

Mical K. Solomon, LMT

Karla Solomon, RN

SAUNDERS

ELSEVIER

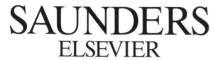

SAUNDERS
ELSEVIER

11830 Westline Industrial Drive
St. Louis, Missouri 63146

STUDY GUIDE FOR INTRODUCTION TO
HUMAN ANATOMY AND PHYSIOLOGY

ISBN: 978-1-4160-4406-2

Notice

ISBN: 978-1-4160-4406-2

or: Jeff Downing
mental Editor: Karen C. Maurer
Services Manager: Deborah Vogel
er: Pat Costigan
Kim Denando

USING THE STUDY GUIDE

Learning anatomy and physiology has been compared to learning a new language. To understand how the body is constructed and how it functions, you must learn the language used by health professionals. The exercises included in the *Study Guide for Introduction to Human Anatomy and Physiology* are designed to help you learn both the words and the concepts presented in the textbook, *Introduction to Human Anatomy and Physiology*, by Eldra Pearl Solomon, PhD. Working through the exercises, diagrams, and crossword puzzles will help you test your mastery of the material and gain both knowledge and confidence.

The following steps will help you use this Study Guide effectively.

1. Read the Outline presented at the beginning of the chapter. The outline reflects the organization of the corresponding textbook chapter and provides you with an overview of the material in the Study Guide chapter.
2. Read the Learning Objectives and refer back to them frequently as you work through the chapter exercises. The Learning Objectives tell you what you need to do to demonstrate mastery of the material.
3. Answer the Study Questions provided for each section. After you complete a section, check your answers in the Answer Key at the back of the book. If one or more of your answers are incorrect, reread the corresponding sections in the textbook.
4. Label the diagrams that are provided in appropriate sections throughout the Study Guide. To check the accuracy of your labels, consult the corresponding labeled diagram presented in the textbook.
5. When you feel confident that you have learned the material in the chapter you are studying, check your level of mastery by completing the Chapter Test at the end of the chapter.
6. To build your confidence even more, complete the Crossword Puzzle provided for the block of chapters you are studying. Answers are provided in the Answer Key.

CONTENTS

Chapter

1

INTRODUCING THE HUMAN BODY

■ ■ ■

Outline

I. Anatomy and physiology are the studies of structure and function.
II. The body has several levels of organization.
III. The body is composed of inorganic compounds and organic compounds.
IV. Metabolism is essential to maintenance, growth, and repair of the body.
V. Homeostatic mechanisms maintain an appropriate internal environment.

VI. The body has a basic plan.
  A. Directions in the body are relative.
  B. The body has three main planes.
  C. We can identify specific body regions.
  D. The body has two main body cavities.
  E. It is important to view the body as a whole.

Learning Objectives

After you have studied this chapter, you should be able to:

1. Define anatomy and physiology.
2. Describe the levels of biological organization in the human body from the simplest (the chemical level) to the most complex (the organism).
3. Describe the principal organ systems.
4. Distinguish between inorganic and organic compounds, and briefly describe four important groups of organic compounds.
5. Define metabolism, and contrast anabolism and catabolism.

6. Define homeostasis, and contrast negative and positive feedback mechanisms.
7. Describe the anatomical position of the human body.
8. Define and properly use the principal directional terms used in human anatomy.
9. Recognize sagittal, transverse, and frontal sections of the body and of body structures.
10. Define and locate the principal regions and cavities of the body.

STUDY QUESTIONS

Within each category, fill in the blanks with the correct response.

I. ANATOMY AND PHYSIOLOGY ARE THE STUDIES OF STRUCTURE AND FUNCTION

~~Adapted~~   **Anatomy**   ~~Biology~~   **Gross**   ~~Physiology~~   **Shape**   **Structure**

1. _Anatomy_ is the science of body structure.

2. _Physiology_ is the science of body function.

3. Each body part is precisely _adapted_ for carrying out its specific function.

4. In the body, the size, ___shape___, and ___structure___ of each part are related to the job the part must perform.

5. ___Biology___ anatomy focuses on structures that can be studied by dissection.

6. Cell ___gross___ is the study of the structure, function, and interaction of cells.

II. THE BODY HAS SEVERAL LEVELS OF ORGANIZATION

Atom	Cells	Cellular	Chemical	Connective	Epithelial
Functions	Microscope	Molecules	Muscle	Nervous	Organ
Organelles	Organism	Organs	Tissue	Water	

1. The simplest level of organization in the body is the ___chemical___ level.

2. A(n) ___Atom___ is the smallest amount of a chemical element that has the characteristic properties of that element.

3. Atoms combine chemically to form ___molecules___.

4. Two atoms of hydrogen combine with one atom of oxygen to form one molecule of ___water___.

5. The level of organization above the chemical level is the ___cellular___ level.

6. In living things, atoms and molecules associate in specific ways to form ___cells___, the building blocks of the body.

7. Although cells vary in size and shape according to their function, most are so small that they can be seen only with a(n) ___microscope___.

8. Each cell consists of specialized cell parts called ___organelles___.

9. The next highest level of organization above the cellular level is the ___tissue___ level.

10. A tissue is a group of closely associated cells specialized to perform particular ___functions___.

11. The four main types of tissue in the body are ___connective___, ___epithelial___, ___muscle___, and ___nervous___.

12. Tissues are organized into ___organs___, such as the brain, stomach, or heart.

13. A group of tissues and organs that work together to perform specific functions makes up a body system, or ___organ___ system.

14. Working together with great precision and complexity, the body systems make up the living ___organism___.

III. THE BODY IS COMPOSED OF INORGANIC COMPOUNDS AND ORGANIC COMPOUNDS

~~Amino~~	Carbohydrates	Chemical	DNA	Enzymes	~~Inorganic~~
~~Ion~~	Nucleic	~~Organic~~	Proteins	RNA	Steroids

1. A(n) _Ion_ is an electrically charged atom or group of atoms.

2. A(n) _____ compound is a molecule that contains two or more different elements combined in a fixed proportion.

3. _Inorganic_ compounds are relatively small, simple compounds such as water, salts, simple acids, and simple bases and are required for many cell activities such as transporting materials through cell membranes.

4. _Organic_ compounds are large, complex compounds containing carbon. They are the chemical building blocks of the body.

5. _____ are sugars and starches; they are used by the body as fuel molecules and to store energy.

6. _____ are an important group of lipids that includes several hormones such as the male and female sex hormones.

7. Proteins are large, complex molecules composed of subunits called _amino_ acids.

8. _____ are catalysts that regulate chemical reactions.

9 The kinds and amounts of _____ in a cell determine to a large extent what a cell looks like and how it functions.

10. Two very important _____ acids are DNA and RNA.

11. _DNA_ makes up the genes, and contains the instructions for making all the proteins needed by the cell.

12. _____ is a type of chemical compound important in the process of manufacturing proteins.

IV. METABOLISM IS ESSENTIAL TO MAINTENANCE, GROWTH, AND REPAIR OF THE BODY

~~Anabolism~~	ATP	~~Breaking down~~	Building	~~Catabolism~~
Cellular respiration	~~Metabolism~~	Nutrients	Oxygen	Synthetic

1. All the chemical processes that take place within the body are referred to as its _Metabolism_.

2. Two phases of metabolism are _Anabolism_ and _Catabolism_.

3. Catabolism is the _Breaking Down_ phase of metabolism.

4. Cells obtain energy from food molecules by a complex series of catabolic chemical reactions referred to as _Cellular Res._.

5. During cellular respiration, nutrients are used as fuel; they are slowly broken down and the energy released is packaged within a special energy storage molecule called _ATP_.

6. Cellular respiration requires _Nutrients_ as well as _Oxygen_.

7. Anabolism is the _Building_ or _Synthetic_ phase of metabolism.

V. HOMEOSTATIC MECHANISMS MAINTAIN AN APPROPRIATE INTERNAL ENVIRONMENT

Homeostasis	Negative	Negative feedback
Positive	Positive feedback	Stressor

1. Metabolic activities occur continuously in every living cell and they must be carefully regulated to maintain _Homeostasis_ —an appropriate internal environment.

2. A _Stressor_ is a stimulus that disrupts homeostasis, and causes stress in the body.

3. In a _Neg_ system, a change in some steady state triggers a response that is opposite to the change.

4. Most homeostatic mechanisms in the body are _Negative_ feedback systems—like the thermostat in your furnace or air conditioning system.

5. In a _pos_ system, the variation from the steady state sets off a series of events that intensify the changes.

6. The delivery of a baby is an example of a _positive_ feedback system.

VI. THE BODY HAS A BASIC PLAN

Bilateral	Cranium	Mirror	Vertebral column

1. The body consists of right and left halves that are _Mirror_ images; that is, it has _Bilateral_ symmetry.

2. Two of the structures that characterize humans as vertebrates are the _Cranium_, or brain case, and the backbone, or _Vertebral Column_.

A. Directions in the Body Are Relative

Anatomical	Anterior	Axis	Caudal	Cephalic	Closer
Deep	Distal	Dorsal	Inferior	Lateral	Medial
Midline	Posterior	Proximal	Superficial	Superior	Ventral

1. In the _Anatomical_ position, the body is standing erect, eyes looking forward, arms at the sides, and the palms and toes are directed forward.

2. The "north pole" of the human body is the top of the head, its most __superior__ point.

3. The "south pole" of the body is represented by the soles of the feet, its most __inferior__ part.

4. The heart is superior to the stomach because it is _____ to the head.

5. The terms _____ and "cranial" are sometimes used instead of "superior."

6. The term _____ is sometimes used instead of "inferior."

7. The front (belly) surface of the body is _____ or _____.

8. The back surface of the body is _____ or _____.

9. The body _____ is an imaginary line extending from the center of the top of the head to the groin.

10. The main superior-inferior body axis is _____, going right through the midline of the body.

11. A structure is said to be medial if it is closer to the _____ of the body than to another structure.

12. A structure is _____ if it is toward one side of the body.

13. When a structure is closer to the body midline or point of attachment to the trunk, it is described as _____.

14. _____ means farther from the midline or point of attachment to the trunk.

15. Structures located toward the surface of the body are _____.

16. Structures located farther inward (away from the surface of the body) are _____.

B.   The Body Has Three Main Planes

Axes   **Frontal plane**   **Midsagittal plane**   **Sagittal plane**   **Transverse plane**

1. The body has three _____, each at right angles to the other two.

2. A(n) _____ divides the body into right and left parts.

3. A(n) _____ passes through the body axis and divides the body into two mirror-image halves.

4. A(n) _____ divides the body into superior and inferior parts.

5. A(n) _____ divides the body into anterior and posterior parts.

C. We Can Identify Specific Body Regions

Appendicular   Axial   Cephalic   Cervical   Cranial   Torso

1. The body may be subdivided into a(n) _____ portion, consisting of the head, neck, and trunk.

2. The _____ portion of the body consists of the limbs.

3. The _____ consists of the thorax, abdomen, and pelvis.

4. The _cranial_ region refers to the head.

5. The _cervical_ region refers to the neck.

6. The _____ region refers to the skull.

D. The Body Has Two Main Body Cavities

Abdominopelvic   Cavities   Cranial   Diaphragm   Dorsal
Pericardial   Thoracic   Ventral   Vertebral

1. The spaces within the body that contain the internal organs are called the body _____.

2. The two principal body cavities are the _____ cavity and the _____ cavity.

3. The dorsal cavity is subdivided into the _____ cavity, which holds the brain, and the _____ canal, which contains the spinal cord.

4. The ventral cavity is subdivided into the _____, or chest cavity, and the _____ cavity.

5. The thoracic and abdominopelvic cavities are separated by a broad muscle, the _____, which forms the floor of the thoracic cavity.

6. The heart is surrounded by the _____ cavity.

E.   It Is Important to View the Body as a Whole

Labeling Exercise

Please fill in the correct labels for Figure 1-1.

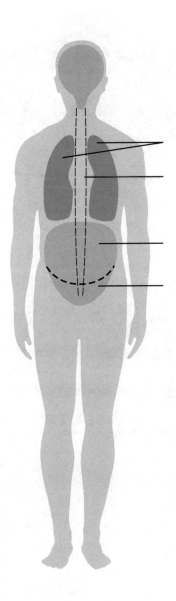

Labeling Exercise

Please fill in the correct labels for Figure 1-2.

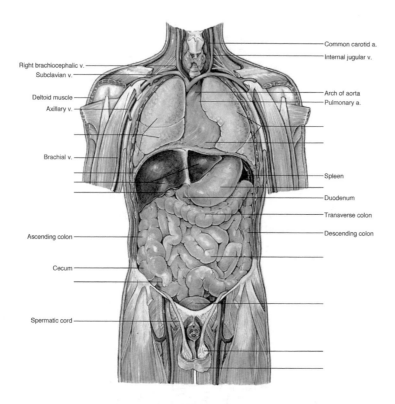

Right brachiocephalic v.
Subclavian v.
Deltoid muscle
Axillary v.
Brachial v.
Ascending colon
Cecum
Spermatic cord

Common carotid a.
Internal jugular v.
Arch of aorta
Pulmonary a.
Spleen
Duodenum
Transverse colon
Descending colon

CHAPTER TEST

Select the correct response.

1. The study of anatomy is the
   a. science of body structure.
   b. science of body function.
   c. science of cell structure.
   d. both a and b.

2. The study of physiology is the
   a. science of body structure.
   b. science of body function.
   c. science of cell structure.
   d. both a and b.

3. Each cell consists of specialized cell parts called
   a. organs.
   b. protons.
   c. organelles.
   d. molecules.

4. The information and control center of the cell is the
   a. cytoplasm.
   b. neutron.
   c. nucleus.
   d. ribosome.

5. An electrically charged atom is called a(n)
   a. proton.
   b. ion.
   c. electron.
   d. molecule.

6. _____ are sugars and starches; they are used by the body as fuel molecules.
   a. Carbohydrates
   b. Fats
   c. Steroids
   d. Proteins

7. Steroids are an important group of _____ which include hormones; for example, male and female sex hormones.
   a. lipids
   b. carbohydrates
   c. glucose
   d. proteins

8. _____ are catalysts that regulate chemical reactions.
   a. Amino acids
   b. Enzymes
   c. Lipids
   d. Carbohydrates

9. Proteins are composed of subunits called
   a. amino acids.
   b. nucleic acids.
   c. carbohydrates.
   d. lipids.

10. _____ is a nucleic acid that makes up the genes (hereditary material).
    a. RNA
    b. DNA
    c. ERA
    d. ATP

11. All of the chemical processes that take place within the body are referred to as its
    a. metabolism.
    b. mitosis.
    c. anabolism.
    d. chemicalism.

12. Cells obtain energy from food molecules by a complex series of catabolic chemical reactions called
    a. homeostasis.
    b. cellular respiration.
    c. anabolism.
    d. catabolic energy production.

13. Metabolic activities occur continuously in every living cell and they must be carefully regulated to maintain
    a. cellular respiration.
    b. positive feedback.
    c. homeostasis.
    d. metabolism.

14. When the body is erect with the eyes looking forward, the arms at the sides, and the palms and toes directed forward, it is said to be in the _____ position.
    a. standing
    b. front
    c. anatomical
    d. physiologic

15. When the body is in the anatomical position, the brain is _____ to the heart.
    a. inferior
    b. superior
    c. superficial
    d. It depends on the individual.

16. The _____ plane divides the body into right and left parts.
    a. sagittal
    b. transverse
    c. frontal
    d. mirror

17. The dorsal cavity is subdivided into the _____ cavity, which holds the brain, and the _____ canal, which contains the spinal cord.
    a. ventral; cranial
    b. vertebral; spinal
    c. cranial; vertebral
    d. ventral; cranial

18. The ventral cavity is subdivided into the _____ cavity and the _____ cavity.
    a. thoracic; chest
    b. thoracic; abdominopelvic
    c. thoracic; diaphragm
    d. dorsal; ventral

Chapter

2

CELLS AND TISSUES

■ ■ ■

Outline

I. The cell contains organelles that perform specific functions.
   A. Membranes surround the cell and divide it into compartments.
   B. The nucleus controls cell activities.
   C. The cytoplasm contains many types of organelles.
II. Materials move through the plasma membrane by both passive and active processes.
III. Cells communicate by signaling one another.

IV. Cells divide by mitosis, forming genetically identical cells.
V. Tissues are the fabric of the body.
   A. Epithelial tissue protects the body.
   B. Connective tissue joins body structures.
   C. Muscle tissue is specialized to contract.
   D. Nervous tissue controls muscles and glands.
VI. Membranes cover or line body surfaces.

Learning Objectives

After you have studied this chapter, you should be able to:

1. Describe the general characteristics of cells.
2. State three functions of cell membranes and describe the structure of the plasma membrane.
3. Describe the structure and functions of the cell nucleus.
4. Describe, locate, and list the functions of the principal cytoplasmic organelles, and label them on a diagram.
5. Explain how materials pass through cell membranes, distinguishing between passive and active processes.
6. Predict whether cells will swell or shrink under various osmotic conditions.

7. Describe the events that take place in cell signaling.
8. Describe the stages of a cell's life cycle and summarize the significance of mitosis with respect to maintaining a constant chromosome number.
9. Define the term *tissue* and describe the structure and functions of the principal types of tissues.
10. Contrast epithelial tissue with connective tissue.
11. Compare the three types of muscle tissue.
12. Identify the main types of membranes and contrast the main types of epithelial membranes.

STUDY QUESTIONS

Within each category, fill in the blanks with the correct response.

I. THE CELL CONTAINS ORGANELLES THAT PERFORM SPECIFIC FUNTIONS

Amino acids	Cell	Cytoplasm	Electron	Functions
Light	Microscope	Organelles	Ovum	

1. The ___Cell___ is a complex structure consisting of a control center, internal transportation system, power plants, and packaging plants.

2. The __Microscope__ is one of the biologist's most important tools for studying the internal structure of cells.

3. Most cell structures were first identified with an ordinary __light__ microscope.

4. The development of the __electron__ microscope enabled researchers to study the fine detail (ultrastructure) of cells and their parts.

5. The size and shape of a cell are related to the specific __Function__ it must perform.

6. The __ovum__ is one of the largest cells in the human body.

7. The jellylike material of the cell is called __cytoplasm__.

8. A great variety of substances needed by the cell are dissolved within the cytoplasm. For example, __amino acids__ found in the cytoplasm are used as subunits of proteins.

9. Scattered throughout the cell are specialized __organelles__ (little organs) that perform different functions within the cell.

A. Membranes Surround the Cell and Divide It into Compartments

Lipids   Plasma

1. Every cell is surrounded by a thin __plasma__ membrane that protects the cell and regulates the passage of materials into and out of the cell.

2. The plasma membrane consists of a double layer of __lipids__ in which a variety of proteins are embedded.

B. The Nucleus Controls Cell Activities

Chromosomes   DNA   Genome   Nucleolus   Nucleus

1. The __Nucleus__, a large, rounded organelle, is the control center of the cell.

2. When a cell prepares to divide, the chromatin in the nucleus becomes more tightly coiled and condenses to form rod-shaped bodies called __Chromosomes__.

3. Genes are composed of the chemical compound __DNA__.

4. The complete set of genes that make up the human genetic material is the human __Genome__.

5. The __Nucleolus__ is a specialized region within the nucleus where ribosomes are assembled.

C.   The Cytoplasm Contains Many Types of Organelles

ATP	Cellular respiration	Cilia	Endoplasmic reticulum
Free radicals	Golgi complex	Lysosomes	Mitochondria
Proteins	Ribosomes	Rough	Smooth
Vesicle			

1.   The __ER__ is a system of membranes that extends throughout the cytoplasm.

2.   There are two types of endoplasmic reticulum: __smooth__ and __rough__.

3.   Rough endoplasmic reticulum has a granular appearance that results from the presence of organelles called __ribosomes__ along its outer walls.

4.   Ribosomes function as factories where __proteins__ are manufactured.

5.   Looking somewhat like a stack of pancakes, the __golgi complex__ is composed of layers of platelike membranes.

6.   An important function of the Golgi complex is to produce __Lysosomes__.

7.   Cells contain power plants called __Mitochondria__.

8.   Mitochondria carry on __cellular respiration__, the process of breaking down fuel molecules and releasing their energy.

9.   Mitochondria can affect health and aging by leaking electrons that form __free radicals__.

10. Some of the energy released during cellular respiration is temporarily stored in __ATP__, a chemical compound that can be used to power chemical reactions in the cell.

11. A(n) __vesicle__ is a small membrane-enclosed structure that holds or transports some type of cargo within the cell.

12. __Cilia__ are tiny hairlike organelles that project from the surfaces of many types of cells; they help move materials outside the cell.

Labeling Exercise

Please fill in the correct labels for Figure 2-1.

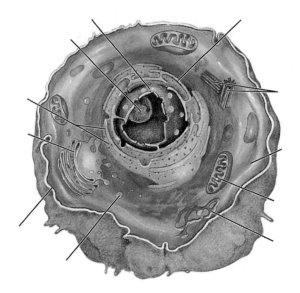

II. MATERIALS MOVE THROUGH THE PLASMA MEMBRANE BY BOTH PASSIVE AND ACTIVE PROCESSES

Active transport   **Diffusion**   **Filtration**   **Osmosis**   **Permeable**   **Phagocytosis**

1. The plasma membrane is selectively _permeable_.

2. _Diffusion_ is the net movement of molecules or ions from a region of higher concentration to a region of lower concentration brought about by the energy of the molecules.

3. _Osmosis_ is the diffusion of water molecules through a selectively permeable membrane from a region in which water molecules are more concentrated to a region in which they are less concentrated.

4. _Filtration_ is the passage of materials through membranes by mechanical pressure.

5. In _Active Transport_, the cell must use some of its stored energy in order to actively move materials from a region of lower concentration to a region of higher concentration.

6. In _phagocytosis_, the cell ingests large, solid particles such as food or bacteria.

III.   CELLS COMMUNICATE BY SIGNALING ONE ANOTHER

Communicate   Receptors   Response   Signaling   Target   Transduction

1. Cells of the body must __Communicate__ with one another in order to carry out essential processes.

2. Cell communication, often referred to as cell __Signaling__, takes place through a series of processes.

3. _____ cells are cells that can receive and respond to a particular signal.

4. In many cases, signal molecules bind to _____, which are specific molecules on the surface of the target cells.

5. The process by which a receptor converts a signal outside the cell into a signal inside the cell that affects some cellular process is called signal _____.

6. The final process in cell communication is the __Response__ by the cell.

IV.   CELLS DIVIDE BY MITOSIS, FORMING GENETICALLY IDENTICAL CELLS

Anaphase   Chromosomes   Five   Interphase   Metaphase
Mitosis   Prophase   Telophase   Two

1. Before a cell divides to form two cells, the chromosomes are precisely duplicated, and the cell undergoes _____.

2. In mitosis, a complete set of _____ is distributed to each end of the parent cell.

3. The life cycle of the cell may be divided into _____ phases.

4. The cell spends most of its life in _____.

5. _____ is the first stage of mitosis.

6. During _____, the chromosomes are positioned along the equator of the cell.

7. During _____, the sister chromatids separate and become independent chromosomes.

8. _____ begins with the arrival of a complete set of chromosomes at each end of the cell.

9. During telophase, the cell divides, forming _____ cells.

Labeling

Label each phase and describe what is happening in Figure 2-2.

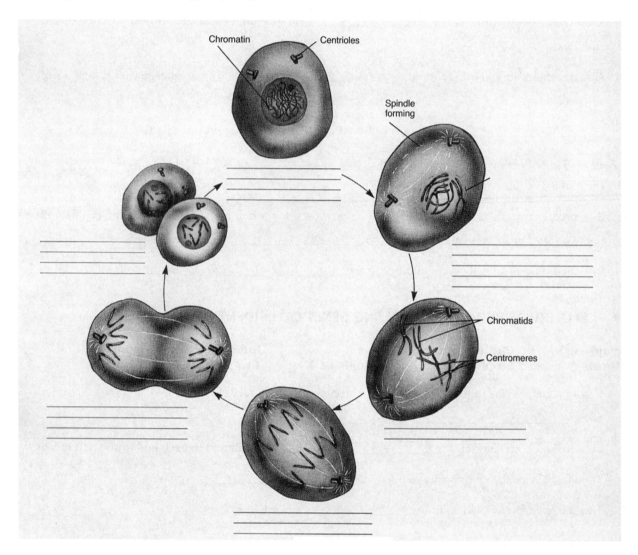

V. TISSUES ARE THE FABRIC OF THE BODY

Connective **Epithelial** **Histology** **Muscle** **Nervous** **Tissue**

1. A _Tissue_ is a group of closely associated cells that work together to carry out a specific function or group of functions.

2. The four principal types of tissue that make up the body are _Muscle_, _Nervous_, _Connective_, and _Epithelial_.

3. The microscopic study of tissues is called _Histology_.

A.   Epithelial Tissue Protects the Body

Absorb	Columnar	Cuboidal	Endocrine	Epithelial	Exocrine
Gland	Pseudostratified	Simple	Squamous	Stratified	Thyroid

1. _Epithelial_ tissue protects the body by covering all of its free surfaces and lining its cavities.

2. In some parts of the body, epithelial tissue is specialized to _absorb_ certain materials.

3. _Squamous_ epithelial cells are thin, flattened cells shaped like pancakes or flagstones.

4. _Cuboidal_ epithelial cells are short cylinders that from the side appear cube-shaped, resembling dice.

5. _Columnar_ epithelial cells look like columns or cylinders when viewed from the side.

6. Epithelial tissue may be _Simpled_, composed of one layer of cells; or _Stratified_, composed of two or more layers.

7. _Pseudostratified_ epithelium appears to be layered, (but isn't) because the cells are of different heights and their nuclei are at different levels in the tissue.

8. A(n) _gland_ consists of one or more epithelial cells specialized to produce and secrete a particular product such as mucus or sweat.

9. Two main types of glands are _endocrine_ and _exocrine_ glands.

10. The _thyroid_ gland is an example of an endocrine gland.

B.   Connective Tissue Joins Body Structures

Adipose	Collagen	Elastic	Fibers	Fibroblasts	Intercellular
Join together	Loose	Macrophages	Organ	Reticular	

1. Connective tissues _____ the other tissues of the body.

2. Almost every _organ_ in the body has a supporting framework of connective tissue.

3. Cells of connective tissue are typically separated by large amounts of _intercellular_ substance, which consists of threadlike microscopic _fibers_ scattered throughout a thick gel or matrix.

4. Three types of connective tissue fibers are _____, _____, and _____.

5. Two types of cells that are common in connective tissues are _Fibroblasts_ and _Macrophages_.

6. _____ connective tissue, or areolar tissue, joins body structures.

7. _____ tissue stores fat and releases it when the body needs energy.

C. Muscle Tissue Is Specialized to Contract

Contract   **Involuntary**   **Skeletal**   **Smooth**

1. Muscle tissue is composed of cells specialized to _____.

2. _____ muscle fibers have a striped, or striated, appearance; are attached to bone; and contract when stimulated by nerves.

3. Cardiac muscle, found in the walls of the heart, is considered _____ because we do not make a conscious decision to contract it.

4. _____ muscle occurs in the walls of the digestive tract, uterus, blood vessels, and other internal organs. Its fibers are not striated and its control is involuntary.

D. Nervous Tissue Controls Muscles and Glands

Axon   **Cell body**   **Dendrites**   **Glial**   **Neurons**   **Sensory**

1. Nervous tissue consists of _____, cells specialized for transmitting nerve impulses, and _____ cells that support and nourish the neurons.

2. Typically, a neuron has a large _____, that contains the nucleus and from which two types of extensions project.

3. _____ are specialized for receiving impulses, whereas the single _____ transmits information away from the cell body.

4. Neurons receive information from _____ receptors—structures that detect changes in the internal or external environment.

VI. MEMBRANES COVER OR LINE BODY SURFACES

Membranes   **Mucous**   **Parietal**   **Serous**   **Synovial**   **Visceral**

1. _____ are sheets of tissue that cover or line body surfaces.

2. A _____ membrane, or mucosa, lines body cavities that open to the outside of the body.

3. A _____ membrane, or serosa, lines a body cavity that does not open to the outside of the body.

4. The portion of the membrane that is attached to the wall of the cavity is the _____ membrane.

5. The part of the membrane that covers the organs inside the cavity is the _____ membrane.

6. A _____ membrane is a connective tissue membrane that lines a joint cavity.

CHAPTER TEST

Select the correct response.

1. Cells associate to form
   a. atoms.
   b. molecules.
   c. tissues.
   d. ribosomes.

2. The _____ is one of the biologist's most important tools for studying the internal structure of cells.
   a. telescope
   b. binoculars
   c. stethoscope
   d. microscope

3. _____ cells look like tiny building blocks.
   a. Bone
   b. Epithelial
   c. Nerve
   d. Muscle

4. The jellylike material of the cell is called
   a. plasma membrane.
   b. cytoplasm.
   c. endoplasmic reticulum.
   d. ribosomes.

5. Every cell is surrounded by a thin membrane, the
   a. plasma membrane.
   b. cytoplasm.
   c. endoplasmic reticulum.
   d. ribosomes.

6. The _____ is a system of membranes that extends throughout the cytoplasm of many cells and through which materials can be transported from one part of the cell to another.
   a. plasma membrane
   b. mitochondria
   c. endoplasmic reticulum
   d. ribosomes

7. _____ function(s) as factories in the cell where proteins are manufactured.
   a. Mitochondria
   b. Endoplasmic reticulum
   c. Ribosomes
   d. Lysosomes

8. Looking like stacks of pancakes, the _____ is composed of layers of platelike membranes. This organelle functions as a protein processing and packaging plant.
   a. Golgi complex
   b. mitochondria
   c. endoplasmic reticulum
   d. ribosomes

9. _____ are little sacs that contain powerful digestive enzymes that destroy bacteria and other foreign matter.
   a. Golgi complex
   b. Mitochondria
   c. Endoplasmic reticulum
   d. Lysosomes

10. Cells contain tiny power plants called
    a. Golgi complex.
    b. mitochondria.
    c. endoplasmic reticulum.
    d. lysosomes.

11. The _____ is the control center of the cell.
    a. Golgi complex
    b. mitochondrion
    c. ribosome
    d. nucleus

12. The nucleus of a cell that is not in the process of dividing contains loosely coiled material called
    a. ATP.
    b. DNA.
    c. chromosomes.
    d. chromatin.

13. When a cell prepares to divide, the chromatin becomes more tightly coiled and condenses, forming rod-shaped bodies called
    a. ATP.
    b. DNA.
    c. chromosomes.
    d. lysosomes.

14. The _____ is a specialized region within the nucleus in which ribosomes are assembled.
    a. Golgi complex
    b. nucleolus
    c. mitochondria
    d. riboplex

15. _____ are tiny cells with long whiplike tails.
    a. Sperm
    b. Egg
    c. Nerve
    d. Muscle

16. _____ is the net movement of molecules or ions from a region of higher concentration to a region of lower concentration.
    a. Diffusion
    b. Osmosis
    c. Filtration
    d. Phagocytosis

17. _____ is the diffusion of water molecules through a selectively permeable membrane from a region in which water molecules are more concentrated to a region in which they are less concentrated.
    a. Diffusion
    b. Osmosis
    c. Filtration
    d. Phagocytosis

18. _____ is the passage of materials through membranes by mechanical pressure.
    a. Diffusion
    b. Osmosis
    c. Filtration
    d. Active transport

19. _____ requires cellular energy for a cell to move material from a region of lower concentration to a region of higher concentration.
    a. Diffusion
    b. Osmosis
    c. Filtration
    d. Active transport

20. In _____, the cell ingests large, solid particles of food or bacteria.
    a. osmosis
    b. filtration
    c. active transport
    d. phagocytosis

21. In _____, a complete set of chromosomes moves to opposite ends of the parent cell.
    a. mitosis
    b. interphase
    c. anaphase
    d. prophase

22. _____ can be considered a phase in the life cycle of the cell.
    a. Interphase
    b. Prophase
    c. Metaphase
    d. All of the above

23. _____ tissue protects the body by covering all of its free surfaces and lining its cavities.
    a. Epithelial
    b. Connective
    c. Muscle
    d. Nervous

24. _____ tissues join the other tissues of the body.
    a. Epithelial
    b. Connective
    c. Muscle
    d. Nervous

25. _____ tissue stores fat and releases it when the body needs energy. It also helps to shape and protect the body and provides insulation.
    a. Areolar
    b. Adipose
    c. Collagen
    d. Cardiac

26. A _____ membrane lines body cavities that open to the outside of the body.
    a. serous
    b. mucous
    c. visceral
    d. tympanic

Chapter

3

THE INTEGUMENTARY SYSTEM

■ ■ ■

Outline

I.   The integumentary system protects the body.
II. The skin consists of epidermis and dermis.
   A. The epidermis continuously replaces itself.
   B. The dermis provides strength and elasticity.
   C. The subcutaneous layer attaches the skin to underlying tissues.
III. The skin has specialized structures.

A. The hair shaft consists of dead cells.
B. Sebaceous glands lubricate the hair and skin.
C. Sweat glands help maintain body temperature.
D. Nails protect the ends of the fingers and toes.
IV. Melanin helps determine skin color.

Learning Objectives

After you have studied this chapter, you should be able to:

1. List six functions of the integumentary system and explain how each is important in maintaining homeostasis.
2. Compare the structure and function of the epidermis with that of the dermis.
3. Describe the subcutaneous layer.

4. Describe the structure of hair.
5. Describe the functions of sebaceous glands.
6. Describe the structure and functions of sweat glands.
7. Describe the structure and function of nails.
8. Explain the function of melanin.

STUDY QUESTIONS

Within each category, fill in the blanks with the correct response.

I. THE INTEGUMENTARY SYSTEM PROTECTS THE BODY

Glands   Homeostasis   Integumentary system   Sensory   Skin   Vitamin D

1. Together with its hair, nails and glands, the skin makes up the _____.

2. The skin is important in maintaining _____—the balanced internal environment.

3. The _____ protects the body against injury and is the body's first line of defense against harmful bacteria and other agents of disease.

4. Located within the skin are _____ receptors that detect touch, pressure, heat, cold, and pain.

5. The skin has sweat _____ that excrete excess water and some wastes from the body.

6. The skin contains a compound that is converted to _____ when the skin is exposed to the ultraviolet rays of the sun.

II. THE SKIN CONSISTS OF THE EPIDERMIS AND DERMIS

Dermis   Epidermis   Subcutaneous

1. The outer layer of the skin is called the _____.

2. The inner layer of the skin is called the _____.

3. Beneath the skin is an underlying _____ layer.

A. The Epidermis Continuously Replaces Itself

Basale   Corneum   Epidermal   Epithelial   Keratin   Outer

1. The epidermis consists of stratified squamous _____ tissue.

2. The _____ cells of the epidermis continuously wear off.

3. New epidermal cells are constantly produced in the deepest sublayer of the epidermis, the stratum _____.

4. _____, a tough, waterproofing protein, gives the skin mechanical strength and flexibility.

5. As _____ cells move through the outer sublayer of epidermis, they die.

6. The outer sublayer of the skin is known as the stratum _____.

B. The Dermis Provides Strength and Elasticity

Collagen   Connective   Fingerprints   Glands
Hair follicles   Papillae   Temperature

1. Dermis consists of dense _____ tissue composed mainly of collagen fibers.

2. _____ is largely responsible for the mechanical strength of the skin.

3. Specialized skin structures such as _____ and _____ are found in the dermis.

4. The upper portion of the dermis has many small, fingerlike extensions called dermal _____ that project into the epidermal tissue.

5. Extensive networks of capillaries in the papillae deliver oxygen and nutrients to the cells of the epidermis, and also function in _____ regulation.

6. _____ result from the patterns of ridges and grooves on the skin of the fingertips.

C.   The Subcutaneous Layer Attaches the Skin to Underlying Tissues

Adipose   Fascia   Muscles   Shock   Subcutaneous

1. The subcutaneous layer beneath the dermis is also known as the superficial _____.

2. The subcutaneous layer attaches the skin to the _____ and other tissues beneath.

3. The thick, fatty, subcutaneous layer helps protect the underlying organs from mechanical _____.

4. Fat stored within the _____ tissue can be mobilized and used as an energy source when adequate food is not available.

5. Distribution of fat in the _____ layer is largely responsible for characteristic male and female body shapes.

III.   THE SKIN HAS SPECIALIZED STRUCTURES

A.   The Hair Shaft Consists of Dead Cells

Capillaries   Contract   Dead   Follicle   Hair
Keratin   Muscle   Nails   Root   Shaft

1. _____ helps protect the body, and is found on all skin surfaces except the palms and the soles.

2. The part of the hair that is visible is called the _____.

3. The part of the hair that is below the skin surface is called the _____.

4. The root together with its epithelial and connective tissue coverings, is called the hair _____.

5. At the bottom of the hair follicle is a little mound of connective tissue containing _____ that deliver nutrients to the cells of the follicle.

6. Each hair consists of cells that manufacture _____ as they move outward, and then die.

7. The shaft of the hair consists of _____ cells and their products.

8. Tiny bundles of smooth _____ are associated with hair follicles.

9. Arrector pili muscles _____ in response to cold or fear, causing the hairs to stand up straight.

B. Sebaceous Glands Lubricate the Hair and Skin

Acne   **Ducts**   **Pimple**   **Sebaceous glands**   **Sebum**

1. _____, also known as oil glands, are generally attached to hair follicles.

2. Sebaceous glands are connected to each hair follicle by little _____ through which they release their secretions.

3. Sebaceous glands secrete an oily substance called _____.

4. Sometimes the duct of a sebaceous gland ruptures, allowing sebum to spill into the dermis. The skin may become inflamed and a _____ may form.

5. At puberty, the stepped-up activity of sebaceous glands can sometimes lead to _____, a condition that is very common during adolescence.

C. Sweat Glands Help Maintain Body Temperature

Armpits   **Body temperature**   **Evaporation**   **Genital**   **Heat**
Nitrogen   **Raise**   **Sweat gland**   **Water**

1. Each _____ is a tiny coiled tube found in the dermis or subcutaneous tissue.

2. About 3 million sweat glands in the skin help maintain _____.

3. Muscle movement and metabolic activity generate _____ and therefore _____ body temperature.

4. Because heat is required for _____, the body becomes cooler as sweat evaporates from the skin.

5. Sweat glands excrete excess water, salts, and small amounts of _____ wastes from the body.

6. The sweat glands excrete about 1 quart of _____ each day.

7. Certain sweat glands found in association with hairs are concentrated in a few specific areas of the body, such as _____ and _____ areas.

D.   Nails Protect the Ends of the Fingers and Toes

Nails   **Corneum**   **Capillaries**   **Lunula**

1. _____ develop from horny epidermal cells and consist mainly of a closely compressed, tough keratin.

2. The nail bed beneath the body of the mail lacks a stratum _____.

3. Nails appear pink because of underlying _____.

4. The actively growing area is the white crescent, or _____, at the base of the nail.

IV.   MELANIN HELPS DETERMINE SKIN COLOR

Albinism	**Cancer**	**Carotene**	**Color**	**Darker**
Epidermis	**Melanin**	**Sun**	**Sunburned**	**Ultraviolet**

1. Scattered throughout the lowest layer of the _____ are cells that produce granules containing pigment.

2. Pigment granules are composed of a type of protein called _____.

3. Melanin gives _____ to hair as well as to skin.

4. Asians have the yellowish pigment _____ in their skin, as well as melanin.

5. _____ is an inherited condition that can occur in a person of any race, where the cells are not able to produce melanin.

6. Melanin is an important protective screen against the _____.

7. Exposure to the sun stimulates an increase in the amount of melanin produced and causes the skin to become _____.

8. A dark tan is a protective response, and is actually a sign that the skin has been exposed to too much _____ radiation.

9. When the melanin is not able to absorb all of the ultraviolet rays, the skin becomes inflamed, or _____.

10. Over a period of years, excessive exposure to the sun can cause wrinkling of the skin, and sometimes skin _____.

Labeling Exercise

Please fill in the correct labels for Figure 3-1.

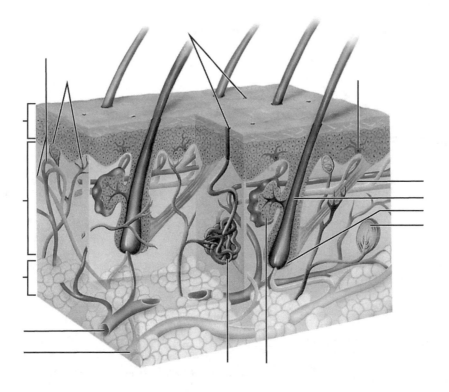

CHAPTER TEST

Select the correct response.

1. The skin, with its glands, hair, and nails, makes up the
   a. dermal system.
   b. epidermal system.
   c. integumentary system.
   d. endocrine system.

2. Oxygen and nutrients are delivered to cells of the epidermis by
   a. arterioles in the superficial fascia.
   b. capillaries in the dermal papillae.
   c. capillaries in the upper sublayer of the epidermis.
   d. hair follicle sinuses.

3. The skin is responsible for
   a. protecting the body against injury.
   b. preventing internal body cells from drying out.
   c. maintaining body temperature.
   d. all of the above.

4. The skin contains a compound that is converted to _____ when the skin is exposed to the ultraviolet rays of the sun.
   a. vitamin A
   b. vitamin C
   c. vitamin D
   d. para-aminobenzoic acid (PABA)

5. The outer layer of the skin is called the
   a. epidermis.
   b. dermis.
   c. subcutaneous layer.
   d. adipose layer.

6. The inner layer of the skin is called the
   a. epidermis.
   b. dermis.
   c. stratum corneum.
   d. adipose layer.

7. The epidermis consists of stratified squamous
   _____ tissue.
   a. nerve
   b. connective
   c. epithelial
   d. muscle

8. The tough, waterproofing protein that fills most
   of each skin cell is called
   a. melanin.
   b. keratin.
   c. hydrotin.
   d. carotene.

9. The dermis consists of dense _____ tissue composed mainly of collagen fibers.
   a. nerve
   b. connective
   c. epithelial
   d. muscle

10. Collagen is largely responsible for the _____ of
    the skin.
    a. color
    b. mechanical strength
    c. cooling
    d. tanning ability

11. The subcutaneous layer beneath the dermis
    consists of loose _____ tissue.
    a. nerve
    b. connective
    c. epithelial
    d. muscle

12. Fat stored within _____ tissue can be mobilized
    and used as an energy source when adequate
    food is not available.
    a. adipose
    b. epithelial
    c. nerve
    d. reserve

13. Sweat glands are tiny coiled tubes in the
    a. epidermis.
    b. dermis.
    c. exoskeleton.
    d. out-skin.

14. There are approximately _____ sweat glands in
    the skin that help maintain body temperature.
    a. 3,000,000
    b. 700
    c. 20,000
    d. too many to count

15. Hair is found on all skin surfaces except the
    a. palms and soles.
    b. palms and fingers.
    c. fingers and soles.
    d. toes and fingers.

16. _____ is caused by the contraction of the arrec-
    tor pili muscles.
    a. Sweat
    b. Body odor
    c. Gooseflesh
    d. Keratin

17. Nails appear pink because of underlying
    a. carotene.
    b. veins.
    c. arteries.
    d. capillaries.

18. In dark-skinned individuals, the pigment cells
    are more active and produce more
    a. blood.
    b. ultraviolet rays.
    c. carotene.
    d. melanin.

19. People who sunbathe are more prone to _____
    than are people who do not stay out in the sun
    very long.
    a. wrinkles
    b. skin cancer
    c. sunburn
    d. all of the above

CROSSWORD PUZZLE FOR CHAPTERS 1, 2, AND 3

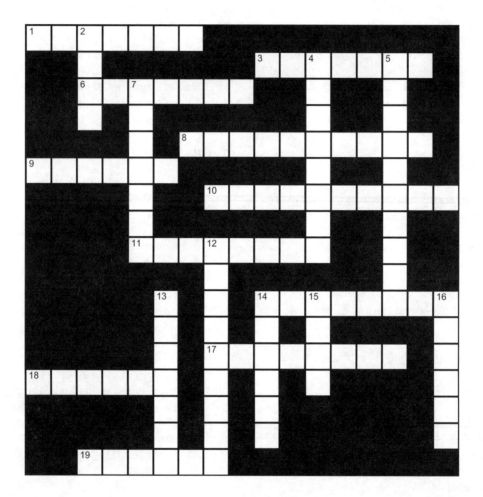

Across
1. Pertains to the skull
3. Science of body structure
6. Movement of water across a cell membrane
8. Tissue that lines body cavities
9. Cell that transmits nerve impulses
10. Science of body function
11. Higher in the body
14. Closer to the body midline
17. Fibrous protein that is the main support of many connective tissues
18. Closer to the body midline
19. Group of cells aggregated to perform a function

Down
2. Smallest unit of an element that retains the chemical properties of that element
4. Ventral
5. Chemical processes that occur within the body
7. Division of the cell nucleus
12. Glands that secrete hormones
13. Control center of a cell
14. The bony ring that supports the lower portion of trunk
15. Relating to the mouth
16. Region of the lower back

Chapter

THE SKELETAL SYSTEM

■ ■ ■

Outline

I. The skeletal system supports and protects the body.
II. A bone consists of compact and spongy bone tissue.
III. Bone develops by replacing existing connective tissue.
IV. The bones of the skeleton are grouped in two divisions.
V. The axial skeleton consists of 80 bones.
   A. The skull is the bony framework of the head.
   B. The vertebral column supports the body.
   C. The thoracic cage protects the organs of the chest.
VI. The appendicular skeleton consists of 126 bones.

A. The pectoral girdle attaches the upper extremities to the axial skeleton.
B. The bones of the upper extremity are located in the arm, forearm, wrist, and hand.
C. The pelvic girdle supports the lower extremities.
D. The bones of the lower extremity are located in the thigh, knee, leg, ankle, and foot.
VII. Joints are junctions between bones.
   A. Joints can be classified according to the degree of movement they permit.
   B. A diarthrosis is surrounded by a joint capsule.

Learning Objectives

After you have studied this chapter, you should be able to:

1. List five functions of the skeletal system.
2. Describe the gross and microscopic structure of a typical bone.
3. Contrast endochondral with intramembranous bone development.
4. Describe the functions of osteoblasts and osteoclasts in bone production and remodeling.
5. Distinguish between the axial skeleton and the appendicular skeleton.
6. Identify the bones of the axial skeleton, and locate each on a diagram or skeleton.
7. Describe and give the function of each of the cranial and facial bones.

8. Describe and give the function of each of the bones of the vertebral column and of the thoracic cage.
9. Identify the bones of the appendicular skeleton, and locate each on a diagram or skeleton.
10. Describe and give the function of each of the bones of the pectoral girdle, upper extremity, pelvic girdle, and lower extremity.
11. Compare the main types of joints.
12. Describe the structure and functions of a diarthrosis.

STUDY QUESTIONS

Within each category, fill in the blanks with the correct response.

I. THE SKELETAL SYSTEM SUPPORTS AND PROTECTS THE BODY

Bones	**Calcium**	**Ligaments**	**Marrow**
Protects	**Supports**	**Tendons**	

1. The skeletal system _____ the body by serving as a bony framework for other tissues and organs.

2. The skeletal system also _____ delicate vital organs.

3. _____ serve as levers that transmit muscular forces.

4. Muscles are attached to bones by bands of connective tissue called _____.

5. Bones are held together at the joints by bands of connective tissue called _____.

6. The _____ within some bones produces blood cells.

7. When the concentration of _____ in the blood increases above normal, it is deposited in the bones where it is stored until needed.

II. A BONE CONSISTS OF COMPACT AND SPONGY BONE TISSUE

Bone	**Bone marrow**	**Canaliculi**	**Cancellous**	**Compact**	**Dense**
Diaphysis	**Endosteum**	**Epiphyseal**	**Epiphyses**	**Haversian canals**	**Hyaline**
Lacunae	**Metaphysis**	**Osteocytes**	**Osteons**	**Periosteum**	**Red**
Spindle	**Spongy**	**Yellow**			

1. The main shaft of a long bone is called its _____.

2. The expanded ends of a long bone are called _____.

3. In children, a disc of cartilage called the _____ is found between the epiphysis and the diaphysis.

4. The metaphyses are growth centers that disappear at maturity, becoming vague _____ lines.

5. At its joint surfaces, the outer layer of a bone consists of a thin layer of _____ cartilage, the articular cartilage.

6. The bone is covered by a layer of specialized connective tissue—the _____.

7. The inner layer of the periosteum contains cells that produce _____.

8. A long bone has a central marrow cavity filled with a fatty connective tissue known as _____ bone marrow.

9. The marrow cavity of the long bone is lined with a thin layer of cells called the

    _____.

10. Two types of bone tissue are _____ bone and _____ bone.

11. Compact bone, which is very _____ and hard, is found near the surfaces of the
    bone where great strength is needed.

12. Compact bone consists of interlocking, _____-shaped units called

    _____, or haversian systems.

13. Within an osteon, _____ (the mature bone cells) are found in small cavities called

    _____.

14. Lacunae are arranged in concentric circles around central _____.

15. Threadlike extensions of the cytoplasm of the osteocytes extend through narrow channels called

    _____. These cellular extensions connect the osteocytes.

16. Spongy bone, or _____ bone, is found within the epiphyses and makes up the
    inner part of the wall of the diaphysis.

17. The spaces within the spongy bone are filled with _____.

18. In an infant, _____ marrow fills the cavities of most bones.

Labeling Exercise

Please fill in the correct labels for Figure 4-1.

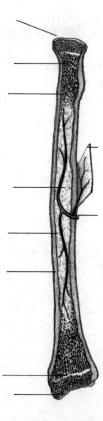

Labeling Exercise

Please fill in the correct labels for Figure 4-2.

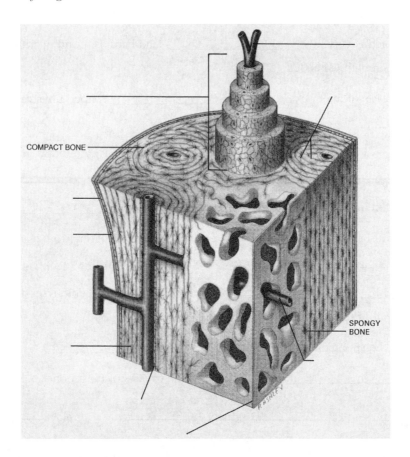

III. BONE DEVELOPS BY REPLACING EXISTING CONNECTIVE TISSUE

Bones	**Diaphysis**	**Endochondral**	**Fetal**	**Hydroxyapatite**
Intramembranous	**Lacunae**	**Marrow**	**Ossification**	**Osteoblasts**
Osteoclasts	**Osteocytes**	**Shape**	**Skeleton**	**Tissue**

1. Bone formation is called _____.

2. During _____ development, bones form in two ways.

3. The long bones develop from cartilage templates, a process called _____ bone development.

4. A bone begins to ossify in its _____.

5. The flat bones of the skull develop from a noncartilage connective tissue scaffold; this is called _____ bone development.

6. _____ are cells that produce bone.

7. The compound _____, composed mainly of calcium phosphate, is present in the tissue fluid.

8. As the bone matrix forms around the osteoblasts, they become isolated within

_____.

9. When osteoblasts become embedded in the bone matrix, they are referred to as

_____.

10. _____ are very large cells that break down bone.

11. Osteoclasts and osteoblasts work side by side to _____ bones and form the precise grain needed.

12. As muscles develop in response to physical activity, the _____ to which they are attached thicken and become stronger.

13. As bones grow, bone _____ must be removed from the interior, especially from the walls of the _____ cavity. This process keeps bones from becoming too heavy.

14. The adult _____ is replaced every ten years.

IV.   THE BONES OF THE SKELETON ARE GROUPED IN TWO DIVISIONS

206   Appendicular   Axial

1. The human skeleton consists of _____ named bones.

2. The _____ skeleton forms the central axis of the body.

3. The _____ skeleton consists of the upper and lower extremities of the body.

V.   THE AXIAL SKELETON CONSISTS OF 80 BONES

A.   The Skull Is the Bony Framework of the Head

Anterior	**Coronal**	**Cranium**	**Face**	**Fontanelles**	**Frontal**	**Lambdoid**
Middle	**Paranasal**	**Sagittal**	**Sinuses**	**Sinusitis**	**Soft spots**	**Sutures**

1. The skull, the bony framework of the head, is divided into the 8 bones of the

_____ and the 14 bones that make up the _____.

2. Contained within the head are six very small bones in the _____ ears.

3. Most of the bones of the skull are joined by the immovable joints called _____.

4. The two parietal bones are joined in the midline by the _____ suture.

5. The coronal suture joins the parietal bones to the _____ bone.

6. The _____ suture is the joint between the parietal bones and the occipital bone.

7. In babies, six joints called _____ occur at the angles of the parietal bone.

8. The largest fontanelle is the _____ fontanelle, and it is found at the junction of the sagittal and _____ sutures.

9. The fontanelles, popularly called _____, permit the baby's head to be compressed slightly as it passes through the mother's bony pelvis during birth.

10. Some cranial bones contain _____, air-filled spaces lined with mucous membranes.

11. Four pairs of sinuses, the _____ sinuses, are continuous with the nose and throat.

12. Sometimes the mucous membranes of the sinuses become swollen and inflamed, producing the condition called _____.

B. The Vertebral Column Supports the Body

5	**24**	**Cervical**	**Coccygeal**	**Coccyx**	**Discs**
Fused	**Intervertebral**	**Sacrum**	**Spine**	**Thoracic**	**Vertebral foramen**

1. The vertebral column, or _____, supports the body and bears its weight.

2. The vertebral column consists of _____ vertebrae.

3. The two fused bones of the vertebral column are the _____ and the _____.

4. The regions of the vertebral column are the _____, which consists of 7 vertebrae; the _____, which consists of 12 vertebrae; the lumbar, which consists of _____ vertebrae; the sacral, which consists of 5 _____ vertebrae; and the _____, which consists of 3-5 fused vertebrae.

5. The vertebrae articulate with each other by means of synovial joints and by means of _____ discs composed of cartilage.

6. The intervertebral _____ are tiny pads that act as shock absorbers.

7. The body and neural arch enclose a large opening called the _____.

Labeling Exercise

Please fill in the correct labels for Figure 4-3.

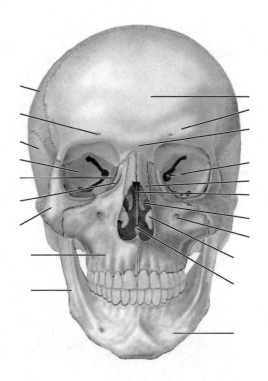

Labeling Exercise

Please fill in the correct labels for Figure 4-4.

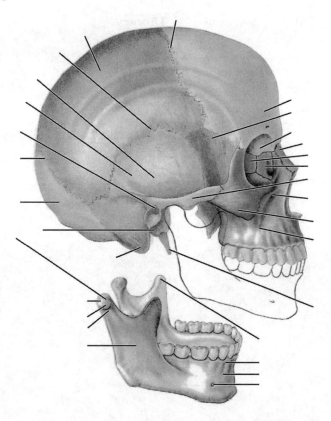

Labeling Exercise

Please fill in the correct labels for Figure 4-5.

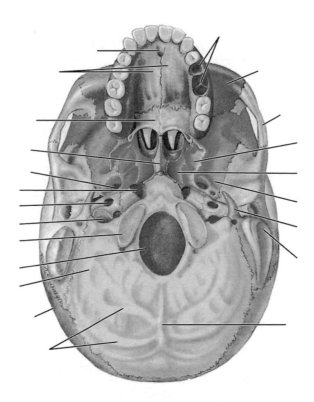

C. The Thoracic Cage Protects the Organs of the Chest

12   Pectoral   Rib   Sternum   Thoracic

1. The thoracic cage, or _____ cage, protects the internal organs of the chest, including the heart and lungs.

2. The thoracic cage is a bony cage formed by the _____, the _____ vertebrae, and _____ pairs of ribs.

3. The thoracic cage provides support for the bones of the _____ girdle and upper extremities.

Labeling Exercise

Please fill in the correct labels for Figure 4-6.

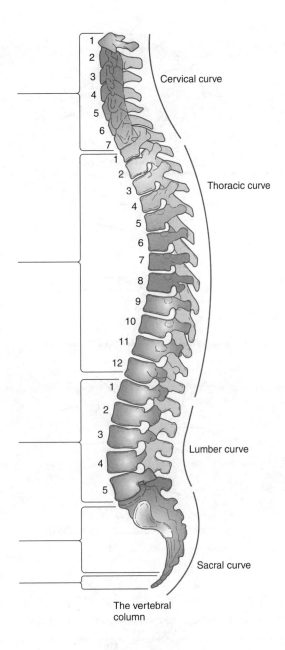

Cervical curve

Thoracic curve

Lumber curve

Sacral curve

The vertebral
column

Labeling Exercise

Please fill in the correct labels for Figure 4-7.

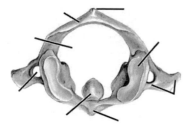

(a) Atlas seen from above

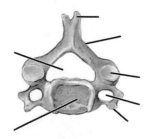

(b) Cervical vertebra seen from above

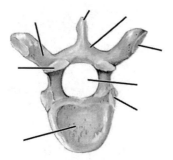

(c) Thoracic vertebra seen from above

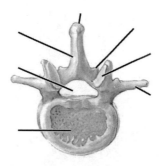

(d) Lumbar vertebra seen from above

VI. THE APPENDICULAR SKELETON CONSISTS OF 126 BONES

A. The Pectoral Girdle Attaches the Upper Extremities to the Axial Skeleton

Clavicle   Sternum

1. Each pectoral girdle consists of a scapula and a _____.

2. The pectoral girdles articulate with the _____ but not with the vertebral column.

B. The Bones of the Upper Extremity Are Located in the Arm, Forearm, Wrist, and Hand

30   Carpal   Humerus   Metacarpal   Phalanges   Radius   Ulna

1. Each upper limb consists of _____ bones.

2. The _____ is the bone in the upper arm.

3. The _____ and the _____ are the bones of the forearm.

4. Eight small _____ bones form the wrist.

5. There are five _____ bones are in the palm of the hand.

6. The _____ are the bones of the fingers.

Labeling Exercise

Please fill in the correct labels for Figure 4-8.

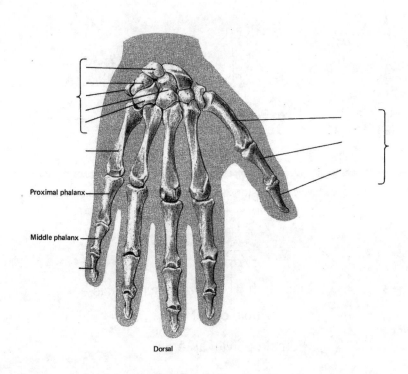

Proximal phalanx

Middle phalanx

Dorsal

C. The Pelvic Girdle Supports the Lower Extremities

Coccyx   **Coxal**   **Ilium**   **Ischium**   **Pelvic**   **Pubis**   **Sacrum**   **Symphysis**

1. The _____ girdle is a broad basin of bone that encloses the pelvic cavity.

2. The hip bones are called _____ bones.

3. The coxal bones together with the _____ and _____ form the pelvic girdle.

4. Each coxal bone is formed from the fusion of three bones. The largest of the three is the _____.

5. The most posterior coxal bone is the _____.

6. The anterior part of the coxal bone is the _____.

7. The joint where the coxal bones come together anteriorly is called the pubic _____.

Labeling Exercise

Please fill in the correct labels for Figure 4-9.

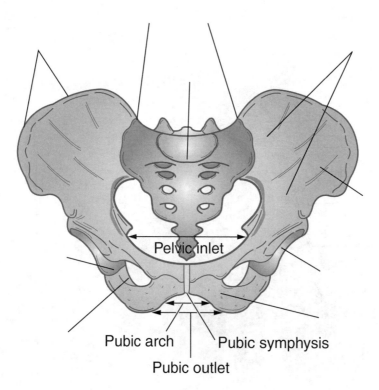

Pelvic inlet

Pubic arch   Pubic symphysis

Pubic outlet

Female pelvis, anterior

D.   The Bones of the Lower Extremity Are Located in the Thigh, Knee, Leg, Ankle, and Foot

30   **Femur**   **Fibula**   **Metatarsal**   **Patella**   **Phalanges**   **Tarsal**   **Tibia**

1.   The lower extremity consists of _____ bones.

2.   The _____ is the bone in the upper leg (thigh).

3.   The _____ is the kneecap.

4.   The _____ and _____ make up the bones of the lower leg.

5.   The bones of the heel and back part of the foot are called _____ bones.

6.   The _____ bones make up the main part of the foot.

7.   The _____ are the bones in the toes.

Labeling Exercise

Please fill in the correct labels for Figure 4-10.

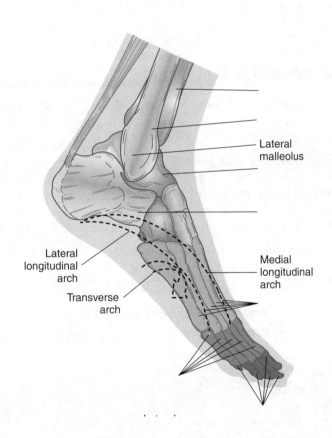

VII. JOINTS ARE JUNCTIONS BETWEEN BONES

A. Joints Can Be Classified According to the Degree of Movement They Permit

Amphiarthroses	Articulation	Cartilage	Diarthroses	Fibrous
Intervertebral	Skull	Synarthroses	Synovial	Three

1. A joint, or _____, is the point of contact between two bones.

2. Joints can be classified into _____ main groups.

3. _____ are joints that do not permit movement. They connect bones by means of _____ connective tissue.

4. The sutures that join the _____ bones are synarthroses.

5. _____ permit slight movement, and are joined by _____.

6. The _____ joints of the vertebral column are examples of amphiarthroses.

7. _____, or synovial joints, are freely movable joints.

8. The six types of _____ joints are gliding, condyloid, saddle, pivot, hinge, and ball-and-socket.

B. A Diarthrosis Is Surrounded by a Joint Capsule

Bursae	Bursitis	Hyaline	Joint	Ligaments	Synovial

1. The ends of the bones forming a diarthrodial joint are covered with _____ cartilage that lacks any sort of covering membrane.

2. The joint is surrounded by a connective tissue capsule, the _____ capsule.

3. The joint capsule is generally reinforced with _____, bands of fibrous connective tissue that connect the bones and limit movement at the joint.

4. The joint capsule is lined with a membrane that secretes a lubricant called _____ fluid.

5. Fluid-filled sacs called _____ are located between bone and tendons.

6. Inflammation of a bursa is a painful condition known as _____.

CHAPTER TEST

Select the correct response.

1. The sternum and ribs protect the
   a. heart.
   b. stomach.
   c. lungs.
   d. both a and c.

2. The _____ within some bones produces blood cells.
   a. osteon
   b. lacuna
   c. marrow
   d. cartilage

3. The main shaft of the long bone is called its
   a. epiphyses.
   b. diaphysis.
   c. endosteum.
   d. periosteum.

4. The thin cellular layer that lines the marrow cavity is the
   a. pericardium.
   b. periosteum.
   c. endosteum.
   d. diaphysis.

5. Osteocytes are found in small cavities (within the osteon) called
   a. lacunae.
   b. canaliculi.
   c. osteoclasts.
   d. osteoblasts.

6. Spongy bone is found within the
   a. canaliculi.
   b. epiphyses.
   c. lacunae.
   d. haversian canals.

7. When osteoblasts become embedded in the bone matrix, they are called
   a. matrix marrow.
   b. lacunae.
   c. osteocytes.
   d. osteoclasts.

8. _____ work side by side to shape bones and form the precise grain needed in the finished bone.
   a. Lacunae and haversian canals
   b. Osteoblasts and osteocytes
   c. Osteoblasts and matrix
   d. Osteoblasts and osteoclasts

9. The axial skeleton consists of the vertebral column, ribs, sternum, and
   a. upper and lower extremities.
   b. pectoral girdle.
   c. pelvic girdle.
   d. skull.

10. The appendicular skeleton consists of the upper and lower limbs, shoulder girdle, and
    a. pelvic girdle.
    b. skull.
    c. ribs.
    d. sternum.

11. The _____ suture is the joint between the parietal bones and the occipital bone.
    a. sagittal
    b. parietal
    c. coronal
    d. lambdoid

12. The paranasal sinuses are located in the
    a. frontal bone.
    b. maxillary bone.
    c. sphenoid bone.
    d. all of the above.

13. The regions of the vertebral column are the cervical, thoracic, lumbar, coccygeal, and
    a. sacral.
    b. centrum.
    c. lamina.
    d. lambdoidal.

14. Vertebrae articulate with each other by means of _____ joints.
    a. inflexible
    b. amphiarthrotic
    c. sacral
    d. thoracic

15. The thoracic cage protects the internal organs of the
    a. reproductive system.
    b. brain.
    c. chest.
    d. all of the above.

16. The thoracic cage contains _____ pairs of ribs.
    a. 24
    b. 6
    c. 12
    d. It depends on the individual.

17. The pectoral girdle attaches the upper limbs to the _____ skeleton.
    a. appendicular
    b. sacral
    c. external
    d. axial

18. Each pectoral girdle consists of a clavicle and a
    s. scalpel.
    b. scapula.
    c. sternum.
    d. pubis.

19. The upper extremity consists of the humerus, ulna, carpals, metacarpals, phalanges, and
    a. tibia.
    b. femur.
    c. sternum.
    d. radius.

20. The pelvic girdle is a broad basin of bone that encloses the _____ cavity.
    a. pelvic
    b. chest
    c. pubic
    d. ischial

21. Two coxal bones together with the sacrum and coccyx form the
    a. pelvic girdle.
    b. pectoral girdle.
    c. ischium.
    d. trunk.

22. The sutures that join skull bones together are an example of
    a. synarthroses.
    b. amphiarthroses.
    c. diarthroses.
    d. synovial joints.

23. The painful condition known as bursitis is a result of
    a. lack of bursae.
    b. too many bursae.
    c. inflammation of a bursa.
    d. the bursting of a bursa.

24. Which of the following joints is considered a ball-and-socket joint?
    a. elbow
    b. hip
    c. carpometacarpal
    d. atlantoaxial

Labeling Exercise

Please fill in the correct labels for Figure 4-11.

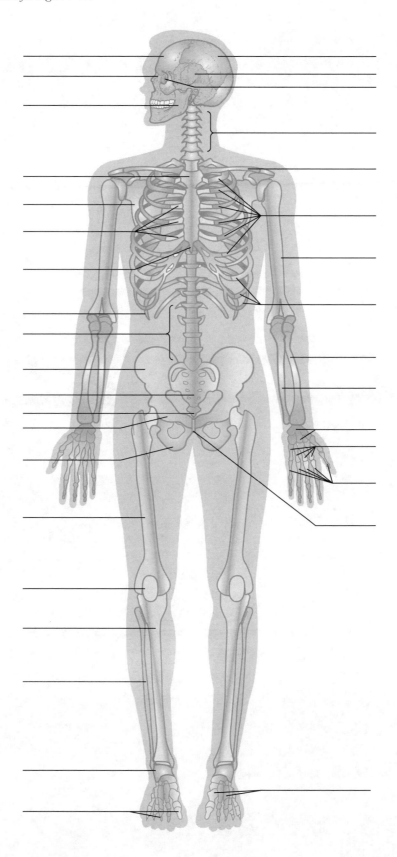

Chapter

5

THE MUSCULAR SYSTEM

■ ■ ■

Outline

Introduction
I.   A skeletal muscle is composed of hundreds of muscle fibers.
II. Muscle fibers are specialized for contraction.
    A. Muscle contraction occurs when actin and myosin filaments slide past each other.
    B. Muscle contraction requires energy.
C. Muscle tone is a state of partial contraction.
D. Two types of contraction are isotonic and isometric.
III. Muscles work antagonistically to one another.
IV. We can study muscles in functional groups.

Learning Objectives

After you have studied this chapter, you should be able to:

1. Describe the structure of a skeletal muscle.
2. Describe the structure of a muscle fiber and relate its structure to its function.
3. List—in sequence—the events that take place during muscle contraction.
4. Compare the roles of glycogen, creatine phosphate, and adenosine triphosphate (ATP) in providing energy for muscle contraction.
5. Define muscle tone and explain why muscle tone is important.
6. Distinguish between isotonic and isometric contraction.
7. Explain how muscles work antagonistically to one another.
8. Locate and give the actions of the principal muscles as described in Table 5-1 in the accompanying textbook.

STUDY QUESTIONS

Within each category, fill in the blanks with the correct response.

INTRODUCTION

Cardiac   **Muscles**   **Skeletal**   **Smooth**   **Striated**

1. Body movements such as walking or talking depend on the action of _____.

2. The three types of muscles are _____, _____, and

   _____.

3. Skeletal muscles are the _____ muscles attached to bones.

I. A SKELETAL MUSCLE IS COMPOSED OF HUNDREDS OF MUSCLE FIBERS

Endomysium   **Fascia**   **Fascicles**   **Fibers**   **Perimysium**   **Tendons**

1. Each skeletal muscle is an organ made up of hundreds, sometimes thousands, of muscle cells, referred to as muscle _____.

2. Individual muscle fibers are surrounded by a connective tissue covering called the _____.

3. The muscle fibers are arranged in bundles called _____.

4. Each fascicle is wrapped by connective tissue known as _____.

5. Extensions of epimysium form tough cords of connective tissue, the _____, that anchor muscles to bones.

6. The muscle is surrounded by fibrous connective tissue called _____ that merges with the tissue of the tendon.

II. MUSCLE FIBERS ARE SPECIALIZED FOR CONTRACTION

Actin   **Contractile**   **Filaments**   **Mitochondria**   **Myofibrils**
Myosin   **Sarcomeres**   **Transverse**   **Z line**

1. Each skeletal muscle fiber is a spindle-shaped cell with several nuclei and numerous _____ that provide energy for muscle contraction.

2. The plasma membrane has many inward extensions that form a set of _____ tubules.

3. Each muscle fiber is almost filled with threadlike structures called _____ that run lengthwise through the muscle fiber.

4. Myofibrils are composed of smaller structures called muscle _____ that are made of protein threads.

5. The thick filaments consisting mainly of the protein myosin are called _____ filaments.

6. The thin filaments consisting of the protein actin are called _____ filaments.

7. Myosin and actin are _____ proteins, which means that they are capable of shortening.

8. Myosin and actin filaments are organized into repeating units called _____, the basic units of muscle contraction.

9. Sarcomeres are joined at their ends by an interweaving of filaments called the _____.

A.   Muscle Contraction Occurs when Actin and Myosin Filaments Slide Past Each Other

Acetylcholine   **Acetylcholinesterase**   **Action**   **Adenosine triphosphate (ATP)**
Bones   **Bridge**   **Calcium**   **Fibers**
Impulses   **Motor**   **Neuromuscular**   **Synaptic**

1. Movement of the body occurs when muscles pull on _____.

2. A muscle contracts when its _____ contract.

3. A(n) _____ nerve is a nerve that controls muscle contraction.

4. Motor neurons (nerve cells) that make up a motor nerve transmit _____ to muscle fibers.

5. The junction of a nerve and muscle fiber is called a(n) _____ junction.

6. A motor neuron releases the neurotransmitter _____.

7. Acetylcholine is released into the _____ cleft between the motor neuron and muscle fiber.

8. Depolarization may cause an electrical impulse, or _____ potential, to be generated in the muscle fiber.

9. Excess acetylcholine is broken down by an enzyme called _____.

10. Depolarization of the T tubules triggers release of stored _____ ions from the endoplasmic reticulum.

11. The energy storage molecule _____ provides the energy for muscle contraction.

12. Energized myosin attaches to the binding site on the actin filament, forming a cross _____ that links the myosin and actin filaments.

B.   Muscle Contraction Requires Energy

ATP   **Creatine phosphate**   **Fuel**   **Glucose**   **Lactic acid**   **Muscle fatigue**   **Oxygen debt**

1. The immediate source of energy for muscle contraction comes from _____.

2. Muscle cells have a backup energy storage compound called _____.

3. The energy for making creatine phosphate and ATP comes from _____ molecules.

4. _____, a simple sugar, is stored in muscle cells in the form of a large molecule called glycogen.

5. The depletion of ATP results in weaker contractions and _____.

6. A waste product called _____ is produced during anaerobic metabolism of glucose.

7. During muscle exertion, a(n) _____ develops.

C. Muscle Tone Is a State of Partial Contraction

Motor nerve   **Muscle tone**   **Posture**   **Unconscious**

1. Even when they are not moving, our muscles are in a state of partial contraction known as

    _____.

2. Muscle tone is a(n) _____ process that helps keep muscles prepared for action.

3. Muscle tone is also responsible for helping the muscles of the abdominal wall hold the internal organs in

    place and is important in maintaining _____.

4. When the _____ to a muscle is cut, the muscle becomes limp, or flaccid.

D. Two Types of Contraction Are Isotonic and Isometric

Isometric   **Isotonic**

1. _____ contraction occurs when muscles shorten and thicken.

2. _____ contraction occurs when muscle length does not appreciably change but

    muscle tension increases.

III. MUSCLES WORK ANTAGONISTICALLY TO ONE ANOTHER

Agonist   **Antagonist**   **Articulates**   **Fixators**   **Insertion**   **Origin**   **Synergists**   **Tendons**

1. Skeletal muscles produce movements by pulling on _____, which in turn pull on

    bones.

2. When the muscle contracts, it draws one bone toward or away from the bone with which it

    _____.

3. The attachment of the muscle to the less movable bone is called its _____.

4. The attachment of the muscle to the more movable bone is called its _____.

5. The muscle that contracts to produce a particular action is known as the _____, or

    prime mover.

6. The muscle that produces the opposite movement is the _____.

7. _____ stabilize joints so that undesirable movement does not occur.

8. _____ stabilize the origin of a prime mover so that its force is fully directed on the bone on which it inserts.

IV.   WE CAN STUDY MUSCLES IN FUNCTIONAL GROUPS

Biceps brachii   **Diaphragm**   **Gastrocnemius**   **Gluteus maximus**
Masseter   **Pectoralis**   **Rectus abdominis**   **Trapezius**

1. The _____ raises the jaw.

2. The _____ draws the shoulder upward.

3. The _____ compresses abdominal contents.

4. The _____ increases the volume of the chest cavity.

5. The _____ rotates the arm medially.

6. The _____ flexes the elbow.

7. The _____ extends and rotates the thigh.

8. The _____ flexes the foot.

Labeling Exercise

Please fill in the correct labels for Figure 5-1.

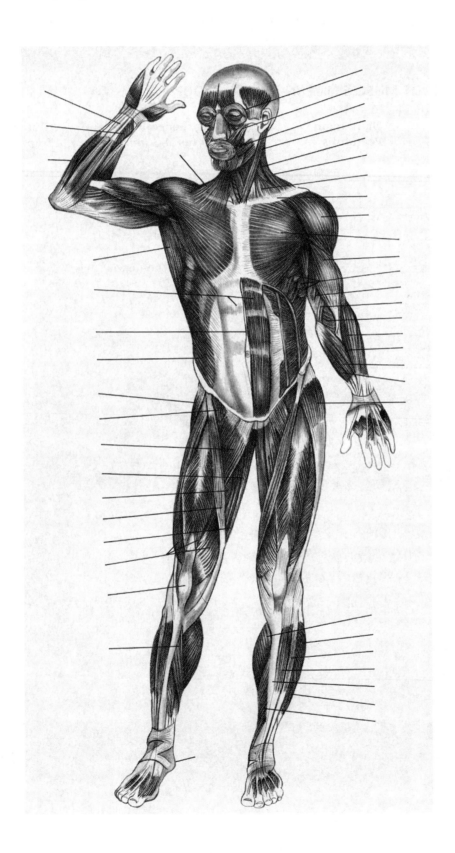

Labeling Exercise

Please fill in the correct labels for Figure 5-2.

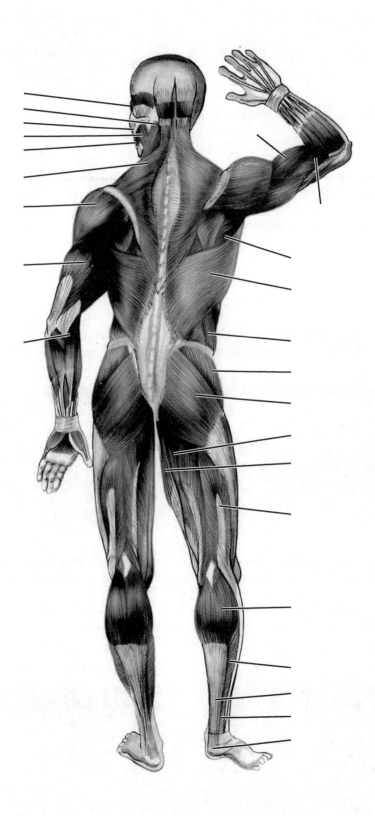

CHAPTER TEST

Select the correct response.

1. _____ depend(s) on muscle action.
   a. Walking
   b. Talking
   c. Breathing
   d. All of the above

2. Each muscle is surrounded by a covering of connective tissue called the
   a. epimysium.
   b. fascicles.
   c. perimysium.
   d. endomysium.

3. The muscle fibers are arranged in bundles called
   a. epimysium.
   b. fascicles.
   c. perimysium.
   d. endomysium.

4. Each fascicle is wrapped by connective tissue called the
   a. epimysium.
   b. myosin.
   c. perimysium.
   d. endomysium.

5. Individual muscle fibers are surrounded by a connective tissue covering called the
   a. epimysium.
   b. fascicles.
   c. perimysium.
   d. endomysium.

6. Extensions of the epimysium form tough cords of connective tissue called _____ that anchor muscles to bones.
   a. fibers
   b. tendons
   c. nerves
   d. anchors

7. Each muscle fiber is a spindle-shaped cell with many control centers called
   a. cell walls.
   b. nuclei.
   c. Golgi complexes.
   d. mitochondria.

8. Each muscle fiber is almost entirely filled with tiny protein threads, or
   a. monofilaments.
   b. striations.
   c. myofibrils.
   d. filaments.

9. Thick filaments consist mainly of the protein
   a. actin.
   b. thicktin.
   c. myosin.
   d. glycogen.

10. Thin filaments consist mainly of the protein
    a. actin.
    b. thicktin.
    c. myosin.
    d. glycogen.

11. A _____ nerve is a nerve that stimulates muscle contraction.
    a. controller
    b. motor
    c. contractor
    d. constrictor

12. The impulse generated during an action potential spreads through the T tubules and stimulates the release of
    a. calcium.
    b. vitamin C.
    c. acetylcholine.
    d. sodium.

13. The immediate source of energy for muscle contraction comes from the energy storage molecule
    a. DNA.
    b. TAP.
    c. PTA.
    d. ATP.

14. Glucose is stored in muscle cells in the form of a large molecule called
    a. glycerol.
    b. glucosis.
    c. glycogen.
    d. ATP.

15. Even when we are not moving, our muscles are in a state of partial contraction called
    a. muscle tone.
    b. muscle contraction.
    c. partial tone.
    d. semicontraction.

16. When the motor nerve to a muscle is cut, the muscle becomes
    a. tight.
    b. limp.
    c. firm.
    d. stiff.

17. When a heavy object is lifted, muscles shorten and thicken as they contract. This kind of muscle contraction is called a(n) _____ contraction.
    a. isotonic
    b. isometric
    c. hypertonic
    d. hypotonic

18. When one pushes against a wall, no movement occurs, and muscle length does not appreciably change, but muscle tension increases. This type of muscle contraction is called _____ contraction.
    a. isotonic
    b. isometric
    c. hypertonic
    d. hypotonic

19. Skeletal muscles produce movements by pulling on tendons, which in turn pull on
    a. ligaments.
    b. joints.
    c. bones.
    d. other muscles.

20. The attachment of a muscle to a less movable bone is called its
    a. insertion.
    b. origin.
    c. root.
    d. inclusion.

21. The attachment of a muscle to a more movable bone is called its
    a. insertion.
    b. origin.
    c. root.
    d. inclusion.

CROSSWORD PUZZLE FOR CHAPTERS 4 AND 5

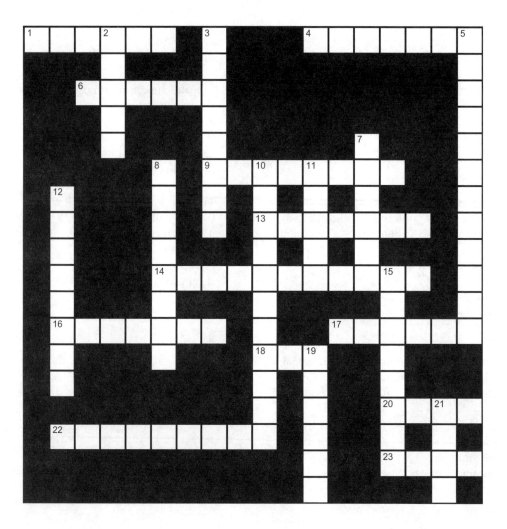

Across

1. A protein that together with actin is responsible for muscle contraction
4. Shoulder blade
6. _____ tone is the state of partial contraction that keeps muscle prepared for action
9. There are 12 _____ vertebrae
13. Three-headed muscle in posterior part of the arm
14. Cells that produce bone
16. The skull is formed by the _____ and facial bones
17. There are five _____ vertebrae
18. Immediate source of energy for muscle contraction
20. There are 12 pairs of _____
22. Each muscle fiber contains thick myosin and thin actin _____
23. A _____ bone consists of a shaft with flared ends

Down

2. Formed by the cranial and facial bones
3. System that supports and protects the body
5. The _____ skeleton consists of the upper and lower limbs, pectoral girdle, and pelvic girdle
7. A skeletal muscle consists of hundreds of _____ arranged in fascicles
8. In _____ contraction, muscles shorten and thicken as they contract
10. Cells that break down bone
11. The _____ skeleton consists of the skull, vertebral column, ribs, and sternum
12. There are seven _____ vertebrae
15. The cranium includes the frontal, occipital, ethmoid, spheroid, and paired parietal and _____ bones
19. The _____ girdle consists of the coxal bones together with the sacrum and coccyx
21. Compact _____ consists of osteons

Chapter

THE CENTRAL NERVOUS SYSTEM

■ ■ ■

Outline

I. The nervous system has two main divisions.
II. Neurons and glial cells are the cells of the nervous system.
III. Bundles of axons make up nerves.
IV. Appropriate responses depend on neural signaling.
V. Neurons transmit information with electrical signals.
  A. The neuron has a resting potential.
  B. An action potential is a wave of depolarization.
VI. Neurons signal other cells across synapses.
  A. Neurons signal other cells with neurotransmitters.
  B. Neurotransmitters bind with receptors on postsynaptic neurons.
  C. Neurotransmitter receptors can send excitatory or inhibitory signals.
VII. Neural impulses must be integrated.
VIII. The human brain is the most complex mechanism known.

A. The medulla contains vital centers.
B. The pons is a bridge to other parts of the brain.
C. The midbrain contains centers for visual and auditory reflexes.
D. The diencephalon includes the thalamus and the hypothalamus.
E. The cerebellum is responsible for coordination of movement.
F. The cerebrum is the largest part of the brain.
G. The limbic system affects emotional aspects of behavior.
H. Learning involves many areas of the brain.
IX. The spinal cord transmits information to and from the brain.
X. The central nervous system is well protected.
  A. The meninges are connective tissue coverings.
  B. The cerebrospinal fluid cushions the CNS.

Learning Objectives

After you have studied this chapter, you should be able to:

1. Distinguish between the central nervous system and the peripheral nervous system, and describe each.
2. Distinguish between neurons and glial cells, describing their structure and functions.
3. Distinguish between nerve and tract, ganglion and nucleus.
4. Briefly describe the basic processes essential for neural signaling—reception, transmission, integration, and response.
5. Contrast an action potential with the resting potential of a neuron, and describe each.

6. Compare continuous conduction and saltatory conduction.
7. Describe the transmission of a signal across a synapse, and draw a diagram to support your description.
8. Describe the actions of the neurotransmitters discussed in this chapter.
9. Define neural integration and describe how a postsynaptic neuron integrates incoming stimuli and "decides" whether to fire.

10. Describe the structure and functions of the main parts of the brain: medulla, pons, midbrain, diencephalon (thalamus and hypothalamus), cerebellum, and cerebrum. Be able to label the main structures of the brain on a diagram.
11. Describe the principal areas and functions associated with the lobes of the cerebrum and the limbic system.

12. List two functions of the spinal cord and describe its structure.
13. Trace in sequence the structures through which signals are transmitted in a withdrawal reflex. Draw and label a diagram of a withdrawal reflex.
14. Describe the structures that protect the brain and spinal cord.

STUDY QUESTIONS

Within each category, fill in the blanks with the correct response.

I. THE NERVOUS SYSTEM HAS TWO MAIN DIVISIONS

Afferent	Autonomic	Brain	Central	Cranial
Efferent	Peripheral	Sensory	Somatic	Spinal

1. The two main divisions of the nervous system are the _____ nervous system and the _____ nervous system.

2. The central nervous system consists of the _____ and spinal cord.

3. The peripheral nervous system is made up of the _____ receptors and the nerves which are the communication lines to and from the central nervous system.

4. Twelve pairs of _____ nerves link the brain and 31 pairs of _____ nerves link the spinal cord with sensory receptors and other parts of the body.

5. The peripheral nervous system may be subdivided into _____ and _____ divisions.

6. _____ (also called sensory) nerves transmit messages from the receptors to the central nervous system.

7. _____ (also called motor) nerves transmit information back from the central nervous system to the structures that must respond.

II. NEURONS AND GLIAL CELLS ARE THE CELLS OF THE NERVOUS SYSTEM

Action	Astrocyte	Axon	Cellular	Dendrites
Glial	Impulses	Myelin	Neural	Neurons
Neurotransmitters	Sheath	Synaptic terminals		

1. _____ are highly specialized to receive and transmit electrical and chemical signals.

2. These signals are called _____ impulses or _____ potentials.

3. _____ are highly branched fibers that extend from the cell body.

4. Typically, a single _____ transmits neural messages from the cell body toward another neuron.

5. At its distal end, the axon divides extensively, forming many terminal branches that end in _____.

6. Synaptic terminals release _____, chemical compounds that transmit signals from one neuron to another.

7. Axons of many neurons of the peripheral nervous system are covered by two sheaths: an inner _____ sheath and an outer _____ sheath called a neurilemma.

8. The cellular _____ is important in the repair of injured neurons.

9. Myelin is an excellent electrical insulator that speeds the conduction of nerve _____.

10. _____ cells protect and support neurons.

11. One type of glial cell, the _____, helps regulate the composition of the extracellular fluid in the CNS by removing excess potassium ions.

Labeling Exercise

Please fill in the correct labels for Figure 6-1.

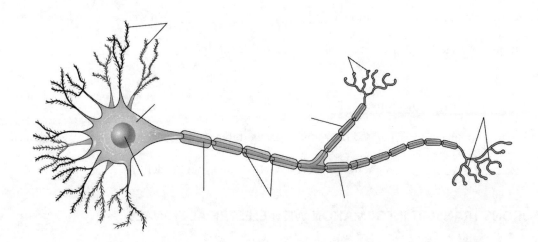

III. BUNDLES OF AXONS MAKE UP NERVES

Axons   Ganglion   Myelin   Nerve   Nuclei   Tracts

1. A(n) _____ is a large bundle of axons wrapped in connective tissue.

2. In comparing a nerve to a telephone cable, the _____ are like the individual wires, and the _____, cellular, and connective tissue sheaths are like the insulation.

3. The cell bodies attached to the axons of a nerve are often grouped together in a mass known as a _____.

4. Within the central nervous system, bundles of axons are called _____, or pathways, instead of nerves.

5. Masses of cell bodies located in the central nervous system are referred to as _____, rather than ganglia.

IV. APPROPRIATE RESPONSES DEPEND ON NEURAL SIGNALING

1. Number the following processes in order of occurrence from 1 to 5.
    _____ Integration
    _____ Reception
    _____ Transmission (to the muscles)
    _____ Transmission (to the central nervous system)
    _____ Actual response

Dendrites   Interneurons   Neurotransmitters   Synapse   Synaptic

2. Afferent neurons transmit information to _____ in the central nervous system.

3. Neurons are arranged so that the axon of one neuron signals the _____ of other neurons.

4. A junction between two neurons is called a(n) _____.

5. At a synapse, neurons are separated by a tiny gap called the _____ cleft.

6. _____ conduct "messages" across the synaptic cleft.

V. NEURONS TRANSMIT INFORMATION WITH ELECTRICAL SIGNALS

Gradient   Plasma   Polarized   Potential

1. Most cells have a difference in electrical charge across the _____ membrane.

2. The plasma membrane is said to be electrically _____.

3. The difference in electrical charge across the plasma membrane produces an electrical

_____.

4. The voltage measured across the plasma membrane is referred to as the membrane

_____.

A.   The Neuron Has a Resting Potential

Millivolts   **Passive ion**   **Potassium**   **Resting**   **Sodium**   **Sodium-potassium**

1. The membrane potential in a resting neuron is its _____ potential.

2. The resting potential is expressed in units called _____.

3. Many types of ions pass through specific _____ channels.

4. The gradients that determine the resting potential are maintained by _____ pumps in the plasma membrane.

5. Sodium-potassium pumps continuously transport _____ ions out of the neuron, and transport _____ ions in.

B.   An Action Potential Is a Wave of Depolarization

Action potential   **Hyperpolarization**   **Impulses**   **Permeability**   **Ranvier**
Repolarization   **Saltatory**   **Unmyelinated**   **Voltage-activated**

1. Neurons have the ability to respond to stimuli and to convert stimuli into nerve

_____.

2. An electrical, chemical, or mechanical stimulus may alter the resting potential by increasing the membrane's _____ to sodium.

3. _____ decreases the ability of the neuron to generate a neural impulse and is described as inhibitory.

4. When a stimulus is sufficiently strong, _____ ion channels in the plasma membrane open.

5. When voltage across the membrane is decreased to a critical point, called the threshold level, a neural impulse, or _____, is generated.

6. As the action potential moves down the axon, _____ occurs behind it.

7. Continuous conduction occurs in _____ neurons.

8. Myelin acts as an effective electrical insulator around the axon. However, the nodes of

_____ are not myelinated.

9. _____ conduction is faster and requires less energy than continuous conduction.

VI. NEURONS SIGNAL OTHER CELLS ACROSS SYNAPSES

Postsynaptic   **Presynaptic**   **Synapse**   **Synaptic cleft**

1. A _____ is a junction between two neurons or between a neuron and a muscle (or gland).

2. A neuron that terminates at a specific synapse is referred to as a _____ neuron.

3. A neuron that begins at a synapse is known as a _____ neuron.

4. A presynaptic neuron is separated from a postsynaptic neuron by a _____.

A. Neurons Signal Other Cells with Neurotransmitters

Adrenergic	**Amino**	**Biogenic**	**Chemical**	**Cholinergic**
Endorphins	**Enkephalins**	**Neuromodulators**	**Neurotransmitters**	**Nitric oxide**

1. _____ are chemical messengers that transmit the neural signal across the synapse and signal other neurons or muscle or gland cells.

2. More than 60 different _____ compounds are now known to function as neurotransmitters.

3. Some neurotransmitters, sometimes called _____, modify the effects of other neurotransmitters.

4. Cells that release the neurotransmitter acetylcholine are referred to as _____ neurons.

5. Neurons that release norepinephrine are called _____ neurons.

6. Norepinephrine, serotonin, and dopamine belong to a class of compounds called _____ amines.

7. Certain _____ acids also serve as neurotransmitters.

8. The body makes its own opioids, called _____ and _____.

9. _____ , which is a gas, is a retrograde messenger at some synapses, transmitting information in the opposite direction of other neurotransmitters.

B. Neurotransmitters Bind with Receptors on Postsynaptic Neurons

Dopamine   **Ion**   **Receptors**   **Reuptake**   **Synaptic vesicles**

1. Neurotransmitters are stored in the synaptic terminals within small membrane-bounded sacs called _____.

2. Neurotransmitter molecules diffuse across the synaptic cleft and combine with specific _____ on the plasma membrane of postsynaptic cells.

3. Many neurotransmitter receptors are chemically activated _____ channels.

4. The process in which catecholamines are actively transported back into the synaptic terminals is called

   _____.

5. Cocaine inhibits the reuptake of _____.

C.   Neurotransmitter Receptors Can Send Excitatory or Inhibitory Signals

Excitatory   Excitatory postsynaptic potential (EPSP)   Inhibitory
Inhibitory postsynaptic potential (IPSP)   Summation

1. Acetylcholine has a(n) _____ effect on skeletal muscle, while it has a(n)

   _____ effect on cardiac muscle.

2. A change in membrane potential that brings the neuron closer to firing is called a(n)

   _____.

3. A neurotransmitter-receptor combination that hyperpolarizes the postsynaptic membrane takes the neu-

   ron farther away from the firing level. This is referred to as a(n) _____.

4. Excitatory postsynaptic potentials may be added together in a process known as

   _____.

VII.   NEURAL IMPULSES MUST BE INTEGRATED

Action potential   Cancel   CNS   Graded   Neural integration

1. _____ is the process of summing incoming signals.

2. EPSPs and IPSPs are produced continually in postsynaptic neurons, and IPSPs

   _____ the effects of some of the EPSPs.

3. IPSPs and EPSPs are _____ responses that may be added to or subtracted from

   other EPSPs and IPSPs.

4. Local responses permit the neuron and the entire nervous system a far greater range of response than

   would be the case if every EPSP generated a(n) _____.

5. Most neural integration takes place in the _____.

VIII.   THE HUMAN BRAIN IS THE MOST COMPLEX MECHANISM KNOWN

Brain stem   Cerebrovascular   Cerebrovascular accident   Glucose   Neural
Oxygen   Ventricles

1. At any moment, millions of _____ messages are flashing through the brain.

2. Brain cells require a continuous supply of _____ and

   _____.

3. The most common cause of brain damage is a(n) _____.

4. In a(n) _____ accident, a portion of the brain is deprived of its blood supply.

5. The medulla, pons, and midbrain make up the _____.

6. The brain is a hollow organ; its fluid-filled spaces are called _____.

A. The Medulla Contains Vital Centers

Cardiac	**Cerebrum**	**Medulla**	**Oblongata**
Respiratory	**Reticular formation**	**Spinal cord**	**Vasomotor**

1. More formally known as the medulla _____, the medulla is the most posterior portion of the brain stem.

2. Because of its position, all nerve tracts carrying messages from the _____ to the brain must pass through the medulla.

3. The _____ is a network of neurons that extends from the spinal cord through the medulla and upward through the brain stem and thalamus.

4. The reticular formation is important in keeping the _____ conscious and alert.

5. _____ centers in the medulla control heart rate.

6. _____ centers in the medulla help regulate blood pressure by controlling the diameter of the blood vessels.

7. _____ centers in the medulla initiate and regulate breathing.

8. Four cranial nerves, designated cranial nerves IX through XII, originate within the _____, and their nuclei are located there.

B. The Pons Is a Bridge to Other Parts of the Brain

Brain	**Cerebellum**	**Medulla**	**Nerve**	**Respiration**	**Pons**

1. The _____ forms a bulge on the anterior (ventral) surface of the brain stem.

2. The pons is just superior to the _____, with which it is continuous.

3. The posterior surface of the pons is hidden by the _____.

4. The pons serves as a link connecting various parts of the _____.

5. The pons consists mainly of _____ fibers passing between the medulla and other parts of the brain.

6. The pons also contains centers that help regulate _____ and sleep.

C. The Midbrain Contains Centers for Visual and Auditory Reflexes

Auditory   **Cerebral aqueduct**   **Midbrain**   **Neurons**   **Pons**   **Visual**

1. The _____ is the shortest portion of the brain stem.

2. The midbrain extends from the _____ to the diencephalon.

3. The cavity of the midbrain, known as the _____, connects the third and fourth ventricles.

4. Anteriorly, the midbrain consists of large bundles of _____ connecting the cerebrum with lower portions of the brain and with the spinal cord.

5. The roof of the midbrain consists of four rounded bodies that serve as centers for _____ and _____ reflexes.

D. The Diencephalon Includes the Thalamus and the Hypothalamus

ADH	Autonomic	Circadian	Diencephalon	Endocrine
Hypothalamus	Motor	Nuclei	Suprachiasmatic	Thalamus

1. The _____ is the part of the brain between the cerebrum and the midbrain.

2. The _____ is a major relay center, consisting of two oval masses, located on each side of the third ventricle.

3. _____ in the thalamus serve as relay stations for all sensory information (except smell) to the cerebrum.

4. The thalamus integrates motor information from the cerebellum and transmits messages to _____ areas in the cerebrum.

5. The _____ lies below the thalamus. Its function is to help regulate homeostasis and reproductive behavior.

6. The hypothalamus is sometimes called the control center of the _____ nervous system because it is the most important relay station between the cerebral cortex and the lower autonomic centers.

7. The hypothalamus is the link between the nervous and _____ systems.

8. _____ produced by cells in the hypothalamus regulates the volume of water excreted by the kidneys.

9. The hypothalamus, along with the brain stem, regulates sleep-wake cycles called _____ rhythms.

10. The _____ nucleus in the hypothalamus is the most important of the body's biological clocks.

E. The Cerebellum Is Responsible for Coordination of Movement

Cerebellum   **Language**   **Motor**   **Movements**   **Muscle**   **Vestibular**

1. The _____ is the second-largest part of the brain, and consists of two lateral masses called hemispheres and a connecting portion.

2. The cerebellum helps make _____ smooth instead of jerky, and steady rather than trembling.

3. The cerebellum helps maintain _____ tone and posture.

4. Impulses from the _____ apparatus in the inner ear are continuously delivered to the cerebellum, which uses that information to help maintain equilibrium.

5. The cerebellum is also important in learning _____ skills.

6. Recent studies indicate that the cerebellum receives information from sensory association areas in the cerebrum and is important in cognitive function, including _____.

F. The Cerebrum Is the Largest Part of the Brain

Association   **Central sulcus**   **Cerebrum**   **Corpus callosum**   **Intellectual**
Motor   **Movement**   **Precentral**   **Primary visual area**   **Postcentral**
Sensory   **Temporal**   **Transverse**

1. The _____ is the largest and most prominent part of the human brain.

2. The functions of the cerebrum can be divided into _____ functions, _____ functions, and _____ functions.

3. The motor areas of the cerebrum are responsible for all voluntary and some involuntary _____.

4. *Association* is a term used to describe all of the _____ activities of the cerebral cortex.

5. The cerebrum is separated from the cerebellum by the _____ fissure.

6. A large band of white matter, the _____, connects the right and left hemispheres of the cerebrum.

7. Each frontal lobe is separated from a parietal lobe by a _____.

8. Just anterior to the central sulcus lies the _____ gyrus of the frontal lobe.

9. The parietal lobe has a primary sensory area, the _____ gyrus, which receives information from the sensory receptors in the skin and joints.

10. The area in the occipital lobe that receives visual information is known as the _____.

11. The _____ lobe is concerned with reception and integration of auditory messages.

G.   The Limbic System Affects Emotional Aspects of Behavior

Amygdala   **Emotional**   **Hippocampus**   **Limbic**   **Memories**   **Motivation**

1.   The _____ system is a group of interconnected nuclei involved in memory and in the regulation of emotion.

2.   The system of neurons of the limbic system evaluates rewards, and is important in _____.

3.   Two very important limbic regions are the _____ and the _____.

4.   The hippocampus is involved in the formation and retrieval of _____.

5.   The amygdala filters incoming sensory information and evaluates its importance in terms of _____ needs and survival.

Labeling Exercise

Please fill in the correct labels for Figure 6-2.

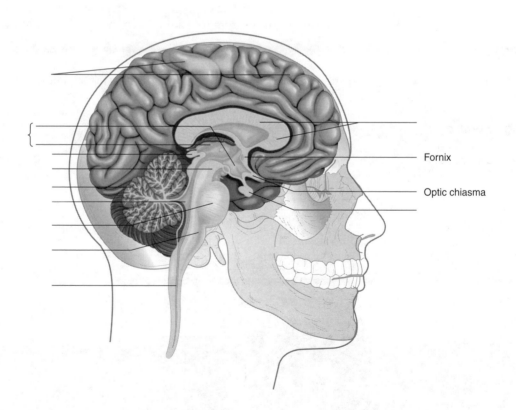

Fornix

Optic chiasma

H. Learning Involves Many Areas of the Brain

Learning   Memory   Synaptic plasticity

1. _____ is the process by which we acquire information as a result of experience.

2. _____ is the process by which information is encoded, stored, and retrieved.

3. _____ refers to the ability of the nervous system to modify synapses during learning and remembering.

IX. THE SPINAL CORD TRANSMITS INFORMATION TO AND FROM THE BRAIN

Ascending   Descending   Fissures   Reflex action   Spinal   Vertebral

1. The _____ cord has two main functions: (1) it transmits information to and from the brain and (2) it controls many reflex activities of the body.

2. The spinal cord occupies the _____ canal of the vertebral column.

3. Several grooves called _____ divide the spinal cord into regions.

4. _____ tracts transmit sensory information up the spinal cord to the brain.

5. _____ tracts transmit impulses from the brain down the spinal cord to the efferent nerves.

6. A _____ is a predictable, automatic response to a specific stimulus.

Labeling Exercise

Please fill in the correct labels for Figure 6-3.

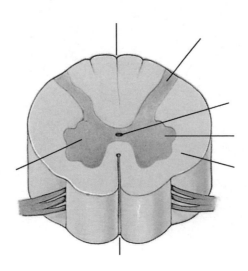

X.   THE CENTRAL NERVOUS SYSTEM IS WELL PROTECTED

A.   The Meninges Are Connective Tissue Coverings

Arachnoid   Dura mater   Encephalitis   Meninges   Meningitis   Pia mater   Sinuses

1.   The three connective tissue layers covering the brain and spinal cord are the

_____.

2.   The outermost of the meninges is the _____, a tough, double-layered membrane.

3.   Inside the skull, the two layers of the dura mater are separated in some regions by large blood vessels called _____. These vessels receive blood leaving the brain and deliver it to the jugular veins in the neck.

4.   The second layer of the meninges is the _____, a thin, delicate membrane.

5.   The innermost meningeal layer is the _____, a very thin membrane that adheres closely to the brain and spinal cord.

6.   _____ is an inflammation of the meninges.

7.   Some viruses that cause meningitis can spread, causing inflammation of the brain itself. This more serious illness is _____.

B.   The Cerebrospinal Fluid Cushions the CNS

Brain   Cerebrospinal fluid   Choroid plexuses   Hydrocephalus   Lumbar

1.   The shock-absorbing fluid that fills the ventricles, the cavities within the brain, and the subarachnoid space is called _____.

2.   Most of the cerebrospinal fluid (CSF) is produced by clusters of capillaries called the _____ which project from the pia mater into the ventricles.

3.   The _____ actually floats in CSF, which protects it against mechanical injury.

4.   Blockage of CSF flow or abnormally rapid production of CSF can result in _____.

5.   A _____ puncture is a procedure that can be used to withdraw small amounts of CSF or measure CSF pressure without damaging the spinal cord.

Labeling Exercise

Please fill in the correct labels for Figure 6-4.

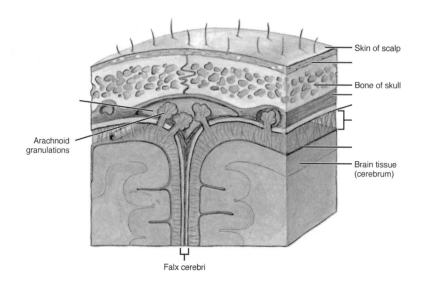

Skin of scalp

Bone of skull

Brain tissue
(cerebrum)

Arachnoid
granulations

Falx cerebri

CHAPTER TEST

Select the correct response.

1. The _____ system serves as the body's link to the outside world.
   a. digestive
   b. nervous
   c. reproductive
   d. circulatory

2. The two principal divisions of the nervous system are the
   a. central and accessory nervous systems.
   b. central and autonomic nervous systems.
   c. central and peripheral nervous systems.
   d. autonomic and peripheral nervous systems.

3. The central nervous system is made up of the
   a. eyes and ears.
   b. brain and spinal cord.
   c. taste buds.
   d. both a and c.

4. The peripheral nervous system includes the
   a. sense organs (i.e., eyes, ears, etc.).
   b. arms and legs.
   c. medulla.
   d. muscles and bones.

5. The correct order of response of the following processes is
   a. reception, transmission, integration, transmission, response.
   b. transmission, reception, transmission, integration, response.
   c. reception, integration, transmission, response, transmission.
   d. response, reception, transmission, integration, transmission.

6. The main divisions of the brain are the
   a. medulla, pons, diencephalon, and cerebrum.
   b. medulla, pons, midbrain, diencephalon, cerebrum, and cerebellum.
   c. medulla, cerebrum, and cerebellum.
   d. thalamus, hypothalamus, medulla, and cerebrum.

7. The brain stem is made up of the
   a. medulla, pons, and cerebrum.
   b. cerebellum, midbrain, and pons.
   c. medulla, pons, and midbrain.
   d. midbrain, pons, and cerebrum.

8. The _____ is a vital center of the medulla.
   a. cardiac center
   b. vasomotor center
   c. respiratory center
   d. all of the above

9. All of the following are functions of the hypo-thalamus *except*
   a. linking nervous and endocrine systems.
   b. helping to maintain fluid balance.
   c. regulating body temperature.
   d. coordination of movement.

10. Functions of the cerebellum include helping to
    a. smooth and coordinate movement.
    b. maintain posture.
    c. maintain equilibrium.
    d. all of the above.

11. All of the following are functions of the cere-brum *except*
    a. controlling motor activities.
    b. interpreting sensation.
    c. serving as the center of intellect.
    d. regulating body temperature.

12. Which of the following processes are compo-nents of a reflex pathway?
    a. reception of the stimulus
    b. transmission of information
    c. integration of the stimulus
    d. all of the above

13. All of the following are true of the limbic sys-tem *except*
    a. helps regulate emotion.
    b. involved in memory processing.
    c. coordinates movement.
    d. important in motivation.

14. The primary visual area is located in the
    a. thalamus.
    b. temporal lobe.
    c. prefrontal area.
    d. occipital lobe.

15. Broca's speech area
    a. is located in the parietal lobe.
    b. directs the formation of words.
    c. is important in learning to make decisions and put them into words.
    d. all of the above.

16. The dura mater is
    a. a tough, double-layered membrane.
    b. the innermost of the meninges.
    c. a large blood sinus.
    d. all of the above.

17. The cerebrospinal fluid
    a. fills the anterior median fissure.
    b. is produced by the choroid plexuses.
    c. contains amino acids used to produce neu-rons.
    d. all of the above.

Labeling Exercise

Please fill in the correct labels for Figure 6-5.

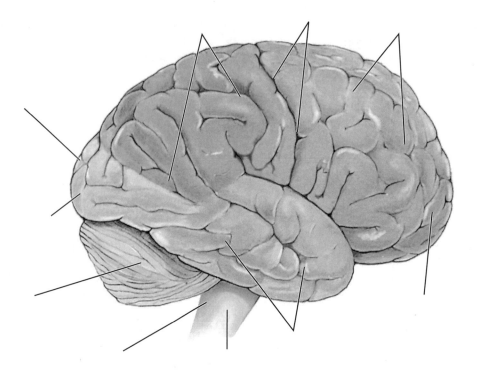

Chapter

7

THE PERIPHERAL NERVOUS SYSTEM

■ ■ ■

Outline

Introduction

I.   The somatic division responds to changes in the outside world.
   A.   The cranial nerves link the brain with sensory receptors and muscles.
   B.   The spinal nerves link the spinal cord with various structures.
      1.   Each spinal nerve divides into branches.
      2.   The ventral branches form plexuses.

II.   The autonomic division maintains internal balance.
   A.   The sympathetic system mobilizes energy.
   B.   The parasympathetic system conserves and restores energy.
   C.   Sympathetic and parasympathetic nerves have opposite effects on many organs.

Learning Objectives

After you have studied this chapter, you should be able to:

1.   Describe the components of the somatic division of the nervous system.
2.   List the cranial nerves and give the functions of each.
3.   Describe the structure of a typical spinal nerve.
4.   Name and describe the major plexuses.
5.   Compare and contrast the autonomic division with the somatic division.
6.   Describe a reflex pathway in the autonomic system.
7.   Compare and contrast the sympathetic with the parasympathetic system.
8.   Compare the effect of sympathetic with that of parasympathetic stimulation on specific organs such as the heart and the digestive tract.

STUDY QUESTIONS

Within each category, fill in the blanks with the correct response.

INTRODUCTION

Autonomic   Sensory   Somatic

1.   The peripheral nervous system is made up of _____ receptors, the nerves that link the sensory receptors with the central nervous system, and the nerves that link the central nervous system with effectors—the muscles and glands.

2. The portion of the peripheral nervous system that keeps the body in adjustment with the outside world is the _____ division.

3. The nerves and receptors that maintain internal balance make up the _____ division.

I. THE SOMATIC DIVISION RESPONDS TO CHANGES IN THE OUTSIDE WORLD

Cranial   Somatic   Spinal

1. The _____ division includes the sensory receptors that react to changes in the outside world.

2. The afferent and efferent neurons of the somatic division, like those of the autonomic division, are part of the _____ and _____ nerves.

A. Cranial Nerves Link the Brain with Sensory Receptors and Muscles

Afferent   CNS   Cranial   Efferent   Sensory

1. Twelve pairs of _____ nerves emerge form the brain.

2. Cranial nerves transmit information to the brain from _____ receptors.

3. Cranial nerves transmit orders in the form of neural signals from the _____ to muscles and glands.

4. Most cranial nerves consist of both sensory (or _____) neurons, and motor (or _____) neurons.

B. The Spinal Nerves Link the Spinal Cord with Various Structures

Coccygeal	Dorsal	Eight	Five	Ganglion
Lumbar	Spinal	Thoracic	Ventral	Vertebral column

1. Thirty-one pairs of _____ nerves emerge form the spinal cord.

2. Spinal nerves are named for the general region of the _____ from which they originate and are numbered in sequence.

3. There are _____ pairs of cervical spinal nerves.

4. There are 12 pairs of _____ spinal nerves.

5. There are five pairs of _____ spinal nerves.

6. There are _____ pairs of sacral spinal nerves.

7. There is one pair of _____ spinal nerves.

8. The _____ root consists only of afferent (sensory) fibers that transmit information from sensory receptors to the spinal cord.

9. Just before the dorsal root joins the spinal cord, it is marked by a swelling called the spinal _____, which consists of the cell bodies of the sensory neurons.

10. The _____ root consists only of efferent (motor) fibers leaving the spinal cord.

1. Each Spinal Nerve Divides Into Branches

Branches   Dorsal   Ventral

1. Just after a spinal nerve emerges form the vertebral column, it divides into _____.

2. The _____ branch of each nerve supplies the muscles and skin of the posterior part of the body in that region.

3. The _____ branch innervates the anterior and lateral body trunk in that area, as well as the limbs.

2. The Ventral Branches Form Plexuses

Brachial   Cervical   Femoral   Innervate   Lumbar
Phrenic   Plexuses   Sacral   Sciatic

1. The ventral branches of several spinal nerves interconnect, forming networks called _____.

2. Nerves that emerge from a plexus may be named for the region of the body that they _____.

3. The main plexuses are the _____ plexus, the _____ plexus, the _____ plexus, and the _____ plexus.

4. The _____ nerve, which sends impulses to the diaphragm, exits from the cervical plexus.

5. The _____ nerve is the largest nerve arising from the lumbar plexus.

6. The main branch of the sacral plexus is the _____ nerve, the largest nerve in the body.

Labeling Exercise

Please fill in the correct labels for Figure 7-1.

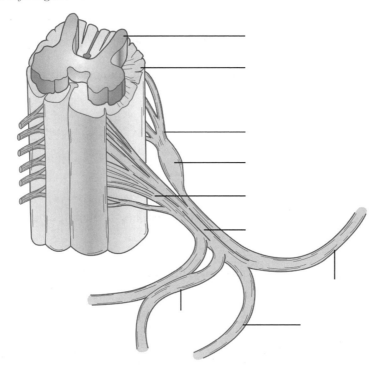

II. THE AUTONOMIC DIVISION MAINTAINS INTERNAL BALANCE

Autonomic   **Efferent**   **Parasympathetic**   **Sympathetic**

1. The _____ division works automatically to maintain homeostasis within the body.

2. The efferent portion of the autonomic division is subdivided into _____ and _____ systems.

3. In the autonomic division, two _____ neurons are found between the central nervous system and the muscle or gland it innervates.

A. The Sympathetic System Mobilizes Energy

Acetylcholine   **Action**   **Adrenergic**   **Cholinergic**   **Collateral**   **Neurons**
Norepinephrine   **Paravertebral** **Postganglionic** **Preganglionic**   **Sympathetic**

1. The sympathetic system prepares the body for _____.

2. The _____ system dominates when you are rushing to class or taking a test.

3. _____ of the sympathetic system emerge from the thoracic and lumbar regions of the spinal cord.

4. Efferent sympathetic neurons pass through the autonomic branch of the spinal nerve, then they pass into the ganglia of the _____ sympathetic ganglion chain.

5. Some of the first efferent neurons pass on to ganglia located in the abdomen, known as

    _____ ganglia.

6. The first efferent neurons are referred to as _____ neurons.

7. The second efferent neurons are referred to as _____ neurons.

8. Preganglionic neurons of the sympathetic system release the neurotransmitter

    _____, and are referred to as _____.

9. Postganglionic neurons release _____, and are referred to as

    _____.

B.   The Parasympathetic System Conserves and Restores Energy

Acetylcholine	**Active**	**Brain**	**Conserving**	**Parasympathetic**
Pelvic	**Terminal ganglia**	**Vagus**		

1. The parasympathetic system is most _____ during periods of calm and physical

    rest.

2. Activities of the parasympathetic system result in _____ and restoring energy.

3. Neurons of the parasympathetic system emerge from the _____ as part of the

    cranial nerves, and from the sacral region of the spinal cord.

4. About 75% of the parasympathetic fibers are in the _____ nerves.

5. The first efferent neurons synapse with the second efferent neurons in _____

    located near or within the walls of the organs they innervate.

6. The parasympathetic nerves that emerge from the sacral region form the _____

    nerves.

7. _____ nerves do not innervate blood vessels or sweat glands.

8. Both preganglionic and postganglionic fibers of the parasympathetic system are cholinergic. They release

    the neurotransmitter _____.

C.   Sympathetic and Parasympathetic Nerves Have Opposite Effects on Many Organs

Decrease	**Increase**	**Parasympathetic**	**Sympathetic**

1. Sympathetic nerves _____ heart rate.

2. Parasympathetic nerves _____ heart rate.

3. Digestive system activity is increased by the _____ system,

4. The _____ system is not necessary for normal digestive system function.

CHAPTER TEST

Select the correct response.

1. The _____ nerves link the brain with sensory receptors and muscles.
   a. cranial
   b. spinal
   c. thalamic
   d. thoracic

2. There are 8 pairs of _____ spinal nerves and 12 pairs of _____ spinal nerves.
   a. cervical; sacral
   b. lumbar; thoracic
   c. cervical; thoracic
   d. thoracic; lumbar

3. The _____ ganglion consists of cell bodies of sensory neurons.
   a. paravertebral
   b. spinal
   c. ventral
   d. collateral

4. The ventral branches of several spinal nerves interconnect, forming networks called
   a. ganglia.
   b. tracts.
   c. cranial nerves.
   d. plexuses.

5. The _____ plexus supplies the thigh, leg, and foot.
   a. brachial
   b. cervical
   c. lumbar
   d. sacral

6. The main branch of the sacral plexus is the _____ nerve.
   a. cardiac
   b. vagus
   c. sciatic
   d. phrenic

7. In the autonomic division, two _____ neurons are found between the central nervous system and the muscle it innervates.
   a. afferent
   b. efferent
   c. sensory
   d. cranial

8. _____ nerves increase heart rate.
   a. Sympathetic
   b. Parasympathetic
   c. Vagus
   d. Spinal

9. In the sympathetic system, some efferent neurons end in _____ ganglia located in the abdomen.
   a. collateral
   b. terminal
   c. paravertebral
   d. spinal

10. Neurons of the sympathetic system emerge from the _____ and _____ regions of the spinal cord.
    a. cervical; thoracic
    b. thoracic; lumbar
    c. lumbar; sacral
    d. cervical; lumbar

11. The _____ system is most active during periods of calm.
    a. somatic
    b. parasympathetic
    c. sympathetic
    d. cranial

12. In the parasympathetic system, the first efferent neurons synapse with the second efferent neurons in _____ ganglia.
    a. collateral
    b. terminal
    c. paravertebral
    d. spinal

Chapter

THE SENSE ORGANS

■ ■ ■

Outline

Introduction
I.   Sensory receptors transduce the energy of a stimulus into electrical signals.
II. Sensory receptors respond to different types of energy.
III. The eye contains photoreceptors.
   A. The eye is well protected.
   B. The eye is enclosed by three specialized tissue layers.
   C. The eyes form a sharp image.
   D. The retina contains light-sensitive rods and cones.
   E. The optic nerves transmit signals to the brain.
IV. The ear functions in hearing and equilibrium.
   A. The outer ear conducts sound waves to the middle ear.
   B. The middle ear amplifies sound waves.

   C. The inner ear contains mechanoreceptors.
     1. The cochlea contains the receptors for hearing.
     2. Sounds differ in pitch, loudness, and quality.
   D. The vestibule and semicircular canals help maintain equilibrium.
V. Chemoreceptors sense smell and taste.
   A. Chemoreceptors in the nasal cavity sense odorants.
   B. Taste buds detect dissolved food molecules.
VI. The general senses are widespread through the body.
   A. Tactile receptors are located in the skin.
   B. Temperature receptors are nerve endings.
   C. Pain sensation is a protective mechanism.
   D. Proprioceptors inform us of our position.

Learning Objectives

After you have studied this chapter, you should be able to:

1. Describe how a sensory receptor functions, including sensory reception, energy transduction, receptor potential, sensory adaptation, and perception.
2. Classify sensory receptors according to the type of energy they transduce.
3. Describe the anatomy of the eye and give the function of each structure. (Include a description of the visual pathway.)
4. Describe the structures and functions of the three major parts of the ear.

5. Trace the transmission of sound through the ear.
6. Describe the functions of the vestibule and semicircular canals.
7. Compare the receptors of smell and taste.
8. Describe the tactile receptors and temperature receptors.
9. Describe the process of pain perception and explain the basis of phantom and referred pain.
10. Locate proprioceptors in the body and describe their functions.

STUDY QUESTIONS

Within each category, fill in the blanks with the correct response.

INTRODUCTION

Homeostasis   **Sensory**   **Stimulus**

1. Any detectable change in the environment is called a _____.

2. We detect stimuli through our _____ receptors.

3. Sensory receptors connect us with the outside environment, and also transmit signals about internal changes that threaten _____.

I. SENSORY RECEPTORS TRANSDUCE THE ENERGY OF A STIMULUS INTO ELECTRICAL SIGNALS

Action	**Brain**	**CNS**	**Decreases**
Ears	**Eyes**	**Graded response**	**Neurons**
Nose	**Perception**	**Receptor potential**	**Sensors**
Sensory adaptation	**Sensory experience**	**Sensory receptors**	**Taste buds**
Transduce			

1. Sensory receptors _____ (convert) the energy of a stimulus into electrical signals.

2. Sensory receptors, along with other types of cells, make up complex sense organs:

   _____, _____, _____, and

   _____.

3. The body has many internal _____ that maintain homeostatic balance.

4. When a change in membrane potential occurs, it produces a(n) _____—a depolarization or hyperpolarization of the membrane.

5. The sensory neuron transmits signals to the _____.

6. A receptor potential is a(n) _____, which means that the extent of change depends on the energy of the stimulus.

7. Each sensory receptor is connected by _____ to a particular area of the brain.

8. The _____ decodes incoming sensory messages.

9. An intense pain would involve a greater frequency of _____ potentials than a mild pain.

10. With time, the response to a continued, constant stimulus _____.

11. The decrease in frequency of action potentials in a sensory neuron even though the stimulus is maintained is called _____.

12. Sensory _____ is the process of selecting, interpreting, and organizing sensory information.

13. The brain interprets sensations by converting them to perceptions of the stimuli received by our _____.

14. We construct sensory perceptions by comparing our _____ with our memories of past experiences.

II.   SENSORY RECEPTORS RESPOND TO DIFFERENT TYPES OF ENERGY

Chemoreceptors   **Mechanoreceptors**   **Photoreceptors**   **Thermoreceptors**   **Transduce**

1. Sensory receptors _____ various types of energy into electrical energy that can result in action potentials.

2. _____ transduce light energy.

3. _____ transduce mechanical energy such as touch, pressure, or gravity.

4. _____ transduce chemical compounds.

5. _____ respond to heat and cold.

III.   THE EYE CONTAINS PHOTORECEPTORS

A.   The Eye Is Well Protected

Blinking   **Eyelashes**   **Eyelids**   **Fat**
Lacrimal duct   **Lacrimal glands**   **Orbit**   **Reflex**

1. The eye and its muscles are set in the _____ formed by the skeletal bones of the face.

2. The eye and its muscles are cushioned by layers of _____.

3. The _____ and _____ help protect the eye anteriorly from foreign objects.

4. The eyelids close by _____ action if danger is perceived.

5. Frequent _____ of the eye lubricates the eye and clears debris.

6. Even though we are not aware of the process, tears flow at all times from the _____.

7. Tears pass out through the _____ and lubricate the surface of the eye.

B. The Eye Is Enclosed by Three Specialized Tissue Layers

| Aqueous humor | Choroid | Conjunctiva | Cornea |
| Retina | Sclera | Vitreous humor | |

1. The eyeball is formed by three layers of tissue: the fibrous sclera and _____, the _____ layer, and the _____.

2. The _____ is known as the "white of the eye."

3. The sclera is covered by the _____, a moist mucous membrane that extends as a continuous lining of the inner layer of the eyelids.

4. The anterior cavity between the cornea and the lens is filled with a watery substance known as the _____.

5. The larger posterior cavity between the lens and the retina is filled with a more viscous fluid known as the _____.

C. The Eyes Form a Sharp Image

| Accommodation | Ciliary | Extrinsic | Iris |
| Lens | Light | Pupil | Suspensory ligament |

1. The _____ is the colored part of the eye.

2. The iris regulates the amount of _____ entering the eye.

3. The black spot, or opening in the center of the circular muscles of the iris, is the _____ of the eye.

4. The _____ of the eye is an adjustable, transparent, elastic ball that lies just behind the iris.

5. The six _____ muscles control the movement of each eye.

6. The eye has the power of _____—the ability to change focus for near or far vision by changing the shape of the lens.

7. The _____ processes are glandlike folds that project toward the lens and secrete the aqueous humor.

8. The lens is attached to the ciliary muscles by tiny fibers that make up the _____.

D. The Retina Contains Light-Sensitive Rods and Cones

| Cones | Fovea | Optic disc | Photoreceptors | Rods |

1. The retina, the innermost layer of the eye, contains the _____—rods and cones.

2. The _____ are responsible for color vision and vision during the daytime.

3. The _____ are responsible mainly for vision in dim light or darkness.

4. Cones are most concentrated in the _____, a small depression in the center of the posterior region of the retina.

5. The area where the optic nerve passes out of the eyeball, the _____, is known as the blind spot because it lacks rods and cones.

E.   The Optic Nerves Transmit Signals to the Brain

Cerebrum   **Optic chiasm**   **Optic nerves**   **Primary visual cortex**

1. Axons of ganglion cells in the retina form the _____, which transmit information to the brain by way of complex, encoded signals.

2. The optic nerves cross in the floor of the hypothalamus, forming an X-shaped structure called the _____.

3. From the thalamus, neurons send signals to the _____ in the occipital lobe of the cerebrum.

4. We know that a large part of the association areas of the _____ are involved in integrating visual input.

Labeling Exercise

Please fill in the correct labels for Figure 8-1.

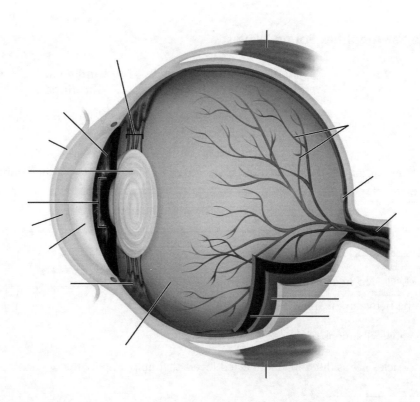

IV. THE EAR FUNCTIONS IN HEARING AND EQUILIBRIUM

Equilibrium   **Middle**   **Outer**   **Sensory**

1. The _____ ear includes the part we see and a canal connecting with the middle ear.

2. The _____ ear contains three small bones (auditory ossicles) that conduct sound waves.

3. The inner ear contains _____ receptors for sound waves and for maintaining the _____ of the body.

A. The Outer Ear Conducts Sound Waves to the Middle Ear

Cerumen   **Ceruminous**   **External auditory meatus**   **Pinna**   **Tympanic membrane**

1. The _____ is the part of the outer ear that projects from the side of the head and surrounds the ear canal.

2. The ear canal, more formally called the _____, leads to the middle ear.

3. The lining of the ear canal contains _____ glands that secrete earwax.

4. _____, commonly called earwax, helps protect the lining of the ear canal from infection.

5. The _____, or eardrum, separates the middle and external ear.

B. The Middle Ear Amplifies Sound Waves

Eustachian   **Incus**   **Malleus**   **Middle ear**   **Ossicles**
Oval window   **Stapes**   **Tympanic membrane**   **Vibrations**

1. The _____ is a small, moist cavity in the temporal bone containing air and three small bones called auditory _____.

2. Under normal circumstances, the air pressure is equalized on the two sides of the tympanic membrane by the _____ tube.

3. The three auditory ossicles are the _____, _____, and _____.

4. The auditory ossicles form a chain from the tympanic membrane to the _____, a small membrane between the middle and inner ear.

5. Sound waves cause vibrations of the _____.

6. The auditory ossicles act as three interconnected levers that help amplify the _____.

C.   The Inner Ear Contains Mechanoreceptors

Cochlea   **Endolymph**   **Equilibrium**   **Labyrinth**   **Mechanoreceptors**
Membranous   **Perilymph**   **Semicircular canals** **Vestibule**   **Vibrations**

1. The inner ear contains _____ that convert sound waves to nerve impulses.

2. The inner ear also contains receptors that enable us to maintain our _____.

3. The inner ear is a bony _____ composed of three compartments.

4. The _____, _____, and _____ make up the three compartments of the inner ear.

5. The bony labyrinth contains a fluid called _____.

6. The perilymph surrounds the _____ labyrinth.

7. The membranous labyrinth contains a fluid called _____.

8. Perilymph and endolymph carry _____ through the system of canals within the inner ear.

1.   The Cochlea Contains the Receptors for Hearing

Basilar   **Cochlea**   **Cochlear**   **Cochlear nerve**   **Glutamate**
Hair   **Organs of Corti** **Perilymph**   **Stereocilia**   **Tectorial membrane**
Tympanic   **Vestibular**

1. The _____ is a snail-shaped portion of the inner ear.

2. The cochlea contains the _____, the sound receptors.

3. Each organ of Corti contains sensory cells that respond to sound waves by stimulating the _____.

4. The _____ canal and the _____ canal are connected at the apex of the cochlea and are filled with _____.

5. The _____ duct is filled with endolymph and contains the organ of Corti.

6. Each organ of Corti contains about 18,000 _____ cells arranged in rows that extend the length of the coiled cochlea.

7. Each hair cell in the organ of Corti is equipped with tiny projections called _____ that extend into the cochlear duct.

8. The _____ membrane separates the cochlear duct from the tympanic canal.

9. Hair cells release the neurotransmitter _____, which binds to receptors on sensory neurons that synapse on each hair cell.

10. The _____ overhangs and is in contact with the hair cells of the organs of Corti.

2. *Sounds Differ in Pitch, Loudness, and Quality*

Amplitude	Cochlear	Deafness	Hair	High-frequency
High-intensity	Low-frequency	Pitch		

1. _____ depends on frequency of sound waves and is expressed as hertz (Hz).

2. _____ vibrations result in the sensation of low pitch.

3. _____ vibrations result in the sensation of high pitch.

4. The brain infers the pitch of a sound from the particular _____ cells that are stimulated.

5. Loud sounds cause resonance waves of greater _____.

6. When the hair cells are more intensely stimulated, the _____ nerve transmits a greater number of impulses per second.

7. _____ may be caused by malformation of or injury to the sound-transmitting mechanism of the outer, middle, or inner ear.

8. Exposure to heavily amplified music or other _____ sound damages the hair cells of the organ of Corti.

D. The Vestibule and Semicircular Canals Help Maintain Equilibrium

Angular acceleration	Crista	Cupula	Endolymph	Otoliths	Saccule
Semicircular	Utricle	Vestibular	Vestibule	Vestibulocochlear	

1. The _____ and _____ canals contain receptor cells that transmit information about the position of the body.

2. Inside the vestibule, the membranous labyrinth is divided into two saclike chambers—the _____ and the _____.

3. _____ are small, calcium carbonate ear stones that act as gravity detectors.

4. Each receptor cell has a group of hair cells surrounded at their tips by a gelatinous mass called a _____.

5. Information about turning movements, referred to as _____, is provided by the three semicircular canals.

6. Within each ampulla lies a clump of hair cells called a _____.

7. The response of the sensory cells in the semicircular canals is produced by the flow of _____ within the canals as the position of the head changes.

8. The _____ nerve joins the cochlear nerve to form the _____ nerve.

Labeling Exercise

Please fill in the correct labels for Figure 8-2.

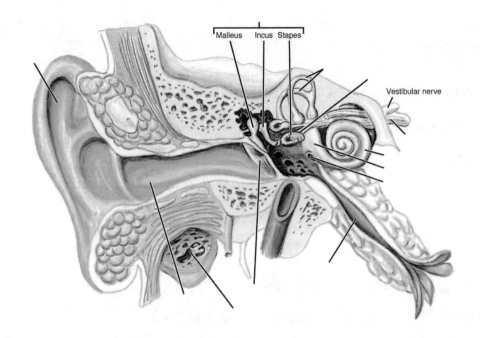

V.   CHEMORECEPTORS SENSE SMELL AND TASTE

A.   Chemoreceptors in the Nasal Cavity Sense Odorants

Chemoreceptors   **Odors**   **Olfaction**   **Olfactory nerve**   **Scents**   **Temporal**

1.   _____ allow us to detect chemical substances in the air and in food and water.

2.   _____, the sense of smell, is the function of chemoreceptor cells in the olfactory epithelium lining the upper part of the nasal cavity.

3.   Odors detected by the olfactory epithelium are transmitted by the _____ to the olfactory cortex in the _____ lobe.

4.   We can detect at least seven main groups of _____, and we can perceive about 10,000 different _____.

B.   Taste Buds Detect Dissolved Food Molecules

Bitter   **Gustation**   **Papillae**   **Salty**   **Smell**
Sour   **Sweet**   **Taste**   **Taste buds**   **Taste receptors**

1.   _____, the sense of taste, is the job of the _____ on the tongue and various parts of the mouth.

2.   Taste buds are found mainly in _____, tiny elevations on the tongue.

3. _____ detect chemical substances dissolved in saliva.

4. Traditionally, four main tastes have been recognized: _____,

   _____, _____, and _____.

5. Both _____ and _____ are important in stimulating appetite and digestive juices.

VI. THE GENERAL SENSES ARE WIDESPREAD THROUGH THE BODY

Muscle   **Nociceptors**   **Pain**   **Pressure**   **Temperature**   **Touch**   **Vibration**

1. The general senses include the receptors that respond to _____,

   _____, _____, _____, changes in

   _____, and _____ stretch.

2. Receptors that sense pain are _____.

A. Tactile Receptors Are Located in the Skin

Mechanoreceptors   **Pressure**   **Tactile**   **Touch**

1. The simplest _____ are free nerve endings in the skin.

2. Free nerve endings in the skin detect _____ and _____ when stimulated by objects that contact the body surface.

3. Some of the more specialized _____ receptors located in the skin can detect light touch and pressure, whereas others inform us of heavy and continuous touch and pressure.

B. Temperature Receptors Are Nerve Endings

Homeostatic   **Hypothalamus**   **Lips**   **Mouth**   **Skin**   **Temperature**   **Thermoreceptors**

1. _____ are free nerve endings that allow us to detect temperature changes.

2. Widely distributed throughout the body, thermoreceptors are especially concentrated in the

   _____ and _____.

3. Thermoreceptors are highly sensitive to differences between _____ temperature and the _____ of objects that come into contact with the body.

4. Thermoreceptors in the _____ detect internal changes in temperature and receive and integrate information from thermoreceptors on the body surface. The hypothalamus then initiates _____ mechanisms that ensure a constant body temperature.

C.   Pain Sensation Is a Protective Mechanism

Acupuncture	Analgesia	Endorphins	Enkephalins	Glutamate	Mechanical
Nociceptors	Pain	Phantom pain	Referred	Substance P	Thermal

1.   The sensation of _____ is a protective mechanism that makes us aware of tissue injury.

2.   Pain receptors, called _____, are free nerve endings of certain sensory neurons found in almost every tissue.

3.   _____ nociceptors respond to temperature extremes.

4.   _____ nociceptors respond to strong tactile stimuli such as penetration by sharp objects or pinching.

5.   Nociceptors transmit signals to sensory neurons that release the neurotransmitter _____ and several other neurotransmitters, including _____.

6.   The body has a variety of mechanisms for _____, or pain control.

7.   _____ and _____ are among the more than 10 opiates that exist in the brain, spinal cord, and pituitary gland.

8.   For years after an amputation, a person may feel _____ in the missing limb.

9.   A person with angina who experiences pain in the left arm is experiencing _____ pain.

10.   During _____, needles are inserted to stimulate afferent neurons that inhibit pain signals.

D.   Proprioceptors Inform Us of Our Position

Equilibrium	Golgi tendon organs	Ligaments	Muscle spindles
Proprioceptors	Semicircular	Vestibule	

1.   _____ help us maintain the position of the body and its parts.

2.   _____ are proprioceptors that detect movement.

3.   _____ are proprioceptors that determine stretch in the tendons that attach muscle to bone.

4.   Joint receptors detect movement in _____.

5.   The brain coordinates information from proprioceptors with input from the _____ and _____ canals in the inner ear to maintain _____ and coordination of muscular activities.

CHAPTER TEST

Select the correct response.

1. A stimulus is
   a. any change in the internal environment of the body.
   b. another name for the olfactory sense.
   c. any change in the external environment.
   d. both a and c.

2. Stimuli are detected through
   a. sensory receptors.
   b. transducers.
   c. stimulus receivers.
   d. sensory detectors.

3. A(n) _____ would not be detected by a sensory receptor.
   a. idea
   b. mosquito bite
   c. sunset
   d. taste of a hot-fudge sundae

4. Sensory _____ is the process of selecting, interpreting, and organizing sensory information.
   a. prevention
   b. perception
   c. deprivation
   d. overload

5. _____ located in the retina of the eye respond to visible wavelengths of light. They transduce light energy.
   a. Thermoreceptors
   b. Chemoreceptors
   c. Photoreceptors
   d. Nociceptors

6. _____ help(s) to protect the eye anteriorly from foreign objects.
   a. Eyelashes
   b. Vitreous humor
   c. Retina
   d. Extrinsic muscles

7. _____ is not one of the layers of tissue that form the eyeball.
   a. Fibrous sclera
   b. Pinna
   c. Retina
   d. Choroid layer

8. The _____ is called the white of the eye.
   a. cornea
   b. sclera
   c. retina
   d. iris

9. The _____ is the colored part of the eye and can appear as blue, green, or brown.
   a. cornea
   b. sclera
   c. retina
   d. iris

10. The _____ is the transparent layer that covers the iris and the pupil at the front of the eye.
    a. cornea
    b. sclera
    c. retina
    d. lens

11. The _____ regulates the amount of light entering the eye.
    a. cornea
    b. sclera
    c. retina
    d. iris

12. The _____ contains sensory receptors called rods and cones.
    a. cornea
    b. sclera
    c. retina
    d. conjunctiva

13. The cones are responsible for
    a. night vision.
    b. color vision.
    c. day vision.
    d. both b and c.

14. The rods are responsible for
    a. night vision.
    b. color vision.
    c. day vision.
    d. both b and c.

15. The _____ is *not* an ossicle.
    a. malleus
    b. eustachian
    c. incus
    d. stapes

16. The _____ is a snail-shaped portion of the inner ear that contains the organs of Corti, the sound receptors.
    a. perilymph
    b. bony labyrinth
    c. cochlea
    d. utricle

17. Hair cells in the organ of Corti
    a. are equipped with tiny projections called flagella.
    b. are equipped with tiny projections called stereocilia.
    c. filter out impurities entering the ear to protect the tympanic membrane.
    d. grow long and need to be cut periodically.

18. The response of the sensory cells in the semicircular canals is produced by the flow of _____ within the canals as the position of the head changes.
    a. polylymph
    b. endolymph
    c. perilymph
    d. otoliths

19. The odors detected by the olfactory epithelium are transmitted by the
    a. olfactory nerve.
    b. auditory nerve.
    c. vestibular nerve.
    d. trigeminal nerve.

20. _____ is the sense of taste.
    a. Gestation
    b. Gustation
    c. Salivation
    d. Gastronomics

21. Which of the following are recognized tastes?
    a. glutamate and sweet
    b. bitter and sour
    c. glutamate and salty
    d. All of the above are recognized tastes.

22. Thermoreceptors are especially concentrated in the
    a. fingertips and toes.
    b. scalp.
    c. lips and mouth.
    d. auditory canal.

23. When stimulated, nociceptors in the skin transmit signals through sensory neurons to interneurons in the
    a. motor cortex.
    b. spinal cord.
    c. visual cortex.
    d. auditory canal.

24. Opiates work by blocking the release of
    a. substance P.
    b. acetylcholine.
    c. gluconate.
    d. endorphins.

25. Which is *not* a type of proprioceptor?
    a. muscle spindles
    b. endorphins
    c. Golgi tendon organs
    d. joint receptors

Chapter

9

ENDOCRINE CONTROL

■ ■ ■

Outline

Introduction
I.   Many tissues secrete hormones or hormone-like substances.
II. Negative feedback systems regulate endocrine glands.
III. Hormones combine with specific receptors on or in target cells.
IV. The hypothalamus regulates the pituitary gland.
   A. The posterior lobe releases two hormones produced by the hypothalamus.
   B. The anterior lobe regulates growth and other endocrine glands.
      1. Growth hormone stimulates protein synthesis.

V.   Thyroid hormones increase metabolic rate.
VI. Parathyroid glands regulate calcium concentration.
VII. The islets of Langerhans regulate glucose concentration.
   A. In diabetes mellitus, glucose accumulates in the blood.
VIII. The adrenal glands function in metabolism and stress.
   A. The adrenal medulla secretes epinephrine and norepinephrine.
   B. The adrenal cortex secretes steroid hormones.
   C. Stress threatens homeostasis.
IX. Many other hormones are known.

Learning Objectives

After you have studied this chapter, you should be able to:

1. Describe the sources, transport, and general functions of hormones and hormone-like substances (for example, neurohormones and prostaglandins).
2. Identify the principal endocrine glands, locate them in the body, and list the hormones secreted by each gland.
3. Describe how endocrine glands are regulated by negative feedback mechanisms.
4. Compare the mechanisms of action of hormones that work through second messengers with those of steroid hormones.
5. Justify the reputation of the hypothalamus as the link between nervous and endocrine systems. (Describe the mechanisms by which the hypothalamus exerts its control.)
6. Compare the functions of the posterior and anterior lobes of the pituitary and describe the actions of their hormones.

7. Summarize the actions of the thyroid hormones and draw a diagram illustrating how they are regulated.
8. Describe how the parathyroid and thyroid glands regulate calcium levels.
9. Contrast the actions of insulin and glucagon and describe the effects of diabetes mellitus.
10. Describe the role of the adrenal medulla in the body's responses to stress.
11. Identify the hormones secreted by the adrenal cortex, and give the actions of glucocorticoids and mineralocorticoids.
12. Describe the actions of hormones secreted by the pineal gland, thymus gland, and atrium of the heart.

STUDY QUESTIONS

Within each category, fill in the blanks with the correct response.

INTRODUCTION

Cells   **Endocrinology**   **Fluid**   **Growth**
Homeostasis   **Metabolic**   **Reproduction**

1. The endocrine system helps regulate _____, _____, use of nutrients by _____, salt and _____ balance, and _____ rate.

2. The endocrine system works with the nervous system to maintain _____, the steady state of the body.

3. _____ is the study of the endocrine system.

I. MANY TISSUES SECRETE HORMONES OR HORMONE-LIKE SUBSTANCES

Blood   **Endocrine**   **Exocrine**   **Hormones**
Neuroendocrine   **Neurohormones**   **Prostaglandins**   **Target**

1. The endocrine system consists of specialized tissues and _____ glands which secrete _____, chemical messengers that can have widespread effects throughout the body.

2. Endocrine glands lack ducts, and differ from _____ glands which release their secretions into ducts.

3. _____ cells, the cells influenced by a particular hormone, may be located in another endocrine gland or in an entirely different type of organ.

4. Certain neurons, known as _____ cells, are an important link between the nervous and endocrine systems.

5. Neuroendocrine cells produce _____ that are transported down axons and released into the interstitial fluid.

6. Neurohormones typically diffuse into capillaries and are transported by the _____.

7. _____ are a group of about 16 closely related lipids that are manufactured by many different tissues in the body.

II. NEGATIVE FEEDBACK SYSTEMS REGULATE ENDOCRINE GLANDS

Endocrine gland   **Homeostasis**   **Hypersecretion**   **Hyposecretion**
Negative feedback   **Parathyroid**

1. _____ depends on normal concentrations of hormones.

2. Hormone secretion is typically regulated by _____ systems.

3. Information about the amount of hormone or of some other substance in the blood or interstitial fluid is fed back to the _____ which then responds to restore homeostasis.

4. The _____ glands regulate the calcium concentration of the blood.

5. In _____, a gland decreases its hormone output to abnormally low levels.

6. In _____, a gland increases its output to abnormally high levels, overstimulating target cells.

III.   HORMONES COMBINE WITH SPECIFIC RECEPTORS ON OR IN TARGET CELLS

Binds **Calcium** **Calmodulin** **Cyclic AMP** **Genes**
Plasma **Receptors** **Second messenger** **Steroid**

1. Specialized proteins on or in the target cell are _____ that bind with the hormone.

2. When a hormone _____ with a receptor, a series of reactions is activated.

3. Hormones that are large molecules, such as proteins, combine with receptors on the _____ membrane of the target cell.

4. A hormone acting as a first messenger relays information to a _____, which may alter the activity of the cell.

5. _____, or cAMP, is a second messenger.

6. _____ ions can act as second messengers.

7. The _____ molecule changes shape and can activate enzymes that regulate certain cellular processes, such as a neurotransmitter release.

8. _____ hormones and thyroid hormones are relatively small molecules that pass easily through the plasma membrane of a target cell.

9. When certain _____ are switched on, specific proteins are synthesized.

IV.   THE HYPOTHALAMUS REGULATES THE PITUITARY GLAND

Anterior **Endocrine** **Hypothalamus** **Inhibiting** **Pituitary gland**
Posterior **Releasing**

1. The _____ links the nervous and endocrine systems.

2. Directly or indirectly, the hypothalamus regulates most _____ activity.

3. Oxytocin is a neurohormone which is stored in the _____.

4. _____ hormones and _____ hormones act on the pituitary gland, regulating secretion of several pituitary hormones.

5. The pituitary gland consists of two main lobes, the _____ lobe and the _____ lobe.

A. The Posterior Lobe Releases Two Hormones Produced by the Hypothalamus

Antidiuretic hormone (ADH)   Diabetes insipidus   Inhibits   Labor   Oxytocin   Posterior lobe

1. The _____ of the pituitary gland secretes two hormones—oxytocin and antidiuretic hormone (ADH).

2. _____ stimulates contraction of smooth muscle in the wall of the uterus and stimulates release of milk from the breast.

3. Oxytocin is sometimes administered clinically to start or speed _____.

4. _____ regulates fluid balance in the body and indirectly helps control blood pressure.

5. Alcohol consumption increases urine output because alcohol _____ ADH secretion.

6. ADH deficiency can lead to the condition known as _____, in which enormous quantities of urine may be excreted.

B. The Anterior Lobe Regulates Growth and Other Endocrine Glands

Adrenal cortex   Anterior lobe   Gonadotropic   Inhibiting   Portal
Prolactin   Releasing   Thyroid   Tropic

1. The _____ of the pituitary gland secretes growth hormone, prolactin, and several other hormones that stimulate other endocrine glands.

2. A(n) _____ hormone stimulates other endocrine glands.

3. Each of the anterior pituitary hormones is regulated in some way by a(n) _____ hormone, and in some cases also by a(n) _____ hormone produced in the hypothalamus.

4. _____ veins are unusual in that they do not deliver blood to a larger vein directly, but connect two sets of capillaries.

5. During lactation, _____ stimulates the cells of the mammary glands to secrete milk.

6. TSH stimulates the _____ gland.

7. ACTH stimulates the _____.

8. Follicle stimulating hormone and luteinizing hormone are _____ hormones, which control the activities of the gonads (sex glands).

1. *Growth Hormone Stimulates Protein Synthesis*

Growth hormone	Hypothalamus	Increases	Insulin-like growth factors
Pituitary	Pituitary dwarfs	Psychosocial dwarfism	Pulses
Sex	Somatomedins		

1. _____ stimulates body growth mainly by stimulating protein synthesis.

2. Growth hormone (GH) stimulates liver cells and cells of many other tissues to produce peptides called
    _____, including _____.

3. A high level of growth hormone in the blood signals the _____ to secrete the
    inhibiting hormone, and the _____ release of growth hormone slows.

4. Secretion of growth hormone _____ during exercise.

5. Growth hormone is released in a series of _____ 2 to 4 hours after a meal.

6. In extreme cases, childhood stress can produce a form of retarded development known as
    _____.

7. _____ hormones must be present for the adolescent growth spurt to occur.

8. _____ are individuals whose pituitary gland did not produce enough growth hor-
    mone during childhood.

V. THYROID HORMONES INCREASE METABOLIC RATE

Goiter	Hypersecretion	Hyposecretion	Hypothyroidism
Negative feedback system	T_3	Thyroid gland	Thyroid hormones
Thyroid-stimulating hormone	Thyroxine		

1. The _____ is shaped somewhat like a shield and is located in the neck.

2. The _____ are essential for normal growth and development and they increase
    metabolic rate in most tissues.

3. The main thyroid hormone is _____, or T_4.

4. A second thyroid hormone, _____ or triiodothyronine, has three iodine atoms in
    its structure.

5. The regulation of thyroid hormone secretion depends on a _____ between the
    anterior pituitary and the thyroid gland.

6. The anterior pituitary secretes _____, which promotes synthesis and secretion of
    thyroid hormones.

7. Extreme _____ during childhood results in low metabolic rate and retarded men-
    tal and physical development.

8. Any abnormal enlargement of the thyroid gland is termed a _____.

9. A goiter may be associated with either _____ or _____.

VI. PARATHYROID GLANDS REGULATE CALCIUM CONCENTRATION

Calcitonin	**Calcium**	**Increases**	**Parathyroid glands**
Parathyroid hormone	**Vitamin D**		

1. The _____ are embedded in the connective tissue that surrounds the thyroid gland.

2. The parathyroid glands secrete _____, a small protein that regulates the calcium level of the blood and tissue fluid.

3. Parathyroid hormone _____ calcium levels by stimulating release of calcium from the bones.

4. Parathyroid hormone also activates _____, which then increases the amount of calcium absorbed from the intestine.

5. The parathyroid glands are regulated by the concentration of _____ in the blood and tissue fluid.

6. When calcium concentration becomes very high, _____ is released from the thyroid gland.

VII. THE ISLETS OF LANGERHANS REGULATE GLUCOSE CONCENTRATION

Antagonistically	**Alpha**	**Beta cells**	**Digestive**	**Endocrine**	**Exocrine**
Glucagon	**Glycogen**	**Insulin**	**Islets of Langerhans**	**Opposite**	**Posterior**

1. The pancreas lies in the abdomen _____ to the stomach.

2. The pancreas has both _____ and _____ functions.

3. The exocrine cells of the pancreas produce _____ enzymes.

4. More than a million small clusters of cells known as the _____ are scattered throughout the pancreas.

5. About 70% of the islet cells are _____ that produce the hormone insulin.

6. _____ cells secrete the hormone glucagon.

7. _____ lowers the concentration of glucose in the blood.

8. Once glucose enters the muscle cells, it is either used immediately as fuel or stored as _____.

9. _____ raises the blood glucose level by stimulating liver cells to convert glycogen to glucose.

10. The effects of glucagon are _____ to those of insulin.

11. Insulin and glucagon work _____ to keep blood glucose concentration within normal limits.

A.   In Diabetes Mellitus, Glucose Accumulates in the Blood

Diabetes mellitus   **Insulin**   **Insulin resistance**   **Urine**   **Type 1**   **Type 2**

1. The main disorder associated with pancreatic hormones is _____.

2. Insulin-dependent diabetes, referred to as _____ diabetes, usually develops before age 20.

3. Type 1 diabetes is clinically treated with _____ injections.

4. About 90% of all cases of diabetes are non-insulin–dependent, or _____ diabetes.

5. In type 2 diabetes, insulin receptors on target cells are not able to bind with the insulin and use it. This condition is known as _____.

6. In diabetics, blood glucose concentration may be so high that glucose is excreted in the _____.

VIII.   THE ADRENAL GLANDS FUNCTION IN METABOLISM AND STRESS

Adrenal cortex   **Adrenal glands**   **Adrenal medulla**   **Metabolism**   **Stress**

1. The paired _____ are small, yellow masses of tissue located above the kidneys.

2. Each adrenal gland consists of a central portion known as the _____, and a larger outer region, the _____.

3. The adrenal medulla and the adrenal cortex function as distinct glands. Both secrete hormones that help regulate _____, and both help the body deal with _____.

A.   The Adrenal Medulla Secretes Epinephrine and Norepinephrine

Adrenal medulla   **Dilate**   **Emergency**   **Epinephrine**
Metabolic   **Neurotransmitter**   **Norepinephrine**

1. The _____ develops from nervous tissue and is sometimes considered part of the sympathetic nervous system.

2. The adrenal medulla secretes two hormones: _____ and _____.

3. Norepinephrine is the same substance that is secreted as a(n) _____ by sympathetic neurons and by some neurons in the central nervous system.

4. The adrenal medulla is the _____ gland of the body; it prepares us to cope with threatening situations.

5. Epinephrine and norepinephrine can increase the _____ rate as much as 100%.

6. Epinephrine and norepinephrine can _____ the airways so that breathing is more effective.

B. The Adrenal Cortex Secretes Steroid Hormones

Adrenal cortex	**Adrenocorticotropic hormone**	**Aldosterone**	**Androgens**
Corticotropin releasing factor	**Cortisol**	**Estrogens**	**Glucocorticoids**
Glucose	**Mineralocorticoids**	**Potassium**	**Sodium**

1. The _____ secretes three different types of steroid hormones.

2. _____ help the body cope with stress.

3. The main glucocorticoid is _____, also called hydrocortisone.

4. The principal action of the glucocorticoids is to promote production of _____ from other nutrients.

5. _____ regulate water and salt balance.

6. _____ is the principal mineralocorticoid.

7. The main function of aldosterone is to maintain homeostasis of _____ and _____ ions.

8. The sex hormones, _____ and _____, are secreted by the adrenal cortex in minute amounts in both sexes.

9. Stress stimulates the hypothalamus to secrete _____, CRF.

10. CRF stimulates the anterior pituitary to secrete _____, ACTH.

C. Stress Threatens Homeostasis

Adrenal   Epinephrine   Homeostasis   Hormones   Norepinephrine   Stressors   Sympathetic

1. Good health and survival depend on maintaining _____.

2. _____ are stimuli that disrupt the steady state of the body.

3. During a stress response, the brain sends messages activating the _____ nervous system and the _____ glands.

4. When the body is reacting to stress, the hormones _____ and

_____ are released, and the body prepares for fight or flight.

5. Chronic stress is harmful because of the effects of long-term elevation of some

_____.

IX. MANY OTHER HORMONES ARE KNOWN

Atrium   Hormones   Melatonin   Thymosin

1. The pineal gland, located in the brain, produces a hormone called _____, which

facilitates the onset of sleep and influences biological rhythms and the onset of sexual maturity.

2. The digestive tract and adipose tissue secrete _____ that regulate digestive pro-

cesses.

3. The thymus gland produces _____, a hormone that plays a role in immune re-

sponses.

4. The _____ of the heart secretes atrial natriuretic factor (ANF) which promotes

sodium excretion and lowers blood pressure.

Labeling Exercise

Please fill in the correct labels for Figure 9-1.

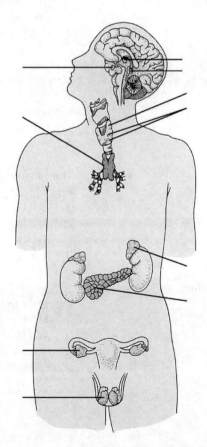

CHAPTER TEST

Select the correct response.

1. The _____ system works with the nervous system to maintain homeostasis of the body.
   a. circulatory
   b. digestive
   c. endocrine
   d. reproductive

2. The endocrine system helps regulate
   a. growth.
   b. reproduction.
   c. metabolic rate.
   d. all of the above.

3. The endocrine system consists of tissues and endocrine glands, which secrete chemical messengers called
   a. hormones.
   b. receptors.
   c. chemical secretors.
   d. capillaries.

4. Hormones are typically transported by the blood and affect the activity of their _____ cells—the specific cells on which they act.
   a. alpha
   b. target
   c. hormonal
   d. glandular

5. _____ are a group of about 16 closely related lipids that are manufactured by many different tissues in the body.
   a. Hormones
   b. Phospholipids
   c. Prostaglandins
   d. Glandular lipids

6. Prostaglandins are manufactured in the
   a. prostate gland.
   b. lungs.
   c. liver.
   d. all of the above.

7. At present, prostaglandins are used to
   a. induce labor.
   b. cure multiple sclerosis.
   c. treat chronic bronchitis.
   d. kill the AIDS virus

8. Hormone secretion is typically regulated by
   a. the digestive system.
   b. the appendix.
   c. positive feedback systems.
   d. negative feedback systems.

9. The _____ glands regulate the calcium concentration of the blood.
   a. parathyroid
   b. pituitary
   c. sebaceous
   d. all of the above

10. Some hormones activate a series of molecular events involving several different kinds of molecules. The first molecule in the series is usually a
    a. C protein.
    b. G protein.
    c. G receptor.
    d. H receptor.

11. Directly or indirectly, the _____ regulates most endocrine activity.
    a. hyperthalamus
    b. hypothalamus
    c. thyroid
    d. target cell

12. The _____ gland is sometimes called the master gland of the body.
    a. thyroid
    b. pituitary
    c. lymph
    d. endocrine

13. The hormone _____ stimulates contraction of smooth muscle in the wall of the uterus.
    a. ADH
    b. ACTH
    c. oxytocin
    d. somatropin

14. _____ regulates fluid balance in the body and indirectly helps control blood pressure.
    a. ADH
    b. ACTH
    c. Oxytocin
    d. Somatropin

15. ADH deficiency leads to the condition called
    _____, in which enormous quantities of dilute
    urine may be excreted.
    a. diabetes mellitus
    b. diabetes insipidus
    c. type 1 diabetes
    d. type 2 diabetes

16. The main thyroid hormone is
    a. ADH.
    b. ACTH.
    c. oxytocin.
    d. thyroxine.

17. Beta cells produce the hormone
    a. glucagon.
    b. ADH.
    c. insulin.
    d. oxytocin.

18. Alpha cells produce the hormone
    a. glucagon.
    b. ADH.
    c. insulin.
    d. oxytocin.

19. The main disorder associated with pancreatic
    hormones is
    a. diabetes insipidus.
    b. diabetes mellitus.
    c. pancreatic cancer.
    d. dwarfism.

20. The normal fasting blood glucose level is about
    a. 10 mg/dl.
    b. 90 mg/dl.
    c. 300 mg/dl.
    d. 1000 mg/dl.

21. Which of the following are actions of epineph-
    rine and norepinephrine?
    a. increase metabolic rate by as much as
        100%
    b. a weakening of muscle contraction
    c. increase blood pressure
    d. a and c

22. Which of the following are stressors?
    a. being sick
    b. taking a test
    c. getting married
    d. all of the above

CROSSWORD PUZZLE FOR CHAPTERS 6, 7, 8, AND 9

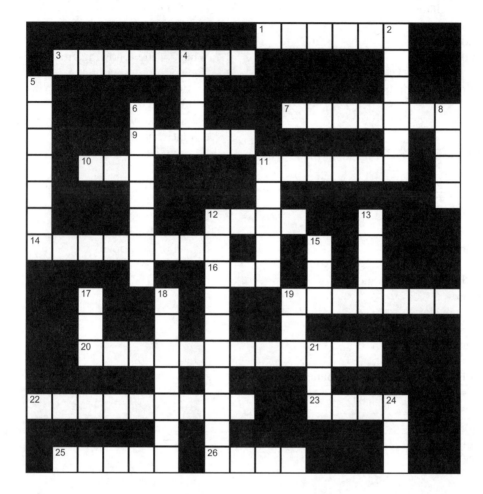

Across

1. Region of spinal cord below the thoracic level
3. Part of the brain that controls voluntary movement
7. Part of the brain that regulates heart rate and blood pressure
9. Second cranial nerve
10. Part of nervous system consisting of brain and spinal cord
11. Gray matter of cerebrum
12. Part of the brain that helps regulate respiration
14. Transmits impulses to cell body
16. An action system of the brain
19. Nerve that supplies the diaphragm
20. Part of the brain that controls body temperature
22. Releases growth hormone
23. Outer layer of the meninges
25. Opening through which light enters the eye
26. Focuses light on retina

Down

2. Automatic sequence of stimulus response
4. Sensory fibers enter the spinal cord through the dorsal
5. Gland that stimulates metabolic rate
6. Controlled by the cerebellum
8. Transmits impulses from the cell body toward the synapse
11. Sensitive to color
12. Part of the nervous system that includes sense organs
13. Each of the six divisions of the cerebral hemisphere is called a _____
15. Hormone that regulates calcium level
17. Tropic hormone released by anterior pituitary gland
18. Lobe where Broca's speech area is located
19. Innermost of the three meninges
21. Visual and auditory reflex centers are located in the _____ brain
24. Hormone that stimulates reabsorption of water

Chapter

10

THE CIRCULATORY SYSTEM: BLOOD

■ ■ ■

Outline

Introduction / I. The circulatory system performs critical functions.
II. Plasma is the fluid component of blood.
III. Red blood cells transport oxygen.
IV. White blood cells defend the body against disease.
V. Platelets function in blood clotting.

VI. Successful blood transfusions depend on blood groups.
    A. The ABO blood groups are based on antigens A and B.
    B. The Rh system consists of several Rh antigens.

Learning Objectives

After you have studied this chapter, you should be able to:

1. List the functions of the circulatory system and describe the composition of blood.
2. Describe the composition of blood plasma and the functions of plasma proteins.
3. Describe the structure, function, and life cycle of red blood cells.
4. Compare the structure and functions of the main types of white blood cells.

5. Describe the structure and function of platelets, and summarize the chemical events of blood clotting.
6. Identify the antigen and antibody associated with each ABO blood type and explain why blood types must be carefully matched in transfusion therapy.
7. Identify the cause and importance of Rh incompatibility.

STUDY QUESTIONS

Within each category, fill in the blanks with the correct response.

INTRODUCTION / I. THE CIRCULATORY SYSTEM PERFORMS CRITICAL FUNCTIONS

Blood	Cardiovascular	Circulatory	Disease	Fluid
Heart	Lymphatic	Plasma	Platelets	

1. The _____ system is the transportation system of the body.

2. The circulatory system consists of two subsystems: the _____ system and the _____ system.

3. In the cardiovascular system, the _____ pumps blood through a vast system of blood vessels.

4. As it circulates, the _____ transports nutrients, oxygen, hormones, and waste products.

5. The lymphatic system helps preserve _____ balance and protects the body against _____.

6. Blood consists of red blood cells, white blood cells, and cell fragments called _____, all suspended in a pale, yellowish fluid called _____.

II. PLASMA IS THE FLUID COMPONENT OF BLOOD

Acid-base	**Albumins**	**Alpha globulins**	**Beta**	**Fibrinogen**
Gamma	**Globulins**	**Interstitial fluid**	**Intracellular fluid**	**Liver**
pH	**Plasma proteins**	**Prothrombin**	**Serum**	**Water**

1. Plasma consists mainly of _____.

2. Plasma is in dynamic equilibrium with the _____, bathing the cells and with the _____ inside cells.

3. Plasma contains several kinds of _____, each with specific properties and functions.

4. Most plasma proteins are manufactured in the _____.

5. Plasma proteins may be divided into three groups, or fractions: _____, _____, and _____.

6. Plasma proteins are important _____ buffers, and help keep the _____ of the blood within a narrow homeostatic range.

7. _____ include certain hormones and proteins that transport hormones.

8. _____ is an alpha globulin involved in blood clotting.

9. _____ globulins include lipoproteins that transport fats and cholesterol, including low-density lipoproteins.

10. The _____ globulin fraction contains many types of antibodies that provide immunity to diseases such as measles and infectious hepatitis.

11. When the proteins involved in clotting have been removed from the plasma, the remaining liquid is called _____.

III.   RED BLOOD CELLS TRANSPORT OXYGEN

Anemia	**Biconcave**	**Erythropoietin**	**Hemoglobin**	**Iron deficiency**	**Kidneys**
Marrow	**Nucleus**	**Oxygen**	**Oxyhemoglobin**	**Red blood cells**	**Stem cells**

1. _____ are one of the most specialized cell types in the body.

2. Red blood cells are adapted for producing and packaging _____, the red pigment that transports oxygen.

3. A mature red blood cell is a tiny, flexible, _____ disk, which provides for a high ratio of surface area to volume, allowing efficient diffusion of _____ and carbon dioxide into and out of the cell.

4. A mature red blood cell lacks a(n) _____ and most other organelles.

5. As blood circulates through the lungs, oxygen combines weakly with hemoglobin to form _____.

6. In children, red blood cells are produced in the red bone _____ of almost all bones.

7. Red bone marrow has immature cells known as _____.

8. Red blood cell production is regulated by the hormone _____.

9. Erythropoietin is secreted by the _____ in response to a decrease in oxygen concentration.

10. A hemoglobin deficiency is called _____.

11. _____ is the most common cause of anemia.

IV.   WHITE BLOOD CELLS DEFEND THE BODY AGAINST DISEASE

Antibodies	**Attack**	**Bacteria**	**Basophils**	**Enzymes**
Eosinophils	**Granular**	**Heparin**	**Histamine**	**Leukocytes**
Lymphocytes	**Lysosomes**	**Macrophages**	**Monocytes**	**Neutrophils**
Phagocytes	**Phagocytosis**	**Tissues**		

1. White blood cells, or _____, are specialized to protect the body against pathogens—harmful bacteria and other microorganisms that cause disease.

2. Whereas red blood cells function within the blood, many white cells leave the circulation and perform their duties in various _____.

3. _____ is the process by which cells engulf microorganisms, foreign particles, or other cells.

4. Cells that are specialized to carry on phagocytosis are called _____.

5. _____ leukocytes have large, lobed nuclei and distinctive granules in their cytoplasm.

6. The kinds of white blood cells that contain granules are _____,
   _____, and _____.

7. Neutrophils are adept at seeking out and ingesting _____.

8. Most of the granules in neutrophils contain _____ that digest ingested material.

9. The _____ of eosinophils contain enzymes that destroy viruses and bacteria.

10. Granules in the cytoplasm of basophils contain _____, a substance that dilates
    blood vessels and makes capillaries more permeable.

11. Other basophil granules contain _____, an anticoagulant that helps prevent blood
    from clotting inappropriately within the blood vessels.

12. Two types of agranular leukocytes are _____ and _____.

14. Some lymphocytes are specialized to produce _____, others
    _____ bacteria or viruses directly.

15. Monocytes migrate into the connective tissues and develop into _____, the large
    scavenger cells of the body.

V.   PLATELETS FUNCTION IN BLOOD CLOTTING

Clotting factors   **Fibrin**   **Fibrinogen**   **Liver**   **Platelet plug**   **Prevent**
Prothrombin activator   **Serum**   **Thrombin**   **Thrombocytes**   **Vitamin K**

1. Platelets, also called _____, are tiny fragments of cytoplasm that are pinched off
   of certain very large cells in the bone marrow.

2. Platelets _____ blood loss.

3. When a blood vessel is cut, platelets stick to the rough, cut edges of the blood vessel, forming a
   _____ that seals the hole in the blood vessel wall.

4. During the clotting process, platelets and injured tissue release substances that activate
   _____ in the blood. A series of reactions takes place that results in formation of
   an enzyme known as _____.

5. Prothrombin activator catalyzes the conversion of prothrombin to its active form,
   _____.

6. Prothrombin is manufactured in the _____ with the help of
   _____.

7. In the presence of calcium ions, thrombin acts as an enzyme that converts the plasma protein _____ to fibrin.

8. _____ threads form the webbing of a blood clot.

9. As a blood clot begins to contract, it squeezes out _____.

VI.   SUCCESSFUL BLOOD TRANSFUSIONS DEPEND ON BLOOD GROUPS

Agglutinate	Antibodies	Centrifuge	Donors	Hemolysis
Plasma	Recipients	Transfusion reaction	Transfusions	

1. Blood _____—the transfer of blood cells, platelets, or plasma from healthy _____ to _____ in need of blood—are routine, lifesaving procedures.

2. Blood components can be separated by a(n) _____.

3. _____ can be used to expand blood volume in patients who are in circulatory shock.

4. If blood is not carefully matched before a transfusion, a(n) _____ may occur.

5. During a transfusion reaction, _____ in the recipient's blood attack the foreign red blood cells in the transfused blood, causing them to _____ or clump.

6. _____ occurs when red blood cells break, releasing hemoglobin into the plasma.

A.   The ABO Blood Groups Are Based on Antigens A and B

Anti-A	Anti-B	Antibodies	Antigens
Repeated	Type O	Universal donors	Universal recipients

1. Red blood cells have specific proteins called _____ on their surfaces.

2. Individuals with type O blood have neither type of antigen on their red cells, and are referred to as _____ because they can donate blood to patients with any blood type.

3. Certain _____ called agglutinins are found in the plasma.

4. People with type A blood have _____ antibodies circulating in their blood.

5. People with Type B blood have _____ antibodies circulating in their blood.

6. People with _____ blood have both anti-A and anti-B antibodies in their blood.

7. Blood mismatching can be fatal, especially if the mistake is ever _____.

8. Because individuals with type AB blood do not have antibodies to either type A or type B blood, they are referred to as _____.

B.   The Rh System Consists of Several Rh Antigens

Antigen D	Exposed	Hemolytic anemia	Red blood cells	Rh antigens
Rh factor	Rh incompatibility	Rh negative	Rh positive	

1. The Rh system consists of more then 40 kinds of _____.

2. Each Rh antigen is referred to as a(n) _____.

3. The most important Rh factor is _____.

4. Most persons of western European descent are _____, which means that they
    have antigen D on the surfaces of their _____.

5. The approximately 15% of the population who are _____ have no antigen D on
    their red blood cell surfaces.

6. Antibody D does not occur in the blood of Rh negative persons unless they have been
    _____ to antigen D.

7. Although several kinds of maternal-fetal blood type incompatibilities are known,
    _____ is probably the most serious.

8. The condition known as _____ occurs in a fetus or newborn when the mother's
    Rh positive antibodies cross the placenta and cause hemolysis of the baby's red blood cells.

CHAPTER TEST

Select the correct response.

1. The circulatory system does all of the following
    except
    a. transport nutrients from the digestive system to all parts of the cells.
    b. move voluntary skeletal muscles.
    c. transport carbon dioxide and other metabolic wastes from the cells to the excretory organs.
    d. transport oxygen from the lungs to all the cells of the body.

2. The circulatory system consists of the
    a. cardiovascular system.
    b. endocrine system.
    c. lymphatic system.
    d. a and c only.

3. Blood consists of
    a. red blood cells.
    b. white blood cells.
    c. platelets.
    d. all of the above.

4. Plasma consists of
    a. salt.
    b. water.
    c. proteins.
    d. all of the above.

5. The _____ serve as antibodies, which provide immunity against disease.
    a. gamma globulins
    b. fibrinogens
    c. albumins
    d. beta globulins

6. Fibrinogen is manufactured in the
    a. liver.
    b. lymph tissues.
    c. lungs.
    d. spleen.

7. _____ are adapted for producing and packaging hemoglobin.
   a. Red blood cells
   b. White blood cells
   c. Eosinophils
   d. Leukocytes

8. Red blood cells are produced in
   a. bone tissue.
   b. muscle tissue.
   c. red bone marrow.
   d. all bone marrow.

9. _____ defend the body against pathogens—harmful bacteria and other microorganisms that cause disease.
   a. White blood cells
   b. Red blood cells
   c. Leukocytes
   d. Both a and c

10. The three types of white blood cells that contain granules are
    a. neutrophils, monocytes, and lymphocytes.
    b. basophils, eosinophils, and neutrophils.
    c. eosinophils, basophils, and lymphocytes.
    d. neutrophils, basophils, and monocytes.

11. The two types of white blood cells that lack specific granules in their cytoplasm are
    a. neutrophils and lymphocytes.
    b. neutrophils and monocytes.
    c. lymphocytes and monocytes.
    d. basophils and monocytes.

12. Prothrombin is a globulin found in plasma; it is manufactured in the _____ with the help of vitamin K.
    a. liver
    b. spleen
    c. stomach
    d. kidneys

13. Individuals with type AB blood have _____ antigens on their red blood cells.
    a. A
    b. B
    c. both A and B
    d. none of the above

14. Individuals with type O blood have _____ antigens on their red blood cells.
    a. A
    b. B
    c. both A and B
    d. none of the above

15. The most important of the Rh factors is
    a. antigen R.
    b. antigen D.
    c. Rh negative.
    d. Rh positive.

Chapter

11

THE CIRCULATORY SYSTEM: THE HEART

■ ■ ■

Outline

Introduction
I.   The heart wall consists of three layers.
II. The heart has four chambers.
III. Valves prevent backflow of blood.
IV. The heart has its own blood vessels.
V.   The conduction system consists of specialized cardiac muscle.

VI. The cardiac cycle includes contraction and relaxation phases.
VII. Cardiac output depends on stroke volume and heart rate.
VIII. The heart is regulated by the nervous and endocrine systems.

Learning Objectives

After you have studied this chapter, you should be able to:

1. Locate the heart and describe the structure of its wall.
2. Identify the chambers of the heart and compare their functions.
3. Locate the atrioventricular and semilunar valves and compare their structures.
4. Identify the principal blood vessels that serve the heart wall.

5. Trace the path of an electrical impulse through the conduction system of the heart.
6. Describe the events of the cardiac cycle, and correlate them with normal heart sounds.
7. Define cardiac output and identify factors that affect it.
8. Describe how the nervous and endocrine systems regulate the heart.

STUDY QUESTIONS

Within each category, fill in the blanks with the correct response.

INTRODUCTION

Blood   **Vessels**   **Nutrients**   **Organ**   **Oxygen**

1. The heart is a hollow, muscular _____ not much bigger than a fist.

2. The heart pumps blood through the complex of blood _____ that bring _____ and _____ to the cells of the body.

3. Depending on the body's changing needs, the heart can vary its output form 5 to 35 liters of _____ per minute.

I. THE HEART WALL CONSISTS OF THREE LAYERS

Blood vessels   **Cardiac**   **Endocardium**   **Endothelial**   **Epicardium**
Heart   **Lymph**   **Midline**   **Myocardium**   **Parietal**
Pericardial cavity   **Pericardium**   **Thorax**   **Visceral**

1. The heart is located in the _____ between the lungs.

2. About two-thirds of the heart lies to the left of the body's _____.

3. The wall of the _____ is richly supplied with nerves, _____, and _____ vessels.

4. From the inside out, the layers of the heart are the _____, _____, and _____.

5. The endocardium consists of a smooth _____ lining resting on connective tissue.

6. The greatest bulk of the heart wall consists of myocardium, the _____ muscle that contracts to pump the blood.

7. The outer layer of the heart is the _____, or _____ pericardium.

8. The pericardium consists of two layers that are separated by a potential space, the _____.

9. The outer layer of the pericardium, the _____ pericardium, forms a strong sac for the heart and helps to anchor it within the thorax.

II. THE HEART HAS FOUR CHAMBERS

Atria   **Auricle**   **Heart**   **Interatrial**   **Interventricular**
Pulmonary   **Septum**   **Ventricles**

1. The _____ is a double pump.

2. The right and left sides of the heart are completely separated by a wall, or _____.

3. The _____ receive blood returning to the heart from the veins and act as reservoirs between contractions of the heart.

4. The _____ pump blood into the great arteries leaving the heart.

5. _____ arteries carry blood to the lungs, where gases are exchanged.

6. The wall between the atria is the _____ septum.

7. The wall between the ventricles is the _____ septum.

8. A small muscular pouch called the _____ increases the surface area of each atrium.

Labeling Exercise

Please fill in the correct labels for Figure 11-1.

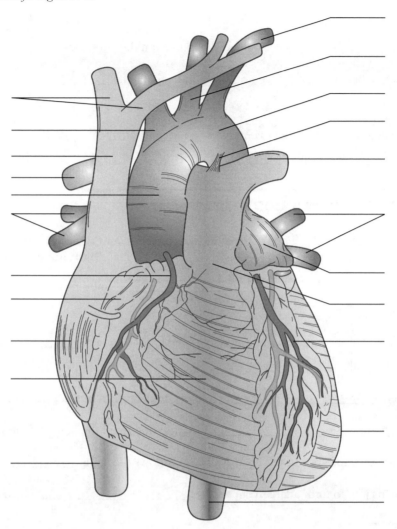

III.   VALVES PREVENT BACKFLOW OF BLOOD

Aortic	**Atrioventricular**	**Bicuspid**	**Cusps**	**Mitral**
Mitral stenosis	**Pulmonary**	**Semilunar**	**Tricuspid**	

1.   To prevent blood from flowing backward into the atrium, a(n) _____ valve guards the passageway between each atrium and ventricle.

2.   The atrioventricular valve consists of flaps or _____ of fibrous tissues that project from the heart wall.

3.   The atrioventricular valve between the right atrium and the right ventricle has three cusps and is called the _____ valve.

4.   The left atrioventricular valve, which has only two cusps, is called the _____ valve.

5. The bicuspid valve is commonly called the _____ valve.

6. _____ is a narrowing of the opening of the mitral valve; a common valve deformity.

7. The _____ valves guard the exits from the ventricles.

8. The semilunar valve between the left ventricle and the aorta is the _____ semilunar valve.

9. The semilunar valve between the right ventricle and the pulmonary artery is the _____ valve.

IV. THE HEART HAS ITS OWN BLOOD VESSELS

Cardiac   **Coronary**   **Coronary arteries**   **Coronary artery disease**
Coronary sinus   **Coronary veins** **Oxygen**   **Right atrium**

1. The wall of the heart is so thick that _____ and nutrients cannot effectively diffuse to all of its cells.

2. Blood vessels must deliver oxygen and nutrients to the hard-working _____ muscle in the heart wall.

3. The right and left _____ arteries branch off from the aorta as it leaves the heart.

4. Branches of the two _____ bring blood to all the tissue of the heart.

5. After passing through capillaries in the heart wall, blood flows through _____.

6. The coronary veins join to form a large vein, the _____, which empties into the _____.

7. _____, a leading cause of death in the United States, develops when the coronary arteries or their branches become thickened or blocked, reducing blood flow.

V. THE CONDUCTION SYSTEM CONSISTS OF SPECIALIZED CARDIAC MUSCLE

Atrioventricular   **Bundle**   **Conduction**   **Intercalated**   **Myocardium**   **Sinoatrial**

1. The heart has its own specialized _____ system and can beat independently from its nerve supply.

2. Each heartbeat is initiated by the _____ node, or pacemaker—a small mass of specialized muscle in the posterior wall of the right atrium.

3. One group of atrial muscle fibers conducts the electrical impulse directly to the _____ node, located in the right atrium along the lower part of the septum.

4. From the atrioventricular node, a muscle impulse spreads into specialized muscle fibers that form the atrioventricular _____.

5. Purkinje fibers end on fibers of ordinary cardiac muscle within the _____.

6. Cardiac muscle fibers are joined at their ends by dense bands called _____ discs.

VI.   THE CARDIAC CYCLE INCLUDES CONTRACTION AND RELAXATION PHASES

Arteries	**Atria**	**Blood**	**Cardiac cycle**	**Diastole**	**Electrocardiogram**
Heart murmurs	**Hissing**	**Lub-dup**	**Semilunar**	**Stethoscope**	**Systole**
Valve	**Veins**	**Ventricles**	**Ventricular**		

1. The events that occur during one complete heartbeat make up the _____.

2. The period of contraction of the heart muscle is known as _____.

3. The period of relaxation of the heart muscle is called _____.

4. Each cardiac cycle begins with an electrical impulse that spreads from the sinoatrial node throughout the atria resulting in the contraction of the _____.

5. As the atria contract, the atrioventricular valves are open, and blood is forced from the atria into the _____.

6. As blood is forced from the atria into the ventricles, the _____ valves close.

7. As the atria relax, they are filled with blood from the _____.

8. As the ventricles contract, blood is forced through the semilunar valves into the _____.

9. The written record produced by using electrodes placed on the body surface on opposite sides of the heart to measure electrical activity in the heart is called a(n) _____.

10. When you listen to the heart through a(n) _____, you can hear certain characteristic sounds, usually described as a(n) _____.

11. The first sound, the "lub," marks the beginning of _____ systole.

12. Abnormal heart sounds called _____ indicate the possibility of valve disorders.

13. When a valve does not close properly, some _____ may flow backward, which may result in a(n) _____ sound.

14. Murmurs can also be detected when a(n) _____ becomes narrowed and rough.

VII. CARDIAC OUTPUT DEPENDS ON STROKE VOLUME AND HEART RATE

Cardiac	Cardiac output	Heart	Heart rate	Starling's
Stroke volume	Venous	Ventricle		

1. The _____ is the volume of blood pumped by the left ventricle into the aorta in one minute.

2. The volume of blood pumped by one ventricle during one beat is called the

   _____.

3. By multiplying the stroke volume by the number of times the left _____ beats per minute, the _____ output can be computed.

4. Cardiac output varies with changes in either stroke volume or _____.

5. The amount of blood delivered to the heart by the veins is _____ return.

6. According to _____ law of the _____, the greater the amount of blood delivered to the heart by the veins, the more blood the heart pumps.

VIII. THE HEART IS REGULATED BY THE NERVOUS AND ENDOCRINE SYSTEMS

Acetylcholine	Autonomic	Beta-adrenergic	Blood pressure	Bradycardia
Cardiac centers	Decreases	Norepinephrine	SA	Tachycardia

1. Sensory receptors in the walls of certain blood vessels and heart chambers are sensitive to changes in

   _____.

2. When stimulated, sensory receptors send messages to _____ in the medulla of the brain.

3. Cardiac centers in the medulla maintain control over two sets of _____ nerves that pass to the _____ node.

4. Parasympathetic nerves release the neurotransmitter _____, which slows the heart.

5. Sympathetic nerves release _____, which speeds the heart rate and increases the strength of contraction.

6. Norepinephrine binds to receptors known as _____ receptors.

7. A fast heart rate of over 100 beats per minute is called _____.

8. A slow heart rate of less than 60 beats per minute is referred to as _____.

9. Heart rate _____ when body temperature is lowered.

Labeling Exercise

Please fill in the correct labels for Figure 11-2.

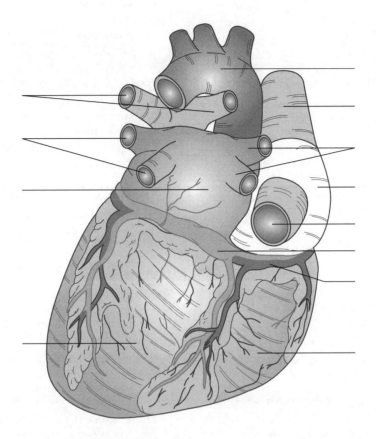

CHAPTER TEST

Select the correct response.

1. The wall of the heart is richly supplied with all but which of the following?
    a. nerves
    b. blood vessels
    c. skeletal muscle
    d. lymph vessels

2. From the inside out, the layers of the heart are
    a. endocardium, myocardium, and pericardium.
    b. myocardium, endocardium, and pericardium.
    c. pericardium, myocardium, and endocardium.
    d. pericardium, endocardium, and myocardium.

3. The inner layer, or _____, consists of a smooth endothelial lining that is resting on connective tissue.
    a. myocardium
    b. pericardium
    c. endocardium
    d. epicardium

4. The greatest portion of the heart wall consists of _____, the cardiac muscle that contracts to pump blood.
    a. myocardium
    b. pericardium
    c. endocardium
    d. epicardium

5. The outer layer of the heart is called the
    a. myocardium.
    b. pericardium.
    c. endocardium.
    d. b and c only.

6. The _____ receive blood returning to the heart from the veins and act as reservoirs between contractions of the heart.
   a. ventricles
   b. atria
   c. arteries
   d. septa

7. The _____ pump blood into the great arteries leaving the heart.
   a. ventricles
   b. atria
   c. capillaries
   d. septa

8. A small muscular pouch called an _____ increases the surface area of each atrium.
   a. interatrial septum
   b. interventricular septum
   c. auricle
   d. atrial pouch

9. The atrioventricular valve between the right atrium and right ventricle is called the _____ valve.
   a. tricuspid
   b. bicuspid
   c. mitral
   d. b and c only

10. The atrioventricular valve between the left atrium and the left ventricle is called the _____ valve.
    a. tricuspid
    b. bicuspid
    c. mitral
    d. both b and c

11. The cusps of each _____ valve are shaped like half-moons.
    a. tricuspid
    b. bicuspid
    c. semilunar
    d. mitral

12. The semilunar valve between the left ventricle and the aorta is called the _____ valve.
    a. ventricular
    b. aortic
    c. pulmonary
    d. mitral

13. The semilunar valve between the right ventricle and the pulmonary artery is called the _____ valve.
    a. ventricular
    b. aortic
    c. pulmonary
    d. mitral

14. Two _____ arteries branch off from the aorta as it leaves the heart.
    a. coronary
    b. pulmonary
    c. aortic
    d. sinoatrial

15. The heart's conduction system is made up of specialized _____ muscle.
    a. smooth
    b. cardiac
    c. pulmonary
    d. skeletal

16. The _____ is a small mass of specialized muscle in the posterior wall of the right atrium.
    a. atrioventricular node
    b. sinoatrial node
    c. sinoatrial bundle
    d. atrioventricular bundle

17. From the AV node, an electrical impulse spreads into specialized muscle fibers that form the
    a. atrioventricular bundle.
    b. cardiac bundle.
    c. sinoatrial bundle.
    d. sinoatrial node.

18. A cardiac cycle occurs approximately _____ times per minute.
    a. 7
    b. 25
    c. 72
    d. 150

19. The period of contraction is known as
    a. diastole.
    b. systole.
    c. fibrillation.
    d. asystole.

20. The period of relaxation is known as
    a. diastole.
    b. systole.
    c. fibrillation.
    d. asystole.

21. The written record produced by an electrocardiograph is called an
    a. ECG.
    b. EKG.
    c. electrocardiogram.
    d. all of the above.

22. Abnormal heart sounds are called
    a. heart mumbles.
    b. valve stenosis.
    c. heart murmurs.
    d. valve murmurs.

23. _____ is the volume of blood pumped by the left ventricle into the aorta in one minute.
    a. Cardiac output
    b. Stroke volume
    c. Cardiac cycle
    d. Ventricular output

24. The volume of blood pumped by one ventricle during one beat is called the
    a. cardiac output.
    b. stroke volume.
    c. cardiac cycle.
    d. ventricular output.

25. Parasympathetic nerves release the neurotransmitter
    a. norepinephrine.
    b. epinephrine.
    c. acetylcholine.
    d. beta blockers.

26. Which of the following does not raise the heart rate?
    a. increased body temperature
    b. exercise
    c. stress
    d. decreased body temperature

Chapter

12

CIRCULATION OF BLOOD AND LYMPH

■ ■ ■

Outline

Introduction
I. Three main types of blood vessels circulate blood.
    A. Arteries carry blood away from the heart.
    B. Capillaries are exchange vessels.
    C. Veins carry blood back to the heart.
II. Blood circulates through two circuits.
    A. The pulmonary circulation carries blood to and from the lungs.
    B. The systemic circulation carries blood to the tissues.
        1. The aorta has four main regions.
        2. The superior and inferior venae cava return blood to the heart.
        3. Four arteries supply the brain.
        4. The liver has an unusual circulation.
III. Several factors influence blood flow.
    A. The alternate expansion and recoil of an artery is its pulse.

B. Blood pressure depends on blood flow and resistance to blood flow.
C. Pressure changes as blood flows through the systemic circulation.
D. Blood pressure is expressed as systolic pressure over diastolic pressure.
E. Blood pressure must be carefully regulated.
IV. The lymphatic system is an accessory circulatory system.
    A. The lymph circulation is a drainage system.
    B. Lymph nodes filter lymph.
    C. Tonsils filter interstitial fluid.
    D. The spleen filters blood.
    E. The thymus gland plays a role in immune function.

Learning Objectives

After you have studied this chapter, you should be able to:

1. Compare the structure and functions of arteries, capillaries, and veins.
2. Trace a drop of blood through the pulmonary and systemic circulations, listing the principal vessels and heart chambers through which it must pass on its journey from one part of the body to another. (For example, trace a drop of blood from the inferior vena cava to an organ such as the brain and then back to the heart.)
3. Identify the main divisions of the aorta and its principal branches.
4. Trace a drop of blood through the brain.
5. Trace a drop of blood through the hepatic portal system.

6. State the physiologic basis for arterial pulse and describe how pulse is measured.
7. State the relationship among blood pressure, blood flow, and resistance, and describe how blood pressure is measured.
8. Compare blood pressure in the different types of blood vessels of the systemic circulation.
9. Describe the mechanisms by which the nervous and endocrine systems regulate blood pressure.
10. Describe the functions, tissues, and organs of the lymphatic system.
11. Trace the flow of lymph from a lymph capillary to the left or right subclavian vein.

STUDY QUESTIONS

Within each category, fill in the blanks with the correct response.

INTRODUCTION

Blood vessels   **Interstitial fluid**   **Nourishes**   **Smaller**   **Tissue**

1. _____ are the tubes that deliver blood to the tissues.

2. The _____ types of blood vessels are quite leaky.

3. When plasma enters the tissues it is called _____ or _____ fluid.

4. Interstitial fluid _____ the cells and keeps them moist.

I. THREE MAIN TYPES OF BLOOD VESSELS CIRCULATE BLOOD

A. Arteries Carry Blood Away From the Heart

Arteries   **Arterioles**   **Collagen**   **Connective**   **Dilate**
Endothelium   **Nervous**   **Pulmonary**   **Tunics**

1. _____ carry blood from the ventricles of the heart to the organs of the body.

2. The _____ arteries are an important exception; they don't carry blood rich in oxygen.

3. The smallest branches of an artery, called _____, are important in regulating blood pressure.

4. The wall of an artery or vein has three layers, or _____.

5. The inner layer of a blood vessel consists of _____ that forms a smooth surface for the blood.

6. The middle layer of a blood vessel consists of _____ tissue and smooth muscle.

7. The outer layer of a blood vessel consists of connective tissue that is rich in elastic and _____ fibers.

8. Changes in blood flow are regulated by the _____ system in response to metabolic needs of the tissue, as well as by the demands of the body as a whole.

9. During exercise, arterioles within the muscles _____, increasing by more than tenfold the amount of blood flowing to the muscle.

B.   Capillaries Are Exchange Vessels

Capillaries	**Exchange**	**Macrophages**	**Metarterioles**
Plasma	**Precapillary sphincter**	**Sinusoids**	

1.   From the arterioles, blood flows through _____, tiny vessels that form extensive networks within each tissue.

2.   Capillary walls are thin and somewhat porous, permitting _____ to pass through them into the tissues.

3.   Capillaries permit the _____ of oxygen, nutrients, and other materials between the blood and tissues.

4.   _____ are small blood vessels that directly link arterioles with venules.

5.   Whenever a capillary branches from a metarteriole, a smooth muscle cell called a _____ is present.

6.   In the liver, spleen, and bone marrow, arterioles and venules are connected by capillary-like vessels called _____, rather than by typical capillaries.

7.   _____ lie along the outer walls of sinusoids; reaching into the vessels to remove worn-out blood cells and foreign matter from circulation.

C.   Veins Carry Blood Back to the Heart

Pulmonary   **Valves**   **Veins**   **Venules**

1.   Blood passes from capillaries into _____.

2.   The smallest veins are called _____.

3.   All veins except the _____ veins carry blood that is poor in oxygen.

4.   Most large veins have _____ that permit the vein to conduct blood toward the heart, even against the force of gravity.

Labeling Exercise

Please fill in the correct labels for Figure 12-1.

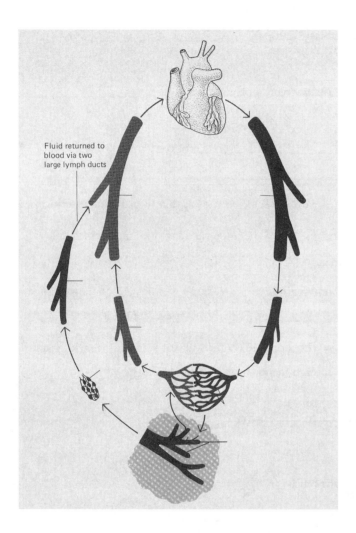

Fluid returned to
blood via two
large lymph ducts

II. BLOOD CIRCULATES THROUGH TWO CIRCUITS

Atrium   **Left**   **Pulmonary**   **Right**   **Systemic**   **Ventricle**

1. The _____ circulation connects the heart with the lungs.

2. The _____ circulation connects the heart with all of the organs and tissues.

3. The left _____ pumps blood into the systemic circulation.

4. The _____ ventricle pumps blood into the pulmonary circulation.

5. From the pulmonary circulation, blood is returned to the left _____, and is then
    pumped into the _____ ventricle.

A.   The Pulmonary Circulation Carries Blood To and From the Lungs

Atrium   Left atrium   Pulmonary   Pulmonary veins

1.   Blood that is poor in oxygen returns from the systemic circulation to the right

     _____.

2.   The _____ arteries deliver blood to the lungs.

3.   The _____ return oxygen-rich blood to the _____.

4.   Place numbers next to each item to indicate the correct sequence for pulmonary circulation.
     _____ Pulmonary arteries
     _____ Right ventricle
     _____ Right atrium
     _____ Pulmonary capillaries
     _____ Left atrium
     _____ Pulmonary veins

B.   The Systemic Circulation Carries Blood to the Tissues

1.   The Aorta Has Four Main Regions

Abdominal   Aortic arch   Ascending   Descending aorta   Thoracic

1.   The _____ aorta is the first part of the aorta which travels upward (superiorly).

2.   The _____ curves from the ascending aorta and makes a U-turn.

3.   The _____ aorta descends from the aortic arch passing through the thorax. It lies
     posterior to the heart.

4.   The _____ aorta is the region of the aorta below the diaphragm and is the longest
     region of the aorta.

5.   The thoracic aorta and the abdominal aorta together make up the _____.

2.   The Superior and Inferior Venae Cava Return Blood to the Heart

Carbon dioxide   Capillaries   Inferior vena cava   Right atrium   Superior vena cava   Veins

1.   As blood circulates through the capillaries in the tissues, it delivers nutrients and oxygen to the cells and
     picks up _____.

2.   _____ deliver blood to venules, which merge to form larger

     _____.

3.   The _____ receives blood from the upper portions of the body.

4.   The _____ receives blood returning from below the level of the diaphragm.

5.   The superior and inferior venae cava return blood to the _____ of the heart.

3. Four Arteries Supply the Brain

Anastomosis	Arteries	Basilar	Brachiocephalic	Circle of Willis
Heart	Internal carotid	Internal jugular	Superior	Venous sinuses
Vertebral				

1. Four _____ bring blood to the brain.

2. The two _____ arteries enter the cranial cavity in the midregion of the cranial floor.

3. The two _____ arteries pass through the foramen magnum and join on the ventral surface of the brain stem. Together, these arteries form the _____ artery.

4. The _____ is the circle of arteries at the base of the brain, formed by branches of the internal carotid arteries and the basilar artery.

5. _____ refers to the joining of two or more arteries.

6. From the brain capillaries, blood drains into large _____ located in the folds of the dura mater.

7. Blood from the venous sinuses empties into the _____ veins at either side of the neck.

8. From the internal jugular veins, blood passes through the _____ veins and into the _____ vena cava, which returns it to the _____.

9. Place numbers next to each item to indicate the correct sequence of blood flow to and from the brain.
   _____ Aorta
   _____ Superior vena cava
   _____ Common carotid artery
   _____ Circle of Willis
   _____ Internal carotid artery
   _____ Venous sinus
   _____ Capillaries in brain
   _____ Brachiocephalic vein
   _____ Internal jugular vein

Labeling Exercise

Please fill in the correct labels for Figure 12-2.

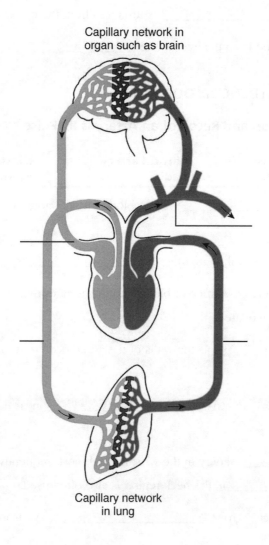

Capillary network in
organ such as brain

Capillary network
in lung

4.   The Liver Has an Unusual Circulation

Hepatic	Homeostatic	Inferior vena cava	Liver
Mesenteric	Portal	Superior mesenteric	Toxic

1.   The body has a few specialized veins that carry blood to a second set of exchange vessels. These veins
are called _____ veins.

2.   The _____ portal vein delivers blood from the organs of the digestive system to
the liver.

3.   Blood is delivered to the intestines by the _____ arteries.

4.   Blood, rich in nutrients, leaves the capillaries in the intestinal wall and flows into the
_____ vein.

5. As blood flows through sinusoids in the liver, _____ cells remove and store nutrients whose concentrations are above _____ levels.

6. Liver cells remove _____ substances from the blood.

7. The hepatic veins carry blood from the liver to the _____.

III. SEVERAL FACTORS INFLUENCE BLOOD FLOW

A. The Alternate Expansion and Recoil of an Artery Is Its Pulse

Arterial	**Artery**	**Carotid artery**	**Diastole**
Left ventricle	**Pulse**	**Radial**	**Systole**

1. Each time the _____ pumps blood into the aorta, the elastic wall of the aorta stretches.

2. The alternate expansion and recoil of an artery is the _____ pulse.

3. As the left ventricle forces a large volume of blood into the aorta during _____, the aorta expands to accommodate it.

4. During _____, as the walls of the aorta recoil to normal size, the blood is kept flowing into the capillaries.

5. When you place your finger over a(n) _____ near the skin surface, you can feel the pulse.

6. The _____ artery in the wrist is used most frequently to measure pulse. The common _____ in the neck region is also often used.

7. Every time the heart contracts, a(n) _____ wave is initiated.

B. Blood Pressure Depends on Blood Flow and Resistance to Blood Flow

Blood	**Blood pressure**	**Diameter**	**Drops**	**Flow**
Peripheral resistance	**Resistance**	**Viscosity**	**Volume**	

1. _____ is the force exerted by the blood against the inner walls of the blood vessels.

2. Blood pressure is determined by the _____ of blood and the _____ to the flow of blood.

3. When cardiac output increases, blood flow increases, causing a rise in _____ pressure.

4. The _____ of blood flowing through the body affects blood pressure.

5. If blood volume is reduced by hemorrhage or by chronic bleeding, the blood pressure

    _____.

6. _____ is the opposing force to blood flow caused by viscosity of the blood and

    by the friction between the blood and the wall of the blood vessel.

7. _____ remains fairly constant in a healthy person and is only a minor factor influ-

    encing changes in blood pressure.

8. A small change in _____ of a blood vessel causes a big change in blood pressure.

C.   Pressure Changes as Blood Flows Through the Systemic Circulation

Arterioles	**Blood**	**Blood flow**	**Blood pressure**
Heart	**Resistance**	**Valves**	**Veins**

1. Because arteries are large, their walls do not present much _____ to blood flow.

2. _____ have a much smaller diameter than arteries, and offer a great deal of resis-

    tance to blood flow.

3. _____ within the arteries is regulated mainly by the degree of constriction or dila-

    tion of the arterioles.

4. As blood flows through the capillaries, most of the pressure caused by the action of the

    _____ is spent.

5. Veins offer little resistance to _____.

6. At any moment, more than 60% of all the blood in circulation can be found within the

    _____.

7. Veins serve as a kind of _____ reservoir.

8. _____ in the veins prevent backflow of blood that would otherwise occur because

    of the force of gravity.

D.   Blood Pressure Is Expressed as Systolic Pressure Over Diastolic Pressure

Blood pressure	**Denominator**	**Diastole**	**Diastolic**
Hypertension	**Left ventricle**	**Normal**	**Numerator**
Sphygmomanometer	**Stethoscope**	**Systole**	**Vascular resistance**

1. In arteries, blood pressure rises during _____ and falls during

    _____.

2. A _____ reading is expressed as systolic pressure over diastolic pressure.

3. _____ blood pressure for a young adult would be about 112/72 mm Hg.

4. In a blood pressure reading, systolic pressure is represented by the _____ and diastolic by the _____.

5. Clinically, blood pressure can be measured with a _____ and _____.

6. When the _____ pressure consistently measures more than 95 mm Hg, a person may be experiencing high blood pressure, or _____.

7. In hypertension, there is usually increased _____.

8. If high blood pressure persists, the _____ enlarges and may begin to deteriorate in function.

E. Blood Pressure Must Be Carefully Regulated

Aldosterone	Angiotensin II	Arterioles	Baroreceptors	Blood pressure
Blood volume	Constrict	Homeostatic	Renin	Vasodilation

1. Blood pressure is kept within normal limits by the interaction of several complex _____ mechanisms.

2. When blood pressure falls, sympathetic nerves signal _____ to constrict, resulting in an increase in blood pressure.

3. When blood pressure increases, specialized receptors called _____ are activated.

4. Cardiac centers in the medulla inhibit sympathetic nerves that constrict arterioles; this action causes _____, which lowers blood pressure.

5. In response to low blood pressure, the kidneys release the enzyme _____.

6. Renin acts on a plasma proteins, which initiates a series of reactions that produces _____, a hormone that acts as a powerful vasoconstrictor.

7. The hormone angiotensin II also acts indirectly to maintain blood pressure by signaling the adrenal glands to increase their output of the hormone _____.

8. Aldosterone increases the retention of sodium ions by the kidneys, resulting in greater fluid retention and increased _____, which results in increased _____.

9. When blood is lost during hemorrhage, special receptors called baroreceptors begin to respond, causing the veins to _____.

IV.   THE LYMPHATIC SYSTEM IS AN ACCESSORY CIRCULATORY SYSTEM

A.   The Lymph Circulation Is a Drainage System

Blood	Drainage	Interstitial	Lymph nodes	Lymph nodules
Lymphatic duct	Lymphatics	Lymphocytes	Thoracic	

1. The lymphatic system consists of the clear, watery lymph that is formed from
    _____ fluid.

2. The lymph tissue is a type of connective tissue characterized by large numbers of
    _____.

3. The lymph system is organized into small masses of tissue called _____ and
    _____.

4. The lymph circulation is a(n) _____ system.

5. The job of the lymphatic system is to collect excess tissue fluid and return it to the
    _____.

6. Lymph capillaries conduct lymph to larger vessels called _____.

7. Lymphatic vessels from throughout the body except the upper right quadrant drain into the
    _____ duct.

8. Lymph from the lymphatic vessels in the upper right quadrant of the body drains into the right
    _____.

B.   Lymph Nodes Filter Lymph

Axillary	Bacteria	Filter	Infection	Lymph nodes	Macrophages

1. _____ are masses of lymph tissue surrounded by a connective tissue capsule.

2. The main function of lymph nodes is to _____ the lymph.

3. Lymph nodes are most numerous in the _____ and groin regions, and many are
    located in the thorax and abdomen.

4. As lymph passes through lymph sinuses in lymph nodes, _____ and other phago-
    cytic cells remove bacteria and other foreign matter.

5. By filtering and destroying bacteria from the lymph, the lymph nodes help prevent the spread of
    _____.

6. When _____ are present, lymph nodes may increase in size and become tender.

C. Tonsils Filter Interstitial Fluid

Adenoids   **Filter**   **Lingual**   **Palatine tonsils**
Pharyngeal   **Tonsillectomy**   **Tonsils**

1. _____ are masses of lymph tissue located under the epithelial lining of the oral

    cavity and pharynx.

2. The major function of the tonsils is to _____ tissue fluid.

3. The _____ tonsils are located at the base of the tongue.

4. The _____ tonsil is located in the posterior wall of the nasal portion of the phar-

    ynx above the soft palate.

5. When enlarged, the pharyngeal tonsil is called the _____.

6. The _____ are prominent oval masses of lymphatic tissue on each side of the

    throat.

7. The process of surgically removing the tonsils is called _____.

D. The Spleen Filters Blood

Bacteria   **Blood**   **Bone marrow**   **Filter**   **Hemorrhage**
Liver   **Macrophages**   **Platelets**   **Spleen**   **Splenectomy**

1. The _____ is the largest organ of the lymphatic system.

2. Because it holds a great deal of _____, the spleen has a distinctive rich purple

    color.

3. One of the main functions of the spleen is to _____ blood.

4. As blood flows slowly through the spleen, _____ and other disease organisms are

    removed.

5. _____ remove worn-out red and white blood cells and platelets in the spleen.

6. A large percentage of the body's _____ are normally found in the spleen.

7. When the spleen is ruptured, extensive—sometimes massive—_____ occurs.

8. The procedure for surgically removing the spleen is called a _____.

9. When the spleen is surgically removed, some of its functions are taken over by the

    _____ and _____.

E.   The Thymus Gland Plays a Role in Immune Function

Hormones   Immune   Lymphocyte   Puberty   Thymus gland

1.   The _____ is a pinkish-gray lymphatic organ located in the upper thorax anterior to the great vessels as they emerge from the heart and posterior to the sternum.

2.   The thymus gland reaches its largest size at _____ and then begins to become smaller with age.

3.   The thymus gland plays a key role in the body's _____ processes.

4.   The thymus gland produces several _____ and also prepares one type of _____ for action.

Labeling Exercise

Please fill in the correct labels for Figure 12-3.

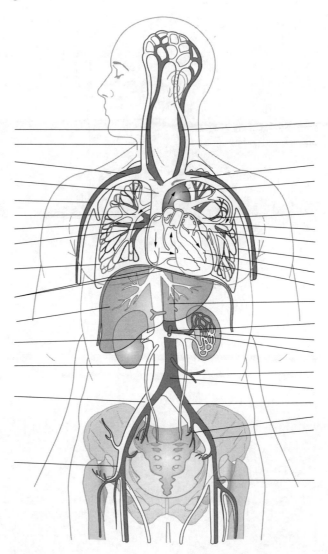

Labeling Exercise

Please fill in the correct labels for Figure 12-4.

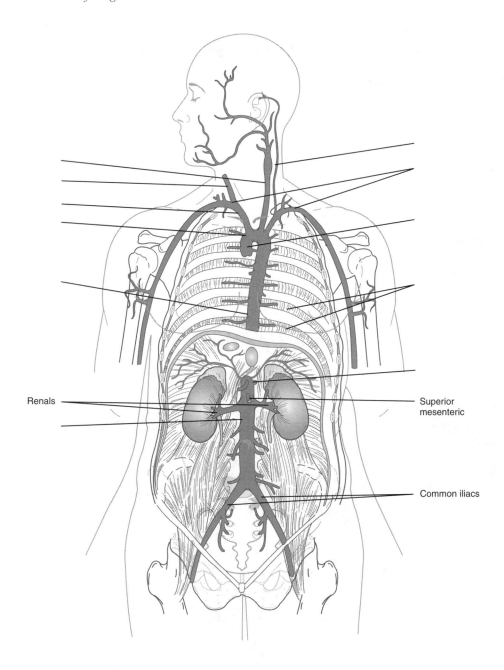

Renals

Superior
mesenteric

Common iliacs

CHAPTER TEST

Select the correct response.

1. _____ carry blood from the ventricles of the heart to each of the organs of the body.
   a. Veins
   b. Arteries
   c. Venules
   d. Capillaries

2. The smallest branches of an artery are called
   a. veins.
   b. arterioles.
   c. venules.
   d. capillaries.

3. Blood flows from arterioles through
   a. arteries.
   b. veins.
   c. venules.
   d. capillaries.

4. The _____ circulation connects the heart with the lungs.
   a. pulmonary
   b. systemic
   c. cardiac
   d. cardiopulmonary

5. The _____ circulation connects the heart with all of the organs and tissues.
   a. pulmonary
   b. systemic
   c. cardiac
   d. cardiopulmonary

6. From the pulmonary circulation, blood is returned to the
   a. left ventricle.
   b. right ventricle.
   c. left atrium.
   d. right atrium.

7. Blood that is poor in oxygen returns from the systemic circulation to the
   a. left ventricle.
   b. right ventricle.
   c. left atrium.
   d. right atrium.

8. Blood is pumped into the right ventricle and then into the
   a. pulmonary veins.
   b. pulmonary arteries.
   c. right atrium.
   d. aorta.

9. Oxygen-rich blood returns from the pulmonary veins to the
   a. left atrium.
   b. pulmonary arteries.
   c. right atrium.
   d. left ventricle.

10. Blood is pumped from the _____ into the aorta, the largest artery in the body.
    a. right ventricle
    b. pulmonary arteries
    c. right atrium
    d. left ventricle

11. The _____ is the first part of the aorta; it travels upward.
    a. thoracic aorta
    b. ascending aorta
    c. abdominal aorta
    d. aortic arch

12. The _____ curves from the ascending aorta and makes a U-turn.
    a. thoracic aorta
    b. superior vena cava
    c. abdominal aorta
    d. aortic arch

13. The _____ descends from the aortic arch, passes through the thorax, and lies posterior to the heart.
    a. thoracic aorta
    b. superior vena cava
    c. abdominal aorta
    d. ascending aorta

14. The basilar artery is formed by
    a. both internal carotid arteries.
    b. pulmonary arteries.
    c. both vertebral arteries.
    d. both a and c.

15. The _____ delivers blood from the organs of the digestive system to the liver.
    a. inferior vena cava
    b. superior vena cava
    c. hepatic portal vein
    d. pulmonary vein

16. Blood is delivered to the intestines by the
    a. mesenteric veins.
    b. mesenteric arteries.
    c. superior vena cava.
    d. carotid artery.

17. When cardiac output increases,
    a. blood flow increases.
    b. blood flow decreases.
    c. blood pressure increases.
    d. both a and c.

18. Blood can flow through the veins against gravity because
    a. a system of valves prevents backflow of blood.
    b. most blood is found in the arteries, not in the veins.
    c. veins are large and elastic and offer little resistance.
    d. there is a lot of pressure in the veins keeping the blood moving at a rapid pace.

19. The function(s) of the lymphatic system is (are) to
    a. collect and return tissue fluid to the blood.
    b. defend the body against disease by producing lymphocytes.
    c. absorb lipids from the intestine and transport them to the blood.
    d. all of the above.

20. Which of the following is *not* part of the lymph system?
    a. tonsils
    b. lungs
    c. thymus gland
    d. spleen

21. Lymph is filtered by
    a. lymphatics.
    b. lymph nodes.
    c. lungs.
    d. liver.

22. The _____ is the largest organ of the lymphatic system.
    a. spleen
    b. liver
    c. lymph node
    d. lymphatics

Chapter

13

INTERNAL DEFENSE: IMMUNE RESPONSES

■ ■ ■

Outline

Introduction

I. Immune responses can be nonspecific or specific.

II. Nonspecific defense mechanisms are rapid.
- A. Mechanical and chemical barriers prevent entry of most pathogens.
- B. Several types of proteins mediate immune responses.
    1. Cytokines are important signaling molecules.
    2. Complement leads to pathogen destruction.
- C. Phagocytes and natural killer cells destroy pathogens.
- D. Inflammation is a protective response.

III. Specific defense mechanisms include cell-mediated immunity and antibody-mediated immunity.

- A. Many types of cells participate in specific immune responses.
    1. Lymphocytes are the principal warriors in specific immune responses.
    2. Macrophages and dendritic cells present antigens.
- B. T cells are responsible for cell-mediated immunity.
- C. B cells are responsible for antibody-mediated immunity.
- D. Long-term immunity depends on memory cells.
- E. Active immunity can be induced by immunization.
- F. Passive immunity is borrowed immunity.

IV. Immune responses are sometimes inadequate or harmful.

Learning Objectives

After you have studied this chapter, you should be able to:

1. Contrast nonspecific and specific immune responses.
2. Describe several nonspecific immune responses including barriers, proteins such as cytokines and complement, phagocytosis, and inflammation.
3. Identify and give the functions of the principal cells of the immune system.
4. Describe cell-mediated immunity, including development of memory cells.

5. Describe antibody-mediated immunity, including the effects of antigen-antibody complex on pathogens both directly and through the complement system.
6. Compare primary and secondary immune responses.
7. Contrast active and passive immunity and give examples of each.
8. Describe several examples of unwanted immune response.

STUDY QUESTIONS

Within each category, fill in the blanks with the correct response.

INTRODUCTION

Immune responses　　　**Immunology**　　　**Pathogens**　　　**Tissues**　　　**Vaccines**

1. Disease-causing organisms or _____, include certain bacteria, viruses, fungi, and protozoa.

2. Some _____ target cancer cells.

3. _____ is the study of internal defense mechanisms.

4. Among the greatest accomplishments of immunologists have been the development of _____ that prevent disease and techniques for transplanting _____ and organs.

I. IMMUNE RESPONSES CAN BE NONSPECIFIC OR SPECIFIC

Antibodies　　　　　　**Antigen**　　　　　　　**Cell signaling**
Immune response　　　**Messenger**　　　　　**Nonspecific immune responses**
Pathogens　　　　　　　**Specific immune responses**

1. A(n) _____ involves recognition of foreign or harmful molecules and an action aimed at eliminating them.

2. Immune responses depend on _____ which is communication among cells.

3. Cells of the immune system communicate directly with their surface molecules and indirectly by releasing _____ molecules.

4. _____ provide general protection against pathogens.

5. Nonspecific immune responses prevent most _____ from entering the body, and rapidly destroy those that do penetrate the outer defenses.

6. _____ are precise responses against specific foreign molecules that have gained entrance to the body.

7. Any molecule that can be specifically recognized as foreign by cells of the immune system is called a(n) _____.

8. An important specific defense mechanism is the production of _____.

II.   NONSPECIFIC DEFENSE MECHANISMS ARE RAPID

Barriers   Immune   Inflammation   Proteins   Skin

1.   Our first line of defense against pathogens is our _____.

2.   Skin and other _____ stop most pathogens from entering the body.

3.   When pathogens succeed in penetrating the body, the _____ system responds quickly to destroy them.

4.   Among the major nonspecific defenses are 1. _____ and cells that destroy patho-gens, and 2. _____.

A.   Mechanical and Chemical Barriers Prevent Entry of Most Pathogens

Acids   Bacteria   Enzymes   Mucous   Nose
Phagocytes   Respiratory   Skin   Sweat

1.   The _____ and _____ membranes are the body's first line of defense against pathogens and other harmful substances.

2.   The skin is populated by large numbers of harmless _____ that inhibit the multi-plication of harmful bacteria that happen to land on it.

3.   _____ and other secretions on the surface of the skin contain chemicals that de-stroy certain types of bacteria.

4.   Pathogens that enter the body with inhaled air may be filtered out by hairs in the _____ or trapped in the sticky mucous lining of the _____ passageway.

5.   Once trapped, pathogens may be destroyed by _____.

6.   Bacteria that enter with food are usually destroyed by the _____ and _____ of the stomach.

B.   Several Types of Proteins Mediate Immune Responses

1.   Cytokines Are Important Signaling Molecules

Antiviral   Cellular   Cytokines   Infecting
Interferons   Interleukins   Lymphocytes

1.   _____ are a large group of peptides and proteins that cells use to signal one an-other.

2.   When infected by viruses or other intracellular parasites, cells respond by secreting cytokines called _____.

3. When viruses infect a cell, they take over the _____ machinery and use it to make more viruses.

4. Interferons signal neighboring cells and stimulate them to produce _____ proteins.

5. Viruses produced in cells exposed to interferon are less effective at _____ new cells.

6. _____ are a diverse group of proteins secreted mainly by macrophages and lymphocytes.

7. Interleukins regulate interaction between _____ and other cells of the body.

2. Complement Leads to Pathogen Destruction

Antigen	Cell wall	Complement
Destroy	Pathogens	Phagocytosis

1. _____ consists of more than 20 proteins present in plasma and other body fluids.

2. Normally, complement proteins are inactive until the body is exposed to a(n) _____ .

3. Certain _____ activate the complement system directly.

4. Once activated, proteins of the complement system work to _____ pathogens.

5. Some complement proteins can rupture the _____ of the pathogen, while others promote _____ and inflammation.

C. Phagocytes and Natural Killer Cells Destroy Pathogens

Bacterium	Macrophages	Natural killer	Neutrophils
Phagocytes	Phagocytosis	Viruses	

1. _____ are cells that ingest bacteria and other foreign matter.

2. In _____, a cell flows around a bacterium and engulfs it.

3. As a _____ is ingested, it is packaged within a vesicle formed by membrane pinched off from the plasma membrane.

4. _____ are the most common type of white blood cell.

5. Neutrophils and _____ are the phagocytes of the nonspecific immune system.

6. _____ cells are large, granular lymphocytes that originate in the bone marrow.

7. Natural killer cells destroy cells infected by _____ and other intracellular pathogens.

D.   Inflammation Is a Protective Response

Edema	Fever	Heat	Histamine	Inflammation	Interstitial
Mast	Pain	Phagocytosis	Plasma	Redness	Serotonin

1.   When pathogens invade tissues, _____ develops within a few hours.

2.   The clinical characteristics of inflammation are _____,

_____, _____, and _____.

3.   Inflammation is regulated by proteins in the _____, by cytokines, and by

_____ cells.

4.   Platelets, basophils, and mast cells release _____ and

_____, compounds that dilate blood vessels in the affected area and increase cap-

illary permeability.

5.   As the volume of _____ fluid increases, swelling, called edema, occurs.

6.   Increased _____ appears to be one of the main functions of inflammation.

7.   _____ is a common clinical sign of widespread inflammatory response.

III.   SPECIFIC DEFENSE MECHANISMS INCLUDE CELL-MEDIATED IMMUNITY AND ANTIBODY-MEDIATED IMMUNITY

Antibody-mediated	Cell-mediated	Lymphatic	Specific

1.   Several days are required to activate _____ immune responses.

2.   Specific immunity is the job of the _____ system.

3.   Two main types of specific immunity are _____ immunity and

_____ immunity.

A.   Many Types of Cells Participate in Specific Immune Responses

Dendritic	Lymphocytes	Macrophages	Neutrophils

1.   The principal warriors in specific immune responses are the million or so _____

stationed strategically in the lymph tissue throughout the body.

2.   Other cell types that participate in specific immune responses are _____,

_____, and _____ cells.

1. Lymphocytes Are the Principal Warriors in Specific Immune Responses

Antibody-mediated	B	Bone marrow	Cell-mediated	Immunologic
Lymph	Mutation	Natural killer	Pathogens	Plasma
Stem cells	T	Thymus	Tumor	Virus

1. Three main types of lymphocytes are _____ lymphocytes,

   _____ lymphocytes, and _____ cells.

2. Natural killer cells kill _____ infected cells and _____ cells.

3. B cells are responsible for _____ immunity; they mature into

   _____ cells that produce specific antibodies.

4. T cells are responsible for _____ immunity.

5. T cells attack body cells infected by invading _____, foreign cells, and cells al-

   tered by _____.

6. B cells are produced in the _____ daily.

7. T cells and B cells originate from _____ in the bone marrow.

8. On their way to the _____ tissues, future T cells stop off in the

   _____ where they mature.

9. The thymus gland makes T cells competent, or capable of _____ response.

2. Macrophages and Dendritic Cells Present Antigens

Antigen-presenting	Bacteria	Dendritic	Digestive	Interferons
Lysosomal	Macrophages	Respiratory	Urinary	Vaginal

1. Macrophages and _____ cells both develop from monocytes.

2. Macrophages secrete about 100 different compounds, including _____ and en-

   zymes that destroy _____.

3. When a macrophage ingests a bacterium, most, but not all, of the bacterial antigens are degraded by

   _____ enzymes.

4. Dendritic cells are strategically stationed in the skin and in the linings of the

   _____, _____, _____, and

   _____ passageways into the body.

5. Like _____, dendritic cells capture foreign antigens and break them down.

6. Macrophages, dendritic cells, and B cells function as _____ cells because they

   display fragments of foreign antigens as well as their own surface proteins.

B.   T Cells Are Responsible for Cell-Mediated Immunity

Antigen	**Cytokines**	**Cytotoxic T cells**	**Enzymes**	**Helper**
Memory	**Mitosis**	**Regulatory**	**T**	

1.   In cell-mediated immunity, _____ cells attack invading pathogens directly.

2.   There are thousands of different types of T cells, each capable of responding to a specific type of _____.

3.   One group of T cells known as _____, or killer T cells, recognizes and destroys cells with foreign antigens on their surfaces.

4.   Killer T cells kill their target cells by releasing a variety of _____ and _____ that destroy cells.

5.   _____ T cells secrete cytokines that activate B cells and enhance immune responses.

6.   _____ T cells suppress immune responses after pathogens have been destroyed.

7.   Once stimulated, a T cell multiplies by _____, giving rise to a sizable clone of cells identical to itself.

8.   Differentiated T cells remain in the lymph tissue as _____ T cells for years or even decades.

C.   B Cells Are Responsible for Antibody-Mediated Immunity

Antibodies	**Antigen**	**Antigen-antibody**	**Antigen-presenting**	**B**
Complement	**Deactivate**	**Helper**	**IgG**	**Memory**
Pathogen	**Phagocytes**	**Plasma**	**Receptor**	

1.   _____ cells produce specific antibodies and send the antibodies out to perform their functions.

2.   Only a B cell displaying a matching _____ on its surface can bind a particular _____.

3.   In most cases, activation of B cells is a complex process that involves _____ cells and helper T cells.

4.   _____ T cells secrete cytokines that help activate the B cells.

5.   _____ cells secrete antibodies, a form of their specific receptor molecule that can be secreted.

6.   Some activated B cells become _____ B cells and continue for years to produce small amounts of antibody.

7. _____ are grouped into five classes according to their structure.

8. Normally, approximately 75% of the antibodies in the body belong in the _____ group.

9. The principal job of an antibody is to identify a(n) _____ as foreign.

10. An antibody usually combines with several antigens, creating a mass of clumped _____ complex.

11. The antigen-antibody complex may _____ the pathogen or its toxin.

12. The antigen-antibody complex stimulates _____ to destroy the pathogen.

13. Antibodies of the IgG and IgM groups work by activating the _____ system.

D. Long-Term Immunity Depends on Memory Cells

Antibodies	**Immunity**	**Killer**	**Memory**
Nonlymphatic	**Primary response**	**Secondary response**	**T**

1. Memory B and memory T cells are responsible for long-term _____.

2. The first time we are exposed to a particular antigen, the body launches a(n)

   _____.

3. Approximately 3 to 14 days are required to mobilize specific _____ cells and

   _____.

4. After an immune response, memory cells group strategically in many _____ tissues, including the lung, liver, kidney, and gut.

5. A second exposure to the same antigen, even years later, results in a(n) _____, which is much more rapid than the primary response.

6. During a secondary response, memory T cells rapidly become _____ T cells that produce interferon and other substances that kill invading cells before we develop the disease.

7. It is because of _____ cells that we do not usually become ill from the same type of infection more than once.

E. Active Immunity Can Be Induced by Immunization

Active immunity	**Antigens**	**Immunization**	**Memory**	**Vaccine**

1. _____ typically develops naturally from exposure to antigens and production of memory cells.

2. Active immunity can be artificially induced by _____; that is, by injection of a

   _____.

3. Immunization causes your body to launch an immune response against the _____ in the vaccine, which then results in the development of _____ cells.

F. Passive Immunity Is Borrowed Immunity

Antibodies	**Effects**	**Immune response**	**Immunity**
Memory	**Milk**	**Passive**	**Pathogens**

1. In _____ immunity, an individual is given antibodies actively produced by other humans or animals.

2. Because passive immunity is borrowed immunity, its _____ do not last.

3. _____ produced by pregnant women can cross the placenta and enter the blood of the fetus, giving the baby some protection for a few months after birth.

4. Babies who are breast-fed receive antibodies in their _____.

5. The antibodies that babies receive during breast-feeding provide _____ to pathogens responsible for gastrointestinal infection, and perhaps to other _____.

6. Passive immunity may only last for a few months because the body has not actively launched a(n) _____ and no _____ cells have been developed.

IV. IMMUNE RESPONSES ARE SOMETIMES INADEQUATE OR HARMFUL

Acquired immunodeficiency syndrome	**Antibodies**	**Antigens**	**Autoimmune**
Helper	**Immune**	**Immune function**	**Rejection**

1. Sometimes pathogens outmaneuver the _____ defenses and cause disease.

2. HIV, the virus that causes _____, infects _____ T cells.

3. Destruction of helper T cells seriously impairs _____ and puts the patient at risk for other infections.

4. Cancer cells have abnormal surface proteins that the immune system targets as foreign _____.

5. During allergic reactions, the body produces _____ against mild antigens that normally do not stimulate an immune response.

6. In some cases, immune responses are directed against the body's own cells resulting in _____ diseases such as rheumatoid arthritis, multiple sclerosis, and insulin-dependent diabetes.

7. Transplanted organs have foreign antigens that stimulate graft _____—an immune response in which T cells destroy the transplant.

CHAPTER TEST

Select the correct response.

1. _____ are organisms that cause disease.
   a. Pathogens
   b. Antigens
   c. Immunogens
   d. Antibodies

2. Which of the following ways can a disease-causing organism enter the body?
   a. wounds in the skin
   b. food
   c. copulation
   d. all of the above

3. Defense mechanisms depend on the body's ability to distinguish between itself and _____ that infect it.
   a. antigens
   b. antibodies
   c. pathogens
   d. lymphocytes

4. Any molecule that can be specifically recognized as foreign by cells of the immune system is called a(n)
   a. pathogen.
   b. antigen.
   c. immunoglobulin.
   d. antibody.

5. Nonspecific defense mechanisms include which of the following?
   a. skin
   b. T cells
   c. inflammation
   d. a and c

6. _____ is (are) important in specific defense.
   a. Skin
   b. Mucus
   c. Stomach acids
   d. Lymphocytes

7. Specific defense is the function of the _____ system.
   a. circulatory
   b. endocrine
   c. lymphatic
   d. reproductive

8. A main type of lymphocyte is a
   a. T cell.
   b. lymph cell.
   c. B cell.
   d. a and c only.

9. In cell-mediated immunity, _____ cells attack invading pathogens directly.
   a. T
   b. B
   c. plasma
   d. red blood

10. T cells multiply by
    a. sexual reproduction.
    b. asexual reproduction.
    c. mitosis.
    d. osmosis.

11. _____ T cells combine with antigens on the surface of an invading cell.
    a. Memory
    b. Combination
    c. Killer
    d. Helper

12. _____ cells produce specific antibodies and send the antibodies out to perform their functions.
    a. T
    b. B
    c. Lymph
    d. Red blood

13. Which is *not* a type of T cell?
    a. memory
    b. killer
    c. helper
    d. antibody

14. Memory cells can develop from
    a. T cells.
    b. monocytes.
    c. B cells.
    d. both T and B cells.

15. _____ is *not* a class of antibodies.
    a. IgN
    b. IgG
    c. IgA
    d. IgM

16. Normally, approximately 75% of the antibodies in the body belong in the _____ group.
    a. IgG
    b. IgM
    c. IgA
    d. IgD

17. The principal function of an antibody is to identify a _____ as a foreign body.
    a. macrophage
    b. pathogen
    c. T cell
    d. B cell

18. Active immunity develops from exposure to
    a. lymph cells.
    b. antigens.
    c. antibodies.
    d. killer T cells.

19. Which of the following is *not* an autoimmune disease?
    a. multiple sclerosis
    b. rheumatoid arthritis
    c. insulin-dependent diabetes
    d. measles

CROSSWORD PUZZLE FOR CHAPTERS 10, 11, 12, AND 13

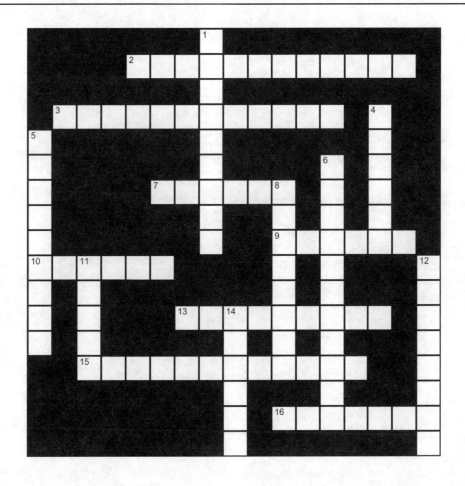

Across
2. Injection of a vaccine
3. Reaction to pathogen invasion
7. Serum plus clotting proteins
9. Function in cell-mediated immunity
10. Largest lymphatic organ
13. Cell fragments in the blood that function in clotting
15. High blood pressure
16. Period of contraction in the cardiac cycle

Down
1. The circulatory system that connects the heart and lungs
4. Artery in wrist commonly used to measure pulse
5. Atrioventricular valve on the right side of the heart
6. Proteins that trigger other cells to produce antiviral proteins
8. Proteins on red blood cell surfaces that determine blood type
11. Clear, watery fluid formed from tissue fluid
12. Vessels that carry blood away from the heart
14. Deficiency of red blood cells

Chapter

14

THE RESPIRATORY SYSTEM

■ ■ ■

Outline

Introduction
I. The respiratory system consists of the airway and lungs.
   A. The nasal cavities are lined with a mucous membrane.
   B. The pharynx is divided into three regions.
   C. The larynx contains the vocal cords.
   D. The trachea is supported by rings of cartilage.
   E. The primary bronchi enter the lungs.
   F. The lungs provide a large surface area for gas exchange.
II. Ventilation moves air into and out of the lungs.
III. Gas exchange occurs by diffusion.
IV. Gases are transported by the circulatory system.
V. Respiration is regulated by the brain.
VI. The respiratory system defends itself against polluted air.

Learning Objectives

After you have studied this chapter, you should be able to:

1. Trace a breath of air through the respiratory system from nose to alveoli.
2. Describe the structure and functions of the respiratory organs, including the lungs.
3. Compare and contrast inspiration and expiration.
4. Compare the process of oxygen and carbon dioxide exchange in the lungs with gas exchange in the tissues.
5. Compare the transport of oxygen and carbon dioxide in the blood.
6. Describe how the body regulates respiration.
7. Describe defense mechanisms that protect the lungs from pollutants in the air and describe some effects of breathing pollutants.

STUDY QUESTIONS

Within each category, fill in the blanks with the correct response.

INTRODUCTION

Carbon dioxide   **Cellular respiration**   **Oxygen**   **Respiration**   **Waste product**

1. _____ is the exchange of gases between the body and its environment.

2. Respiration supplies the cells of the body with _____ and rids them of

   _____ .

3. _____ is the process by which cells capture energy from nutrients that serve as fuel molecules.

4. Oxygen is required for cellular respiration and carbon dioxide is produced as a(n) _____.

I. THE RESPIRATORY SYSTEM CONSISTS OF THE AIRWAY AND LUNGS

Alveoli	Bronchioles	Bronchus	Larynx	Lung
Nostrils (nares)	Oxygen	Respiratory system	Trachea	

1. The _____ consists of the lungs and the airway.

2. A breath of air enters the body through the _____, the openings into the nose.

3. The _____ is also known as the voicebox.

4. The _____ is also known as the windpipe.

5. In order to enter the lungs, air must pass through the right or left _____.

6. After passing through smaller branches of the bronchi, air flows into _____ of the lungs, which divide again and again until the air reaches the microscopic air sacs called _____.

7. _____ diffuses from the air sacs into the blood.

8. One bronchus enters each _____.

9. Trace the path that a breath of air would travel as it enters the body through the nose. Place a number next to each step in sequence starting with 1.
_____ Pharynx
_____ Nasal cavities
_____ Trachea
_____ Nostrils (nares)
_____ Larynx
_____ Alveoli
_____ Bronchioles
_____ Bronchus

A. The Nasal Cavities Are Lined with a Mucous Membrane

Conchae	Filtered	Hairs	Moistened	Mucous
Nares	Nasal septum	Receptors	Sinuses	Throat

1. Air passes into the nose through its two openings, the nostrils, also called _____.

2. Coarse _____ in the nostrils prevent large particles from entering the nose.

3. The _____ is the partition that separates the nasal cavities.

4. The septum and walls of the nose consist of bone covered with a _____ membrane.

5. Three bony projections, the nasal _____, project from the lateral walls of the nose.

6. As air passes through the nose, it is _____, _____, and brought to body temperature.

7. The nasal cavity contains the _____ for the sense of smell.

8. Ciliated epithelial cells of the membrane push a steady stream of mucus, along with its trapped particles, toward the _____.

9. Several paranasal _____ in the bones of the skull communicate with the nasal cavities through small channels.

B.   The Pharynx Is Divided Into Three Regions

Esophagus   Laryngopharynx   Larynx   Mouth   Nasopharynx   Oropharynx   Pharynx

1. Posteriorly, the nasal cavities are continuous with the _____.

2. Air enters the _____, the superior part of the pharynx.

3. From the nasopharynx, air moves down into the _____ behind the mouth.

4. The oropharynx receives food from the _____.

5. From the oropharynx, air passes through the _____ and enters the _____.

6. Posterior to the opening into the larynx, a second opening in the laryngopharynx leads into the _____.

C.   The Larynx Contains the Vocal Cords

Adam's apple   Cough   Epiglottis   Glottis   Laryngitis   Larynx   Lungs   Vocal cords

1. The _____, or voicebox, contains the vocal cords.

2. The opening into the larynx is called the _____.

3. The wall of the larynx is supported by cartilage that protrudes from the midline of the neck and is some times referred to as the _____.

4. Inflammation of the larynx, or _____, is most often caused by a respiratory infection or by irritating substances such as cigarette smoke.

5. The _____ are muscular folds of tissue that project from the lateral walls of the larynx.

6. The vocal cords vibrate as air from the _____ rushes past them during expiration.

7. During swallowing, a flap of tissue called the _____ automatically closes off the larynx so food and water cannot enter the lower airway.

8. When the epiglottis fails to close properly, foreign matter comes into contact with the sensitive larynx, which causes a(n) _____ reflex to expel the material from the respiratory system.

D. The Trachea Is Supported by Rings of Cartilage

Cartilage   Larynx   Lungs   Mucous   Pharynx   Trachea

1. The _____, or windpipe, is located anterior to the esophagus.

2. The trachea extends from the _____ to the middle of the chest.

3. The trachea is kept from collapsing by rings of _____ in its wall.

4. The larynx, trachea, and bronchi are lined by a _____ membrane that traps dirt and foreign matter.

5. Ciliated cells in the mucous linings of the larynx, trachea, and bronchi continuously beat a stream of mucus upward to the _____, where it is swallowed.

6. The cilia-propelled mucus "elevator" keeps foreign material out of the _____.

E. The Primary Bronchi Enter the Lungs

Bronchi   Bronchial tree   Bronchioles   Lung

1. The trachea divides into right and left _____.

2. Each bronchus branches again and again, giving rise to smaller and smaller bronchi, and finally to very small _____.

3. Each _____ has more than a million bronchioles.

4. The network of branching air passageways within the lungs is referred to as the _____.

F. The Lungs Provide a Large Surface Area for Gas Exchange

Alveoli   Diaphragm   Hilus   Lobes   Lungs   Mediastinum
Parietal   Pleural   Pleural cavity   Pulmonary surfactant   Thoracic   Visceral

1. The _____ are large, paired organs that occupy the thoracic cavity.

2. The lungs are separated medially by the _____.

3. The right lung is divided into three _____.

4. Each primary bronchus enters its lung at a depression called the _____.

5. Each lung is covered with a(n) _____ membrane, which forms a sac enclosing the lung, and continues as the lining of the _____ cavity.

6. The part of the pleural membrane that covers the lung is the _____ pleura; the portion that lines the thoracic cavity is the _____ pleura.

7. Between the visceral and parietal pleura is a potential space, the _____.

8. The floor of the thoracic cavity is a strong, dome-shaped muscle, the _____.

9. Each bronchiole leads into a cluster of microscopic air sacs, the _____.

10. Alveoli are coated with a thin film of _____—a substance that prevents the alveoli from collapsing.

II.   VENTILATION MOVES AIR INTO AND OUT OF THE LUNGS

Breathing   Collapsed lung   Diaphragm   Expiration   Inspiration   Intercostal   Pulmonary

1. _____ ventilation is the movement of air into and out of the lungs.

2. In general, we carry on pulmonary ventilation by _____.

3. _____ is the process of taking air into the lungs, or breathing in.

4. _____ is the process of breathing out.

5. During inspiration, the diaphragm contracts and flattens, and the external _____ muscles contract.

6. Expiration occurs when the _____ and external intercostal muscles relax.

7. A(n) _____ occurs when the chest is punctured and the air sacs in the lungs collapse.

III.   GAS EXCHANGE OCCURS BY DIFFUSION

Alveolus   Breathing   Carbon dioxide   Circulatory   Diffuse   Expired   Oxygen

1. _____ delivers oxygen to the alveoli of the lungs.

2. The vital link between the alveoli and the body cells is the _____ system.

3. Each _____ serves as a depot from which oxygen is loaded into the blood of the pulmonary capillaries.

4. The alveoli contain a greater concentration of _____ than the blood entering the pulmonary capillaries.

5. _____ moves from the blood, where it is more concentrated, to the alveoli, where it is less concentrated.

6. Oxygen and carbon dioxide _____ through the thin linings of the capillary and the alveolus.

7. _____ air contains 100 times more carbon dioxide than air from the environment.

IV. GASES ARE TRANSPORTED BY THE CIRCULATORY SYSTEM

Bicarbonate ions   **Chemical buffer**   **Hemoglobin**   **Oxygen**   **Plasma**

1. When _____ diffuses into the blood, it enters the red blood cells and forms a weak chemical bond with hemoglobin, forming oxyhemoglobin.

2. Because the chemical bond linking oxygen with _____ is weak, this reaction is readily reversible.

3. Most of the carbon dioxide that is transported in the blood is transported as

_____.

4. In the _____, carbon dioxide slowly combines with water to form carbonic acid.

5. Most of the hydrogen ions released from carbonic acid combine with hemoglobin, which is a very effective _____.

V. RESPIRATION IS REGULATED BY THE BRAIN

Blood   **Breathing**   **Cardiopulmonary resuscitation**
Cellular respiration   **Chemoreceptors**   **Forcefully**
Hyperventilate   **Oxygen**   **Respiratory centers**
Respiratory failure   **Ventilation**

1. Breathing is a rhythmic, involuntary process regulated by _____ in the brain stem.

2. Groups of neurons in the dorsal region of the medulla regulate the basic rhythm of

_____.

3. A group of neurons in the ventral region of the medulla becomes active only when we need to breathe

_____.

4. Overdose of certain medications such as barbiturates depresses the respiratory centers and may lead to

_____.

5. During exercise, the rate of _____ increases, producing more carbon dioxide. The body must dispose of this carbon dioxide through increased _____.

6. Specialized _____ in the medulla and in the walls of the aorta and carotid arteries are sensitive to changes in arterial carbon dioxide concentration.

7. An increase in carbon dioxide concentration results in an increase in hydrogen ions from carbonic acid; these hydrogen ions lower the pH of the _____.

8. Surprisingly, _____ concentration generally does not play an important role in regulating respiration.

9. In order to stay under water longer, swimmers and some Asian pearl divers voluntarily _____ before going under water in order to decrease the carbon dioxide content of the alveolar air and of the blood.

10. _____ is a method for aiding victims who have suffered respiratory and/or cardiac arrest.

VI.   THE RESPIRATORY SYSTEM DEFENDS ITSELF AGAINST POLLUTED AIR

Bronchial	**Carbon**	**Cilia**	**Disease**	**Hair**
Lung	**Lymph**	**Macrophages**	**Mucous lining**	**Respiratory**

1. The _____ system has a number of defense mechanisms that help protect the delicate lungs from damage.

2. The _____ in the nose and the ciliated _____ of the respiratory passageways help trap foreign particles in inspired air.

3. When we breathe dirty air, the _____ tubes narrow.

4. The smallest bronchioles and the alveoli are not equipped with cells with _____, or mucus.

5. Foreign particles that slip through the respiratory defenses and find their way into the alveoli may remain there indefinitely, or they may be engulfed by _____.

6. Macrophages may accumulate in the _____ tissue of the lungs.

7. Lung tissue of chronic smokers and those who work in dirty industrial environments contains large blackened areas where _____ particles have been deposited.

8. Continued insult to the respiratory system results in _____.

9. Cigarette smoking is the main cause of _____ cancer.

Labeling Exercise

Please fill in the correct labels for Figure 14-1.

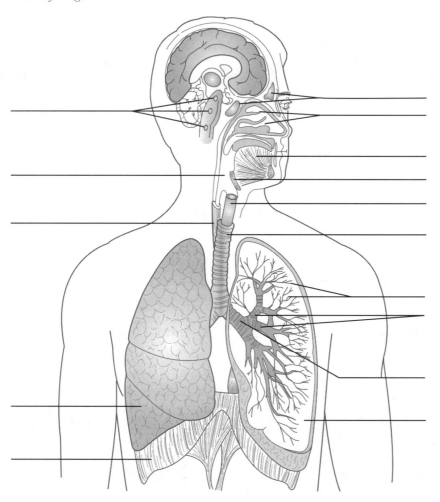

CHAPTER TEST

Select the correct response.

1. The process of respiration includes all of the following *except*
   a. breathing.
   b. gas exchange between the lungs and the blood.
   c. the formation of carbon deposits on the lungs.
   d. gas exchange between the blood and the cells.

2. The respiratory system consists of all of the following *except*
   a. lungs.
   b. esophagus.
   c. nose.
   d. trachea.

3. The correct order in which oxygen passes through the respiratory system is
   a. nasal cavities, larynx, pharynx, trachea, lungs.
   b. nasal cavities, trachea, larynx, pharynx, lungs.
   c. nasal cavities, pharynx, larynx, trachea, lungs.
   d. nasal cavities, pharynx, trachea, lungs, larynx.

4. Cells in the mucous lining of the nose
   a. produce about 1 half pint of mucus a day when there is a respiratory infection.
   b. trap dirt and particles that are inhaled through the nose.
   c. are swallowed with saliva.
   d. all of the above.

5. The pharynx consists of the
   a. nasopharynx.
   b. oropharynx.
   c. laryngopharynx.
   d. all of the above.

6. The inside of the lungs consists of all of the following *except*
   a. bronchi.
   b. bronchioles.
   c. alveoli.
   d. villi.

7. The surface area of the lungs through which gases can be exchanged is about the size of
   a. an average-size computer screen.
   b. a tennis court.
   c. a soccer field.
   d. a football field.

8. During expiration, _____ does not occur.
   a. diaphragm and intercostal muscle contraction
   b. decrease of volume of thoracic cavity
   c. lung recoil
   d. decrease of lung volume

9. Carbon dioxide is transported in the blood
   a. as a compound called bicarbonate.
   b. attached to hemoglobin.
   c. by dissolving in the plasma.
   d. all of the above.

10. The normal adult breathing rate is approximately _____ breaths per minute.
    a. 1 to 10
    b. 12 to 20
    c. 20 to 28
    d. 28 to 35

11. Respiratory centers in the pons and the medulla regulate the
    a. rate of breathing.
    b. depth of breathing.
    c. rhythm of breathing.
    d. all of the above.

12. Cardiopulmonary resuscitation (CPR) must be started immediately because brain damage may occur within _____ minutes of respiratory arrest.
    a. 4
    b. 12
    c. 20
    d. 60

13. Which of the following are pulmonary diseases that have been linked to smoking and breathing dirty air?
    a. emphysema
    b. chronic bronchitis
    c. lung cancer
    d. all of the above

Chapter

15

THE DIGESTIVE SYSTEM

■ ■ ■

Outline

Introduction

I. The digestive system processes food.
   A. The wall of the digestive tract has four layers.
   B. Folds of the peritoneum support the digestive organs.
II. Specific structures of the digestive system have specific functions.
   A. The mouth ingests food.
      1. The teeth break down food.
      2. The salivary glands produce saliva.
   B. The pharynx is important in swallowing.
   C. The esophagus conducts food to the stomach.
   D. The stomach digests proteins.
   E. Most digestion takes place in the small intestine.

F. The pancreas secretes enzymes.
G. The liver secretes bile.
III. Digestion occurs as food moves through the digestive tract.
   A. Glucose is the main product of carbohydrate digestion.
   B. Bile emulsifies fat.
   C. Proteins are digested to free amino acids.
IV. Absorption takes place through the intestinal villi.
V. The large intestine eliminates wastes.
VI. A balanced diet is necessary to maintain health.
VII. Energy metabolism is balanced when energy input equals energy output.

Learning Objectives

After you have studied this chapter, you should be able to:

1. Describe in general terms the following steps in processing food: ingestion, digestion, absorption, and elimination.
2. List in sequence each structure through which a bite of food passes on its way through the digestive tract. Label a diagram of the digestive system.
3. Describe the wall of the digestive tract. Distinguish between the visceral peritoneum and the parietal peritoneum, and describe their major folds.
4. Describe the structures of the mouth (including the teeth) and give their functions.
5. Describe the structure and function of the pharynx and esophagus.
6. Describe the structure of the stomach and its role in processing food.

7. Identify the three main regions of the small intestine and describe the functions of the small intestine.
8. Summarize the functions of the pancreas and liver.
9. Summarize carbohydrate, lipid, and protein digestion.
10. Describe the structure of an intestinal villus and explain the role of villi in absorption of nutrients.
11. Describe the structure and functions of the large intestine.
12. Describe the components of a balanced diet and summarize the functions of each.
13. Contrast basal metabolic rate with total metabolic rate, and write the basic energy equation for maintaining body weight.
14. Define malnutrition and give two examples.

STUDY QUESTIONS

Within each category, fill in the blanks with the correct response.

INTRODUCTION

Digestive   **Energy**   **Nutrients**   **Nutrition**

1. _Nutrients_ are the substances in food that are used as building blocks to make new cells and tissues.

2. Some nutrients serve as a(n) _energy_ source to run the machinery of the body.

3. The process of taking in and using food is called _Nutrition_.

4. The _Digestive_ system processes food and breaks it down into a form that can be delivered to and then used by the cells.

I. THE DIGESTIVE SYSTEM PROCESSES FOOD

~~Absorption~~   ~~Alimentary~~   ~~Anus~~   ~~Chemical~~   Circulatory   ~~Digestion~~
~~Elimination~~   ~~Gastrointestinal~~   ~~Ingestion~~   Liver   ~~Mechanical~~   ~~Mouth~~
Pancreas   Salivary

1. _Ingestion_ involves taking food into the mouth, chewing it, and swallowing it.

2. _Digestion_ is the breakdown of food into smaller molecules.

3. _Mechanical_ digestion is the process of breaking down pieces of food by chewing and by churning and mixing movements in the stomach.

4. _Chemical_ digestion is the process of breaking down large molecules including carbohydrates, proteins, and fats into smaller molecules that can be absorbed from the digestive tract and used by the cells of the body.

5. _Absorption_ is the transport of digested food through the wall of the stomach or intestine and into the circulatory system.

6. The _____ system transports nutrients to the liver where many are removed and stored.

7. _Elimination_ removes undigested and unabsorbed food from the body.

8. The digestive tract, also called the _alimentary_ canal, is a tube approximately 4.4 m long.

9. The digestive tract extends from the _Mouth_, where food is taken in, to the _Anus_, through which unused food is eliminated.

10. Below the diaphragm, the digestive tract is often referred to as the _gastrointestinal_ tract.

11. Place the correct number next to each choice to indicate the proper sequence.

_____ Esophagus

_____ Mouth

_____ Stomach

_____ Pharynx

_____ Large intestine

_____ Small intestine

12. Three types of accessory digestive glands are the _____ glands,

_____, and _____. These are not part of the digestive tract,

but they secrete digestive juices into it.

A. The Wall of the Digestive Tract Has Four Layers

Connective	Digestion	Digestive	Epithelial	Mucosa
Parietal peritoneum	Peristalsis	Peritoneal cavity	Peritonitis	Submucosa

1. From the esophagus to the anus, the wall of the _____ tract consists of four layers.

2. The _____ is the lining of the digestive tract. It consists of

_____ tissue resting on a layer of loose connective tissue.

3. In the stomach and small intestine, the mucosa is compressed into folds, which greatly increase its surface area for _____ and absorption.

4. Beneath the mucosa lies a layer of connective tissue called the _____, which is rich in blood vessels and nerves.

5. The third layer of the digestive system consists of muscle. This muscle contracts in a wavelike motion called _____, which pushes food along through the digestive tract.

6. The outer coating of the wall of the digestive tract consists of _____ tissue.

7. The _____ is the sheet of connective tissue that lines the walls of the abdominal and pelvic cavities.

8. Between the visceral and parietal peritoneum is a potential space called the

_____.

9. Inflammation of the peritoneum, called _____, can have very serious consequences, because infection can easily spread to adjoining organs.

B. Folds of the Peritoneum Support the Digestive Organs

Greater omentum   Intestine   Lesser omentum   Mesocolon   Mesentery   Peritoneum

1. A large double-fold of peritoneal tissue, the _____ extends from the parietal peritoneum and attaches to the small intestine.

2. The mesentery anchors the _____ to the posterior abdominal wall.

3. Other important folds of the _____ are the greater omentum, the lesser omentum, and the mesocolon.

4. The _____, also known as the "fatty apron," is a large double-fold of peritoneum attached to the stomach and intestine.

5. The _____ suspends the stomach and duodenum from the liver.

6. The _____ is a fold of peritoneum that attaches the colon to the posterior abdominal wall.

II. SPECIFIC STRUCTURES OF THE DIGESTIVE SYSTEM HAVE SPECIFIC FUNCTIONS

A. The Mouth Ingests Food

Mechanical   Oral cavity   Taste buds   Tongue

1. The mouth, or _____, ingests food and begins the process of digestion.

2. _____ digestion begins as you bite, grind, and chew food with your teeth.

3. The flexible, muscular _____ on the floor of the mouth pushes the food around, which aids in chewing and swallowing.

4. _____ on the tongue enable us to taste foods as sweet, sour, salty, or bitter.

1. The Teeth Break Down Food

Alveolar   Canines   Crown   Deciduous   Dentin   Enamel
Incisors   Pulp   Pulp cavity   Root canals   Roots

1. The teeth are rooted in sockets of the _____ processes.

2. Each tooth consists of a(n) _____, the region above the gum, and one or more _____, the portion beneath the gum line.

3. Teeth are composed mainly of _____, a calcified connective tissue that imparts shape and rigidity to the tooth.

4. In the crown region of the tooth, the dentin is protected by a tough covering of _____.

5. The dentin encloses a(n) _____ filled with _____, an extremely sensitive connective tissue containing blood vessels and nerves.

6. Narrow extensions of the pulp cavity, called _____, pass through the roots of the tooth.

7. By about 6 months of age, the first of the temporary _____ teeth, also called baby teeth, show their crowns above the gums.

8. The _____ are teeth specialized for biting and cutting.

9. Lateral to the incisors are the _____, which assist humans in biting, but are enlarged in many mammals and are adapted for stabbing and tearing prey.

Labeling Exercise

Please fill in the correct labels for Figure 15-1.

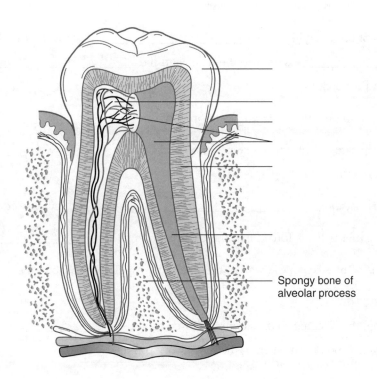

Spongy bone of alveolar process

2. The Salivary Glands Produce Saliva

Bolus   **Parotid**   **Saliva**   **Salivary amylase**   **Sublingual**   **Submandibular**

1. The _____ glands are the largest salivary glands.

2. The _____ glands lie below the jaw.

3. The _____ glands are located under the tongue.

4. _____ consists of two main components: (1) a thin, watery secretion containing

   _____, a digestive enzyme, and (2) a mucous secretion that lubricates the mouth.

5. By moistening food, saliva helps the tongue convert a mouthful of food to a semisolid mass called a(n)

   _____ that can be swallowed easily.

B. The Pharynx Is Important in Swallowing

Epiglottis	**Esophagus**	**Hard palate**	**Laryngopharynx**	**Nasopharynx**	**Oropharynx**
Pharynx	**Soft palate**	**Swallowing**	**Tongue**	**Uvula**	

1. _____ moves the bolus from the mouth through the pharynx and down the

   esophagus.

2. The _____, or throat, is a muscular tube about 12 cm long that serves as the hall-

   way of both the respiratory and digestive systems.

3. The three regions of the pharynx are the _____, posterior to the mouth; the

   _____, posterior to the nose; and the _____, which opens

   into the larynx and esophagus.

4. The oropharynx and the nasopharynx are partitioned by the _____.

5. The muscular soft palate is a posterior extension of the bony _____, which serves

   as the roof of the mouth.

6. A small mass of tissue, the _____, hangs from the lower border of the soft palate.

7. During swallowing, the bolus is forced into the oropharynx by the _____.

8. Reflex contractions of muscles in the wall of the pharynx propel the food into the

   _____.

9. During swallowing, the opening to the larynx is closed by the _____, a small flap

   of tissue that prevents food from entering the respiratory passageways.

C. The Esophagus Conducts Food to the Stomach

Esophagus	**Heartburn**	**Peristaltic**	**Pharynx**	**Sphincter**	**Stomach**

1. The esophagus extends from the _____ through the thoracic cavity.

2. The esophagus passes through the diaphragm and empties into the _____.

3. The bolus is swept through the pharynx and into the esophagus by _____ waves

   of muscle contraction.

4. At the lower end of the esophagus is a circular muscle called a(n) _____ muscle.

5. Normally, because of the closed cardiac sphincter, the highly acidic gastric juice does not splash up into the _____.

6. In gastroesophageal reflux disease (GERD), gastric juice spurts up into the esophagus, irritating its wall and causing spasms. A common symptom of this condition is _____.

D.   The Stomach Digests Proteins

Cardiac	**Chyme**	**Contractions**	**Glands**	**Mucus**	**Pepsinogen**
Peristalsis	**Pyloric**	**Rugae**	**Small intestine**	**Stomach**	

1. When a peristaltic wave passes down the esophagus, the _____ sphincter relaxes, permitting the bolus to enter the _____.

2. When empty, the lining of the stomach has many folds, which are called _____.

3. _____ of the stomach mix the food thoroughly.

4. The stomach mashes and churns food and moves it along by _____.

5. The stomach is lined with simple epithelium that secretes large amounts of _____.

6. Parietal cells in the gastric _____ in the wall of the stomach secrete hydrochloric acid and a substance known as intrinsic factor.

7. Chief cells in the gastric glands secrete _____, an inactive form of the enzyme pepsin, which begins the digestion of proteins.

8. As food is digested over a period of 3 to 4 hours, it is converted into a soupy mixture called _____.

9. The exit of the stomach is guarded by the _____ sphincter, a strong ring of muscle.

10. When the pyloric sphincter relaxes, chyme passes into the _____.

E.   Most Digestion Takes Place in the Small Intestine

Absorption	**Digestion**	**Duodenum**	**Goblet cells**	**Ileum**
Intestinal glands	**Jejunum**	**Pancreas**	**Small intestine**	**Villi**

1. The _____ is a long, coiled tube more than 5 m long by 4 cm in diameter.

2. The first 22 cm or so of the small intestine make up the _____, which is curved like the letter C.

3. As the small intestine turns downward, it is called the _____, which extends for about 2 m; the third part of the small intestine, called the _____, is about 3.5 m long.

4. The lining of the small intestine has millions of tiny fingerlike projections called

   _____.

5. The villi increase the surface area of the small intestine providing a greater surface area for digestion and

   _____ of nutrients.

6. _____ secrete large amounts of fluid that help keep the chyme in a fluid state so

   that nutrients can be easily absorbed.

7. _____ in the mucosa secrete alkaline mucus that helps protect the intestinal wall

   from the acidic chyme and from the action of digestive enzymes.

8. Most _____ takes place in the duodenum rather than in the stomach.

9. The liver and _____ release digestive juices into the duodenum; these secretions

   act on the chyme.

F. The Pancreas Secretes Enzymes

Acute pancreatitis   Duodenum   Enzymes   Exocrine   Pancreas   Pancreatic

1. The _____ is a large, long gland that lies in the abdomen posterior to the stom-

   ach.

2. The pancreas is both an endocrine and a(n) _____ gland.

3. The exocrine portion of the pancreas secretes _____ juice, which contains a num-

   ber of digestive _____.

4. The pancreatic duct from the pancreas joins the common bile duct coming from the liver, forming a

   single duct that passes into the _____.

5. If the pancreatic ducts are blocked, the pancreas may be digested by its own enzymes. This condition,

   called _____, is frequently associated with alcoholism.

G. The Liver Secretes Bile

Bile   Common bile duct   Detoxifies   Gallbladder   Hepatic
Intestine   Liver   Liver cell   Lobe   Portal

1. The _____ is the largest and one of the most complex organs in the body.

2. The right _____ of the liver is larger than its left one and has three main parts.

3. Oxygen-rich blood is brought to the liver by the _____ arteries.

4. The liver also receives blood from the hepatic _____ vein.

5. The hepatic portal vein delivers nutrients absorbed from the _____.

6. Bile is stored and concentrated in the pear-shaped _____.

7. The cystic duct from the gallbladder joins the hepatic duct from the liver to form the _____, which opens into the duodenum.

8. A single _____ can carry on more than 500 separate metabolic activities.

9. The liver produces and secretes _____, which is important in the mechanical digestion of fats.

10. The liver _____ alcohol and many other drugs and toxins that enter the body.

III. DIGESTION OCCURS AS FOOD MOVES THROUGH THE DIGESTIVE TRACT

Chyme   **Gastrin**   **Reflexes**

1. Secretion of digestive juices is stimulated by hormones and by _____.

2. The hormone _____, which is released by the stomach mucosa, stimulates the gastric glands to secrete.

3. The intestinal glands are stimulated to release their fluid mainly by local _____ that occur when the small intestine is stretched by chyme.

A. Glucose Is the Main Product of Carbohydrate Digestion

| Carbohydrate | Glucose | Lactose | Maltase | Maltose |
| Mouth | Pancreatic amylase | Salivary amylase | Sucrose | |

1. Large carbohydrates such as starch and glycogen consist of long chains of _____ molecules.

2. Starch digestion begins in the _____.

3. In the mouth, the enzyme _____ begins breaking down some of the long starch molecules to smaller compounds and then to the sugar _____.

4. In the duodenum, _____, an enzyme in the pancreatic juice, splits the remaining starch molecules to maltose.

5. The enzyme _____ breaks down each maltose molecule to two molecules of glucose.

6. _____, the sugar we use in our coffee, and _____ (milk sugar), are also broken down to simple sugars in the duodenum.

7. Glucose is the major product of _____ digestion.

B. Bile Emulsifies Fat

Bile   **Duodenum**   **Fatty acids**   **Glycerol**   **Lipase**   **Triglycerides**

1. Digestion of fat takes place mainly in the _____.

2. _____ emulsifies fat by a detergent action that breaks down large fat droplets into smaller droplets.

3. Small fat droplets are acted on by an enzyme in the pancreatic juice called _____.

4. Pancreatic lipase breaks down _____ to free _____ and _____.

C. Proteins Are Digested to Free Amino Acids

Amino acids   **Pepsin**   **Peptide**   **Polypeptides**   **Protein**   **Stomach**   **Trypsin**

1. Proteins consist of smaller molecules called _____.

2. Amino acid subunits are linked together by chemical bonds called _____ bonds.

3. During _____ digestion, peptide bonds are broken, and free amino acids are released.

4. Protein digestion begins in the _____, with the enzyme _____.

5. Pepsin breaks down most proteins to smaller molecules called _____.

6. In the duodenum, the enzyme _____ in the pancreatic juice breaks down proteins and polypeptides.

IV. ABSORPTION TAKES PLACE THROUGH THE INTESTINAL VILLI

Absorbed   **Fatty acids**   **Lacteal**   **Liver**   **Villi**   **Villus**

1. After food has been digested, the nutrients are absorbed by the intestinal _____.

2. Within each _____ is a network of capillaries that branches from an arteriole and empties into a venule.

3. Each villus also has a central lymph vessel called a _____.

4. Amino acids and simple sugars are _____ into the blood.

5. Amino acids and simple sugars are transported directly to the _____ by the hepatic portal vein.

6. _____ are absorbed into the lacteals.

V.   THE LARGE INTESTINE ELIMINATES WASTES

Anal canal	**Appendicitis**	**Ascending colon**	**Cecum**	**Chyme**
Colon	**Defecate**	**Feces**	**Ileocecal**	**Peristaltic**
Rectum	**Sigmoid colon**	**Transverse colon**	**Vermiform appendix**	

1. After the _____ has moved through the stomach and small intestine, it consists mainly of water and indigestible wastes such as cellulose.

2. The small intestine is normally shut off from the large intestine by a sphincter muscle called the _____ valve.

3. When a(n) _____ contraction brings chyme toward it, the ileocecal valve opens, allowing the chyme to enter the large intestine.

4. The small intestine joins the large intestine about 7 cm above the end of the large intestine; this creates a pouch called the _____.

5. The _____, a worm-shaped blind tube, hangs down from the end of the cecum.

6. Inflammation of the appendix, called _____, can lead to peritonitis and other complications if not diagnosed and treated promptly.

7. From the cecum to the rectum, the large intestine is known as the _____.

8. The _____ extends from the cecum straight up to the lower border of the liver.

9. As the ascending colon turns horizontally, it becomes the _____.

10. On the left side of the abdomen, the descending colon turns downward and forms the S-shaped _____, which empties into the short _____.

11. The last 4 cm of the rectum are called the _____.

12. As chyme slowly passes through the large intestine, water and sodium are absorbed from it; what remains becomes _____.

13. After meals, contractions of the large intestine increase. This stimulates the desire to _____.

VI.   A BALANCED DIET IS NECESSARY TO MAINTAIN HEALTH

Antioxidants	**Carbohydrates**	**Energy sources**	**Essential amino acids**	**Lipids**
Minerals	**Oxidants**	**Proteins**	**Vitamins**	**Water**

1. Carbohydrates, lipids, and proteins are nutrients that can be used as _____.

2. _____, one of the main components of the body, is used by the body to transport materials.

3. _____ are inorganic nutrients ingested in the form of salts dissolved in food and water.

4. _____ are organic compounds required for certain reactions to take place. Many of these serve as coenzymes, compounds that work with enzymes to regulate chemical reactions.

5. _____ are ingested mainly as starch or cellulose.

6. Most of the _____ we ingest are fats—mainly triglycerides.

7. _____ are digested into their component amino acids.

8. Of the 20 or so amino acids, 9 are considered _____ because they must be provided in the diet.

9. _____ are highly reactive molecules produced during cell activities; they can damage DNA and other cell molecules by snatching electrons.

10. Some phytochemicals function as _____—substances that destroy oxidants.

VII. ENERGY METABOLISM IS BALANCED WHEN ENERGY INPUT EQUALS ENERGY OUTPUT

Basal metabolic rate	**Decreases**	**Heat**	**Malnutrition**
Metabolic rate	**Obesity**	**Stored fat**	**Total metabolic rate**

1. The amount of energy released by the body per unit of time is a measure of

   _____.

2. Much of the energy expended by the body is ultimately converted to _____.

3. The _____ is the rate at which the body releases heat under resting conditions.

4. An individual's _____ is the sum of the basal metabolic rate and the energy used to carry on all daily activities.

5. When energy output is greater than energy input, _____ is burned and body weight _____.

6. _____, or poor nutritional status, can result from dietary intake that is either above or below required needs.

7. _____ is a serious nutritional problem in which energy imbalance results in the deposit of an excess amount of fat in fat tissues.

Labeling Exercise

Please fill in the correct labels for Figure 15-2.

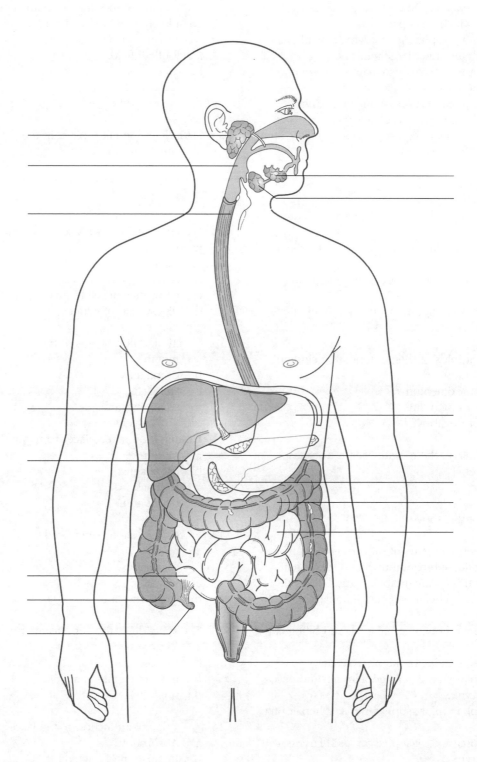

CHAPTER TEST

Select the correct response.

1. The sequence of the parts of the digestive tract through which food passes is
   a. mouth, esophagus, pharynx, stomach, small intestine, large intestine.
   b. mouth, pharynx, esophagus, stomach, small intestine, large intestine.
   c. mouth, esophagus, stomach, pharynx, small intestine, large intestine.
   d. mouth, pharynx, esophagus, stomach, large intestine, small intestine.

2. The sequence of the four major processes of the digestive system is
   a. digestion, absorption, ingestion, elimination.
   b. digestion, indigestion, absorption, elimination.
   c. ingestion, indigestion, digestion, elimination.
   d. ingestion, digestion, absorption, elimination.

3. Important folds of the peritoneum include the
   a. mesentery.
   b. greater omentum.
   c. lesser omentum.
   d. all of the above.

4. Taste buds on the tongue enable us to taste
   a. sweet.
   b. sour.
   c. salty.
   d. all of the above.

5. The three main pairs of salivary glands are
   a. parotid, submandibular, and sublingual.
   b. parotid, inframandibular, and bilingual.
   c. submandibular, supramandibular, and sublingual.
   d. submandibular, sublingual, and bilingual.

6. The three regions of the pharynx are
   a. oropharynx, esophagopharynx, and nasopharynx.
   b. oropharynx, nasopharynx, and hepatopharynx.
   c. oropharynx, nasopharynx, and laryngopharynx.
   d. laryngopharynx, nasopharynx, and esophagopharynx.

7. If the lining of the small intestine could be completely unfolded and spread out, its surface would approximate the size of a
   a. football field.
   b. tennis court.
   c. basketball court.
   d. racquetball court.

8. Most digestion takes place in the
   a. small intestine.
   b. stomach.
   c. large intestine.
   d. esophagus.

9. Which of the following is *not* a function of the liver?
   a. secretes bile
   b. removes nutrients from blood
   c. converts glucose to glycogen
   d. digests carbohydrates

10. Starch digestion begins in the
    a. mouth.
    b. esophagus.
    c. stomach.
    d. small intestine.

11. Fat digestion takes place mainly in the
    a. mouth.
    b. esophagus.
    c. stomach.
    d. duodenum.

12. Protein digestion begins in the
    a. mouth.
    b. esophagus.
    c. stomach.
    d. small intestine.

13. The function of the vermiform appendix is
    a. to store bile.
    b. to store fats.
    c. to store certain vitamins.
    d. unknown.

14. _____ is *not* a function of the large intestine.
    a. Absorption
    b. Incubation of bacteria
    c. Digestion
    d. Elimination of wastes

15. Nutrients required for good health include all of the following *except*
    a. water.
    b. lipids.
    c. vitamins.
    d. alcohol.

16. In order for a person to lose weight, which of the following must happen?
    a. Calories taken in must be greater than calories expended.
    b. Calories taken in must be fewer than calories expended.
    c. Calories taken in must be exactly equal to calories expended.
    d. Calories play very little role in weight loss.

CROSSWORD PUZZLE FOR CHAPTERS 14 AND 15

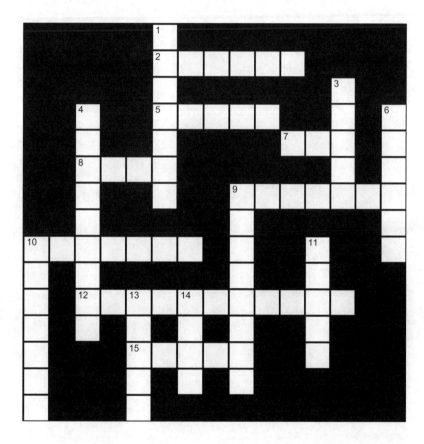

Across
2. Contains vocal cords
5. Large intestine from cecum to rectum
7. Number of bronchi
8. Opening for elimination of feces
9. Windpipe
10. Large salivary gland
12. Stores bile
15. Absorb nutrients

Down
1. During digestion, many carbohydrates are broken down into these components
3. Consists of crown and roots
4. Large muscle that functions in breathing
6. Digests fat
9. Cavity in which lungs are located
10. Throat
11. Terminal part of small intestine
13. Large organ that lies inferior to diaphragm
14. Produced by liver

Chapter

16

THE URINARY SYSTEM AND FLUID BALANCE

■ ■ ■

Outline

Introduction
I.   Metabolic waste products include water, carbon dioxide, and nitrogenous wastes.
II.   The urinary system has many regulatory functions.
III. The urinary system consists of the kidneys, urinary bladder, and their ducts.
    A. The kidney has an outer cortex and inner medulla.
    B. The nephrons are the functional units of the kidney.
    C. Urine is transported by ducts and stored in the bladder.
    D. Urination empties the bladder.
IV.   Urine is produced by filtration, reabsorption, and secretion.
    A. Glomerular filtration is not selective with regard to small molecules and ions.
    B. Tubular reabsorption is highly selective.
    C. Some substances are secreted from the blood into the filtrate.

    D. Urine consists mainly of water.
V.   Hormones regulate kidney function.
    A. Antidiuretic hormone increases water reabsorption.
    B. The renin-angiotensin-aldosterone pathway increases sodium reabsorption.
    C. Atrial natriuretic peptide inhibits sodium reabsorption.
VI.   The volume and composition of body fluid must be regulated.
    A. The body has two main fluid compartments.
    B. Fluid intake must equal fluid output.
    C. Electrolyte balance and fluid balance are interdependent.
    D. Electrolytes serve vital functions.
VII. Acid-base homeostasis depends on hydrogen ion concentration.

Learning Objectives

After you have studied this chapter, you should be able to:

1. Identify the principal metabolic waste products and the organs that excrete them.
2. Summarize the functions of the urinary system in maintaining homeostasis.
3. Describe the anatomy of the urinary system and give the function of each of its structures.
4. Describe the structure and function of a nephron. Be able to label a diagram of a nephron.
5. Trace a drop of filtrate from glomerulus to urethra, listing in sequence each structure through which it passes.

6. Describe the process of urine formation and give the composition of urine.
7. Summarize the regulation of urine volume including the actions of antidiuretic hormone (ADH), renin, aldosterone, angiotensin II, and atrial natriuretic peptide (ANP).
8. Identify the fluid compartments of the body.
9. Summarize the mechanisms that regulate fluid intake and fluid output.

10. Define electrolyte balance and summarize the functions and regulation of five major electrolytes.

11. Describe the mechanisms that maintain acid-base balance and identify causes of acidosis and alkalosis.

STUDY QUESTIONS

Within each category, fill in the blanks with the correct response.

INTRODUCTION

Elimination	Excesses	Excretion	Homeostatic	Urinary	Water

1. The _____ system helps regulate the volume and composition of body fluids.

2. _____ is an excellent solvent.

3. Regardless of how much of it you eat or drink, the fluid and salt content of your body must be kept within _____ limits.

4. The body must replace water and salt losses and excrete _____.

5. _____ is defined as the discharge of metabolic byproducts and wastes, as well as excess solutes and other substances, from the body.

6. Excretion is different from _____, the discharge of undigested or unabsorbed food from the digestive tract.

I. METABOLIC WASTE PRODUCTS INCLUDE WATER, CARBON DIOXIDE, AND NITROGENOUS WASTES

Ammonia	Hemoglobin	Kidneys	Liver	Lungs	Nitrogen
Nitrogenous wastes	Sweat glands	Urea	Uric acid	Urine	

1. The principal metabolic byproducts are water, carbon dioxide, and _____ .

2. Amino acids and nucleic acids contain _____.

3. The amino group is chemically converted to _____, which is then converted to _____.

4. _____ is formed from the breakdown of nucleic acids.

5. Urea and uric acid are transported from the liver to the _____ by the circulatory system.

6. _____ in the skin excrete 5% to 10% of all metabolic wastes.

7. Sweat contains the same substances as _____, but is much more dilute.

8. The _____ excrete carbon dioxide and water (in the form of water vapor).

9. The _____ excretes bile pigments, which are products of the breakdown of _____.

II.   THE URINARY SYSTEM HAS MANY REGULATORY FUNCTIONS

Blood   **Body fluids**   **Erythropoietin**   **Excretes**   **Renin**   **Urine**

1.   The urinary system maintains homeostasis by adjusting the salt and water content of the

   _____.

2.   The urinary system _____ metabolic waste products such as urea.

3.   The urinary system regulates the acid-base (pH) level of the _____ and other

   _____.

4.   The urinary system secretes the enzyme _____, which is important in regulating

   blood pressure.

5.   The urinary system secretes the hormone _____, which regulates production of

   red blood cells.

III.   THE URINARY SYSTEM CONSISTS OF THE KIDNEYS, URINARY BLADDER, AND THEIR DUCTS

Bladder   **Kidneys**   **Ureters**   **Urethra**   **Urinary bladder**   **Urine**

1.   The principal organs of the urinary system are the paired _____, which play a

   vital role in regulating the volume and consumption of body fluid.

2.   The kidneys remove metabolic byproducts and wastes from the blood and produce

   _____.

3.   From the kidneys, urine is conducted to the urinary _____ by the paired

   _____.

4.   The single _____ temporarily stores urine.

5.   Eventually, urine is discharged from the body through the single _____.

A.   The Kidney Has an Outer Cortex and Inner Medulla

Calyx   **Cortex**   **Hilus**   **Kidney**   **Major calyx**   **Medulla**
Renal artery   **Renal capsule**   **Renal papilla**   **Renal pelvis**   **Renal vein**   **Retroperitoneal**

1.   The kidneys are located behind the peritoneum lining the abdominal cavity, and so are described as

   _____.

2.   Each kidney receives blood from a _____, and is drained by a

   _____.

3.   Each _____ resembles a large, dark-red lima bean about the size of a fist.

4. The ureters and blood vessels connect with the kidney at its _____, the notch on its medial border.

5. Covering the kidney is a strong capsule of connective tissue, the _____.

6. The kidney consists of an outer renal _____ and an inner renal _____.

7. The tip of each renal pyramid is called a _____.

8. Urine passes from a collecting duct through a renal papilla and into a small tube called a minor _____.

9. Several minor calyces unite to form a _____.

10. The major calyces join to form a large cavity, the _____.

11. Place the correct number next to each choice to indicate the proper sequence.
_____ Calyx
_____ Renal pelvis
_____ Ureter
_____ Collecting duct
_____ Renal papilla

B. The Nephrons Are the Functional Units of the Kidney

Afferent arteriole	Blood	Bowman's capsule	Collecting ducts	Corpuscle
Efferent arteriole	Filtrate	Glomerulus	Juxtaglomerular	Nephrons
Peritubular	Tubule	Urine		

1. Each kidney contains more than 1 million microscopic units called _____.

2. Nephrons filter the blood and produce _____.

3. Blood is filtered in the renal _____, then the filtered fluid, referred to as _____, passes through the long renal _____.

4. As the filtrate moves through the renal tubule, substances needed by the body are returned to the _____. Waste products, excess water, and other solutes that are not needed by the body pass into the _____ and exit as urine.

5. Each renal corpuscle consists of a cluster of capillaries, the _____, surrounded by a cuplike structure known as _____, or glomerular capsule.

6. Blood from the renal artery flows into the glomerulus through a small _____, and leaves the glomerulus through an _____.

7. The _____ capillaries surround the renal tubule.

8. Part of the distal convoluted tubule curves upward and contacts the afferent arteriole. The cells that make this contact form the _____ apparatus.

9. Place the correct number next to each choice to indicate the proper sequence.

_____ Loop of Henle

_____ Collecting duct

_____ Bowman's capsule

_____ Distal convoluted tubule

_____ Proximal convoluted tubule

C.   Urine Is Transported by Ducts and Stored in the Bladder

Bladder	Penis	Peristaltic	Prostate	Ureters
Urethra	Urinary bladder	Vagina		

1. Urine passes from the kidneys through the paired _____.

2. Urine is forced along through the ureter by _____ contractions.

3. The _____ is a temporary storage sac for urine.

4. When urine leaves the bladder, it flows through the _____, a duct leading to the outside of the body.

5. In the male, the urethra is lengthy and passes through the _____ gland and the _____.

6. In the female, the urethra is short and is found just above the opening into the _____.

7. _____ infections are more common in females than males because the long male urethra is a barrier to bacterial invasion.

D.   Urination Empties the Bladder

External urethral sphincter	Micturition	Nervous system	Urinate	Urination reflex

1. Urination, or _____, is the process of emptying the bladder and expelling urine.

2. The _____ contracts smooth muscle fibers in the bladder wall and also relaxes the internal urethral sphincter.

3. When the time and place are appropriate, the _____ is voluntarily relaxed, allowing urination to occur.

4. Voluntary control of urination cannot be exerted by an immature _____.

5. Most babies under the age of about 2.5 years automatically _____ every time the bladder fills.

IV. URINE IS PRODUCED BY FILTRATION, REABSORPTION, AND SECRETION

A. Glomerular Filtration Is Not Selective with Regard to Small Molecules and Ions

Amino acids   **Blood cells**   **Blood plasma**   **Body**   **Bowman's capsule**
Glomerular filtration   **Glucose**   **Proteins**

1. The first step in urine production is _____.

2. Blood flows through glomerular capillaries under high pressure, forcing more than 10% of the plasma out of the capillaries and into _____.

3. Glomerular filtrate consists of _____ containing ions and small, dissolved molecules.

4. Substances needed by the body, such as _____, _____, and salts, are present in the glomerular filtrate.

5. When _____ or _____ appear in the urine, they signal a problem with glomerular filtration.

6. Every 4 minutes, the kidneys receive a volume of blood equal to the volume of blood in the _____.

B. Tubular Reabsorption Is Highly Selective

Ducts   **Renal tubules**   **Selective**   **Tubular reabsorption**   **Urine**

1. The threat to homeostasis caused by the vast amounts of fluid filtered by the kidneys is avoided because _____ returns about 99% of the filtrate to the blood.

2. Tubular reabsorption is the job of the _____ and collecting _____.

3. Unlike glomerular filtration, tubular reabsorption is highly _____.

4. Wastes, surplus salts, and excess water are kept as part of the filtrate and are excreted as _____.

C. Some Substances Are Secreted from the Blood Into the Filtrate

Creatinine   **Homeostatic**   **Penicillin**   **Renal tubules**   **Tubular secretion**

1. In _____, certain substances are actively transported from the blood in the peritubular capillaries into the filtrate in the _____.

2. Potassium, hydrogen ions, ammonium ions, and some organic ions such as the waste product _____ are secreted into the filtrate.

3. Secretion of hydrogen ions is an important _____ mechanism for regulating the pH of the blood.

4. Certain drugs such as _____ are also removed from the blood by secretion.

D.   Urine Consists Mainly of Water

Ammonia	**Bacterial action**	**Nitrogen wastes**	**Renal pelvis**
Salts	**Sterile**	**Urine**	**Water**

1. By the time the filtrate reaches the _____, its composition has been carefully adjusted.

2. The adjusted filtrate is called _____.

3. Urine is composed of about 96% _____, 2.5% _____, 1.5% _____, and traces of other substances.

4. Healthy urine is _____, and has been used to wash battlefield wounds when clean water was not available.

5. Urine rapidly decomposes when exposed to _____, forming ammonia and other products.

6. It is the _____ in urine that causes diaper rash in infants.

V.   HORMONES REGULATE KIDNEY FUNCTION

A.   Antidiuretic Hormone Increases Water Reabsorption

ADH	**Dehydrate**	**Diabetes insipidus**	**Diuretics**
Greater	**Hypothalamus**	**Osmotic pressure**	**Reabsorption**

1. When fluid intake is low, the body begins to _____.

2. When the volume of blood decreases, the concentration of dissolved salts is _____, causing an increase in the _____ of the blood.

3. Specialized receptors in the _____ are sensitive to increased osmotic pressure.

4. _____ transmits information from the brain to the distal convoluted tubules and collecting ducts of the kidneys.

5. When the pituitary gland does not produce enough ADH, water is not efficiently reabsorbed from the ducts. This results in the production of a large volume of urine. This condition is called _____.

6. Coffee, tea, and alcoholic beverages contain chemicals called _____ that increase urine volume.

7. Diuretics inhibit _____ of water.

B. The Renin-Angiotensin-Aldosterone Pathway Increases Sodium Reabsorption

ADH   **Aldosterone**   **Angiotensin I**   **Angiotensin II**
Blood pressure   **Juxtaglomerular**   **Renin-angiotensin-aldosterone**

1. _____ regulates the excretion of water by the kidneys.

2. Salt excretion is regulated mainly by _____, secreted by the adrenal glands.

3. Aldosterone secretion can be stimulated by a decrease in _____.

4. When blood pressure falls, cells of the _____ apparatus secrete the enzyme renin, activating the _____ pathway.

5. Renin acts on a plasma protein converting it to a prehormone called _____.

6. An enzyme known as ACE converts angiotensin I into its active form _____.

C. Atrial Natriuretic Peptide Inhibits Sodium Reabsorption

ANP   **Blood pressure**   **Blood volume**   **Decreases**   **Fluid**   **Salt**

1. An increase in fluid intake can cause an increase in _____, which results in an increase in blood pressure.

2. When blood pressure increases, the atria of the heart are stretched, and in response, they secrete _____.

3. ANP increases sodium excretion and _____ blood pressure.

4. The renin-angiotensin-aldosterone system and ANP work antagonistically in regulating _____ balance, _____ balance, and _____.

VI. THE VOLUME AND COMPOSITION OF BODY FLUID MUST BE REGULATED

Chemical reactions   **Solutes**   **Solvent**   **Transport**   **Water**

1. The human body is about 60% _____ by weight.

2. Water is used to _____ materials throughout the body.

3. All of the _____ in the body take place in a watery medium.

4. Water serves as an important _____ and is an essential part of many metabolic reactions.

5. The substances dissolved in a solution are called _____.

A.   The Body Has Two Main Fluid Compartments

Blood pressure   Cells   Extracellular   Intracellular   Lymphatic   Osmotic   Volume

1.   Body fluid is distributed in two principal compartments: the _____ compartment and the _____ compartment.

2.   About two-thirds of the body fluid is found within _____.

3.   Fluid constantly moves from one compartment to another. However, in a healthy person, the _____ of fluid in each compartment remains about the same.

4.   The movement of fluid from one compartment to another depends on _____ and _____ concentration.

5.   Excess interstitial fluid is returned to the blood by the _____ system.

B.   Fluid Intake Must Equal Fluid Output

Dehydration   Fluid output   Hypothalamus   Ingested   Kidneys   Metabolism   Thirst center

1.   Normally, fluid intake equals _____ so that the total amount of fluid in the body remains constant.

2.   The average daily fluid intake is about 2500 ml, most of which is _____ in the foods we eat and liquids we drink.

3.   Water is produced during cellular _____.

4.   Fluid is excreted primarily by the _____.

5.   When fluid output is greater than fluid intake, _____ occurs.

6.   Fluid intake is regulated by the _____.

7.   Dehydration causes increased osmotic pressure, which stimulates the _____ in the hypothalamus.

C.   Electrolyte Balance and Fluid Balance Are Interdependent

Anions   Cations   Electrolyte balance   Electrolytes
Glucose   Ions   Nonelectrolytes   Urea

1.   Among the most important components of body fluids are _____.

2.   Electrolytes are compounds such as inorganic salts, acids, and bases that form _____ in solution.

3.   Most organic compounds dissolved in the body fluid are _____—compounds that do not form ions.

4. Examples of nonelectrolytes in the body fluid are _____ and

    _____.

5. Positively charged ions are referred to as _____.

6. Negatively charged ions are referred to as _____.

7. When the amounts of the various electrolytes taken into the body equal the amounts lost, the body is in

    _____.

D. Electrolytes Serve Vital Functions

Acid-base (pH)	Aldosterone	Chloride	Coma	Heart failure
Magnesium	Muscle	Neurons	Osmotic pressure	Phosphate
Potassium	Sodium	Urine	Water	

1. About 90% of the extracellular cations are _____ ions.

2. Sodium ions are needed to transmit impulses in _____ and

    _____ fibers.

3. Severe sodium depletion may result in circulatory shock and _____.

4. Sodium ion concentration is adjusted mainly by regulating the amount of _____ in

    the body.

5. _____ stimulates the distal convoluted tubules and collecting ducts to increase

    their reabsorption of sodium ions.

6. Most of the cations in the intracellular fluid are _____ ions.

7. Potassium ions help regulate _____ levels.

8. A high potassium ion concentration can weaken the heart and lead to death from abnormal heart

    rhythm, or _____.

9. Loss of potassium ions in the _____ brings the potassium concentration in the

    body back to normal.

10. _____ ions are the most abundant intracellular anions.

11. _____ ions are the most abundant extracellular anions.

12. Chloride ions help regulate differences in _____ between fluid compartments and

    are also important in pH balance.

13. _____ ions are important in development of bones and teeth and play a role in

    neural transmission and muscle contraction.

VII.   ACID-BASE HOMEOSTASIS DEPENDS ON HYDROGEN ION CONCENTRATION

Acid-base	**Acidity**	**Acidosis**	**Alkalinity**	**Alkalosis**
Basic	**Bicarbonate**	**Blood**	**Chemical buffer**	**Hemoglobin**
Higher	**Lower**	**Neutral**	**pH**	**Phosphate**
Protein	**Respiratory acidosis**	**Respiratory alkalosis**		

1. _____ balance depends on the concentration of hydrogen ions.

2. _____ is a measurement of the hydrogen ion concentration of a solution.

3. A(n) _____ pH is 7.

4. Lower pH values indicate a(n) _____ hydrogen ion concentration or a greater

   _____.

5. Higher pH values indicate a(n) _____ hydrogen ion concentration or greater

   _____.

6. An alkaline solution is also referred to as _____.

7. _____ and most other body fluids are slightly alkaline.

8. The term _____ refers to any condition in which the hydrogen ion concentration

   of plasma is elevated above the homeostatic range.

9. _____ is any condition in which the hydrogen ion concentration is below the

   homeostatic range.

10. A(n) _____ is a substance that minimizes changes in pH when an acid or base is

    added to a solution.

11. The main buffering systems in the body are the _____ buffer system, the

    _____ buffer system, and the _____ buffer systems.

12. _____ is an example of a protein that is a very effective buffer.

13. _____ develops when carbon dioxide is produced more rapidly than it is excreted

    by the lungs.

14. _____ occurs when the respiratory system excretes carbon dioxide more quickly

    than it is produced.

Labeling Exercise

Please fill in the correct labels for Figure 16-1.

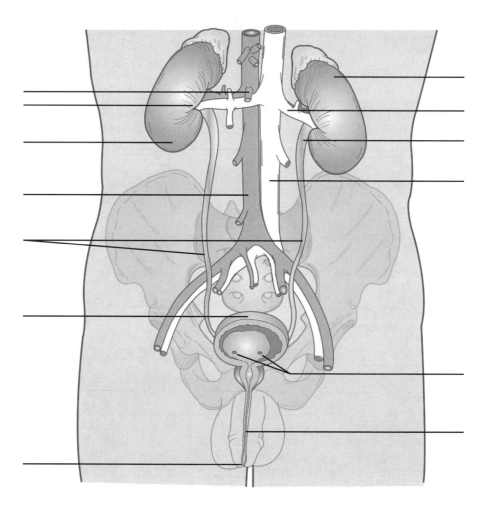

Labeling Exercise

Please fill in the correct labels for Figure 16-2.

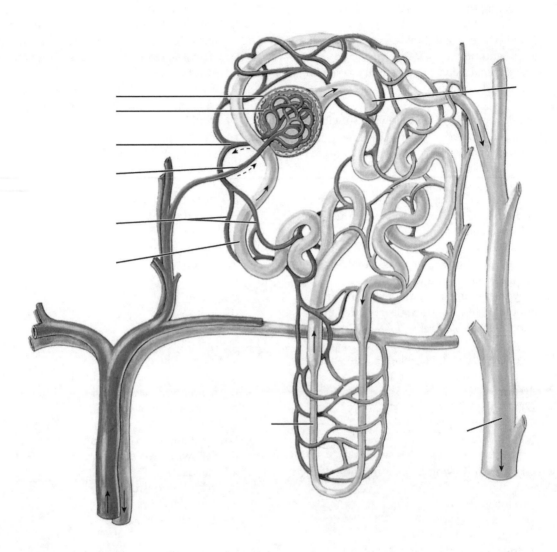

CHAPTER TEST

Select the correct response.

1. Which of the following is *not* a metabolic waste product?
    a. water
    b. glucose
    c. wastes that contain nitrogen
    d. carbon dioxide

2. Organs that function in waste disposal include the
    a. urinary system.
    b. skin.
    c. lungs.
    d. all of the above.

3. Organs of the urinary system include all of the following *except*
    a. kidneys.
    b. spleen.
    c. ureters.
    d. urethra.

4. The correct order of urine flow through the urinary system is
    a. kidney, ureter, bladder, and urethra.
    b. bladder, ureter, kidney, and urethra.
    c. kidney, urethra, bladder, and ureter.
    d. bladder, urethra, kidney, and ureter.

5. Urine flows through the following structures in which sequence?
   a. renal papilla, collecting duct, calyx, renal pelvis, and ureter
   b. collecting duct, renal papilla, calyx, renal pelvis, and ureter
   c. renal pelvis, renal papilla, calyx, collecting duct, and ureter
   d. calyx, renal pelvis, renal papilla, collecting duct, and ureter

6. Filtrate flows through the following structures in which sequence?
   a. loop of Henle, Bowman's capsule, proximal convoluted tubule, collecting duct, and distal convoluted tubule
   b. Bowman's capsule, proximal convoluted tubule, loop of Henle, collecting duct, distal convoluted tubule
   c. Bowman's capsule, proximal convoluted tubule, loop of Henle, distal convoluted tubule, collecting duct
   d. Bowman's capsule, proximal convoluted tubule, collecting duct, distal convoluted tubule, loop of Henle

7. The average adult urinary bladder can stretch so it can hold up to _____ of urine.
   a. 100 ml
   b. 800 ml
   c. 100 L
   d. 800 L

8. Which of the following is *not* a function of the kidney?
   a. produces renin
   b. produces aldosterone
   c. produces erythropoietin
   d. helps regulate the pH of the blood

9. Urine production involves all of the following *except*
   a. glomerular filtration.
   b. tubular reabsorption.
   c. renal acidosis.
   d. tubular secretion.

10. The first step in urine production is
    a. tubular reabsorption.
    b. glomerular filtration.
    c. tubular secretion.
    d. Bowman's capsule.

11. Which of the following is *not* a factor that contributes to the large amount of glomerular filtrate?
    a. The afferent arteriole is smaller in diameter than the efferent arteriole.
    b. The highly coiled glomerular capillaries provide a large surface area for filtration.
    c. The glomerular capillaries are greatly permeable.
    d. Blood flow through glomerular capillaries is at much higher pressure than in other capillaries.

12. _____ is a selective process.
    a. Tubular reabsorption
    b. Glomerular filtration
    c. Tubular secretion
    d. a and c only

13. Urine consists mainly of
    a. blood.
    b. sugar.
    c. water.
    d. salt.

14. Dehydration can result from
    a. profuse sweating.
    b. not drinking enough fluids.
    c. vomiting or diarrhea.
    d. all of the above.

15. Low sodium ion concentration can cause all of the following *except*
    a. headache.
    b. high blood pressure.
    c. low blood pressure.
    d. mental confusion.

16. Calcium ions are essential in which of the following?
    a. blood clotting
    b. regulation of pH
    c. muscle contraction
    d. both a and c

17. Acid ingested in foods but not neutralized by the ingestion of alkaline foods is neutralized by all of the following *except*
    a. muscular system.
    b. respiratory system.
    c. chemical buffers.
    d. kidneys.

Chapter

17

REPRODUCTION

■ ■ ■

Outline

Introduction
I. The male produces sperm.
    A. The testes produce sperm and hormones.
    B. The conducting tubes transport sperm.
    C. The accessory glands produce semen.
    D. The penis delivers sperm into the female reproductive tract.
    E. Hormones regulate male reproduction.
II. The female produces ova and incubates the embryo.
    A. The ovaries produce ova and hormones.
    B. The uterine tubes transport ova.
    C. The uterus incubates the embryo.
    D. The vagina functions in sexual intercourse, menstruation, and birth.
    E. The external genital structures are the vulva.
    F. The breasts contain the mammary glands.
    G. Hormones regulate female reproduction.

1. The preovulatory phase consists of the first two weeks of the menstrual cycle.
2. The corpus luteum develops during the postovulatory phase.
3. The menstrual cycle stops at menopause.
III. Fertilization is the fusion of sperm and ovum.
IV. The zygote gives rise to the new individual.
    A. The embryo develops in the wall of the uterus.
    B. Prenatal development requires about 266 days.
    C. The birth process includes labor and delivery.
    D. Multiple births may be fraternal or identical.
V. The human life cycle extends from fertilization to death.

Learning Objectives

After you have studied this chapter, you should be able to:

1. Describe the anatomy of the male reproductive system and describe the functions of each structure.
2. Trace the passage of sperm cells from the tubules in the testes through the conducting tubes and to their ejaculation from the body in semen.
3. Describe the actions of the male gonadotropic hormones and testosterone.
4. Describe the anatomy of the female reproductive system and describe the functions of each structure.
5. Trace the development of an ovum and its passage through the female reproductive system.

6. Describe the principal events of the menstrual cycle and summarize the interactions of hormones that regulate the cycle.
7. Describe the process of fertilization.
8. Summarize the course of development from fertilization to birth.
9. Describe the functions of the amnion and placenta.
10. Identify the three stages of the birth process.
11. List the stages of human development from fertilization to death.

STUDY QUESTIONS

Within each category, fill in the blanks with the correct response.

INTRODUCTION

Gametes   **Gonads**   **Lactation**   **Reproduction**

1. _____ involves several processes including preparation of the female body for

    pregnancy, sexual intercourse, fertilization, pregnancy, and lactation.

2. Eggs and sperm are specialized sex cells called _____.

3. The mother's production of milk for nourishing her infant is called _____.

4. The sex glands are referred to as _____.

I. THE MALE PRODUCES SPERM

Egg   **Penis**   **Scrotum**   **Sex**   **Sperm**   **Testes**

1. The male's function in reproduction is to produce _____ cells and deliver them

    into the female reproductive tract.

2. The sperm that combines with a(n) _____ contributes half the genes of the off-

    spring and determines the _____ of the baby.

3. Male reproductive structures include the _____ and _____,

    the conducting tubes that lead from the testes to the outside of the body, the accessory glands, and the

    _____.

A. The Testes Produce Sperm and Hormones

Chromosomes   **Inguinal**   **Inguinal hernia**   **Scrotum**
Seminiferous   **Sperm**   **Spermatogenesis**   **Testes**

1. In the adult male, millions of sperm cells are manufactured each day within the paired male gonads, the

    _____.

2. The _____ tubules are the sperm cell factories, and they also produce male hor-

    mones.

3. The process of sperm production is called _____.

4. During fertilization, one set of 23 _____ is contributed by the mother's ovum and

    the other set by the father's sperm.

5. The mature _____ is a tiny, elongated cell with a tail (flagellum) that is used for

    moving toward an egg.

6. The testes develop in the abdominal cavity of the male embryo. About 2 months before birth, they descend into the _____, a skin-covered bag suspended from the groin.

7. As the testes descend, they move through the _____ canals.

8. Straining the abdominal muscles by lifting a very heavy object may result in a tear in the inguinal wall, through which a loop of intestine can bulge into the scrotum. This is called a(n) _____.

B. The Conducting Tubes Transport Sperm

Ejaculatory   Epididymis   Sperm   Spermatic cord   Urethra   Urine   Vas deferens

1. From the tubules inside the testes, sperm pass into a large, coiled tube, the _____.

2. The epididymis empties into a straight tube, the _____, or sperm duct.

3. The vas deferens passes from the scrotum through the inguinal canal as part of the _____.

4. The vas deferens is joined by the duct from the seminal vesicles to become the _____ duct.

5. The ejaculatory duct passes through the prostate gland, and then opens into the _____.

6. The single urethra, which conducts both _____ and _____, passes through the penis to the outside of the body.

7. Place the correct number next to each choice to indicate the proper sequence.
    _____ Vas deferens
    _____ Urethra
    _____ Tubules in the testis
    _____ Epididymis
    _____ Ejaculatory duct

C. The Accessory Glands Produce Semen

Bulbourethral   Ejaculation   Prostate   Semen   Sperm cells   Sterile

1. _____ is a thick, whitish fluid consisting of sperm cells suspended in secretions of the accessory glands.

2. The single _____ gland surrounds the urethra as the urethra emerges from the urinary bladder.

3. The _____ (or Cowper's) glands are about the size and shape of two peas, one on each side of the urethra.

4. Semen is discharged from the penis during _____.

5. Semen consists of about 40 million _____ suspended in the secretions of the accessory glands.

6. Men with fewer than 20 million sperm/ml of semen may be _____.

D. The Penis Delivers Sperm Into the Female Reproductive Tract

Circumcision	Corpus	Ejaculation	Erect	Glans
Penis	Prepuce	Reflex	Shaft	Sinusoids

1. The _____ is the male copulatory organ.

2. The penis consists of a long _____ that enlarges to form an expanded tip, the

    _____.

3. Part of the loose-fitting skin of the penis folds down and covers the proximal portion of the glans, forming a cuff called the _____, or foreskin.

4. The foreskin is removed during _____.

5. Under the skin, the penis consists of three cylinders of spongy tissue called erectile tissue. Each cylinder, referred to as a _____, contains blood vessels called _____.

6. When the male is sexually stimulated, spongy tissue in the penis fills with blood and the penis becomes

    _____.

7. When the level of sexual excitement reaches a peak, _____ occurs.

8. Both erection and ejaculation are _____ actions.

E. Hormones Regulate Male Reproduction

Androgens	Development	Follicle-stimulating hormone (FSH)
Gonadotropic	Hypothalamus	Luteinizing hormone (LH)
Negative feedback	Primary	Puberty
Secondary	Testosterone	

1. Male hormones are referred to as _____.

2. Interstitial cells produce the principal male hormone _____.

3. Testosterone is responsible for the _____ of both primary and secondary sex characteristics in the male.

4. _____ sex characteristics include the growth and activity of the reproductive structures, including the penis and scrotum.

5. _____ sex characteristics include deepening of the voice; muscle development; and growth of pubic, facial, and underarm hair.

6. _____ is the period of sexual maturation that typically begins between age 10–12 years, and continues until age 16–18 years.

7. At puberty, the _____ begins to secrete gonadotropin-releasing hormones (GnRH) that stimulate the anterior lobe of the pituitary gland to secrete _____ hormones.

8. The gonadotropic hormone _____ stimulates sperm production.

9. The gonadotropic hormone _____ stimulates the testes to secrete testosterone.

10. Reproductive hormone concentrations are regulated by _____ mechanisms.

Labeling Exercise

Please fill in the correct labels for Figure 17-1.

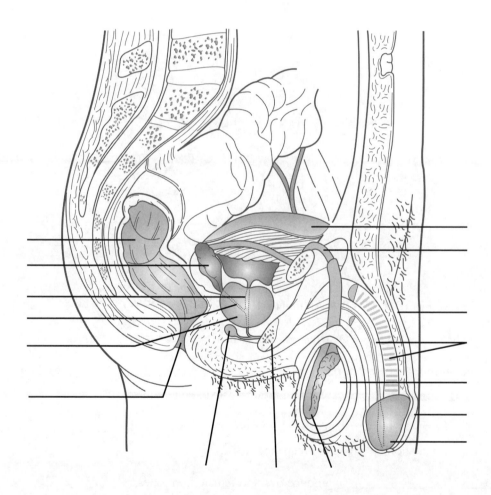

Labeling Exercise

Please fill in the correct labels for Figure 17-2.

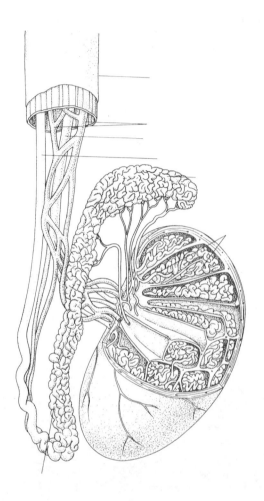

II. THE FEMALE PRODUCES OVA AND INCUBATES THE EMBRYO

Menstrual cycle   **Ova**   **Ovaries**   **Sperm**   **Uterus**   **Vagina**

1. The female reproductive system produces _____, and receives the penis and the _____ released from it during sexual intercourse.

2. Much of the activity of the female reproductive system centers about the _____, the monthly preparation for possible pregnancy.

3. The _____ produce ova and female hormones.

4. The _____ is the incubator for the developing child.

5. The _____ receives the penis during intercourse and serves as a birth canal.

A. The Ovaries Produce Ova and Hormones

Corpus luteum	Estrogen	Female hormones	Follicle	Graafian	Oogenesis
Ova	Ovarian	Ovaries	Ovulation	Progesterone	Puberty

1. The paired _____ are the female gonads.

2. The ovaries produce _____ and the female sex hormones,

   _____ and _____.

3. The _____ ligament anchors the medial end of the ovary to the uterus.

4. The process of ovum development is called _____.

5. The ovum and its surrounding sac make up a(n) _____.

6. With the onset of _____, a few follicles develop each month.

7. Cells of the follicle secrete _____, called estrogens.

8. Mature follicles are called _____ follicles.

9. During _____, the ovum is ejected through the wall of the ovary and into the

   pelvic cavity.

10. The part of the follicle that remains behind in the ovary develops into an important temporary endocrine

   structure, the _____.

B. The Uterine Tubes Transport Ova

Fallopian	Fertilization	Fimbriae	Oviduct
Ovum	Pelvic	Uterus	Zygote

1. Each uterine tube, also called the _____ or _____ tube, is

   about 12 cm long.

2. The free end of the fallopian tube is shaped like a funnel and has long, fingerlike projections called

   _____.

3. During ovulation, the mature ovum is released into the _____ cavity.

4. Action of the cilia in the lining of the uterine tube helps move the ovum toward the

   _____.

5. Normally, _____ takes place in the upper third of the uterine tube.

6. The fertilized egg, or _____, begins its development as it is moved along toward

   the uterus.

7. If fertilization does not occur, the _____ degenerates in the uterine tube.

C. The Uterus Incubates the Embryo

Cervix   **Corpus**   **Embryo**   **Endometrium**
Fundus   **Menstruation**   **Papanicolaou (Pap)**   **Uterus**

1. Each month during a woman's reproductive life, the _____, or womb, prepares for possible pregnancy.

2. When pregnancy occurs, the uterus serves as the incubator for the developing _____.

3. If pregnancy does not occur, the inner lining of the uterus sloughs off each month and is discarded. This process is called _____.

4. The main portion of the uterus is its _____, or body.

5. The rounded part of the uterus above the level of the entrance of the uterine tubes is the _____.

6. The lower, narrow portion of the uterus is the _____, which projects into the vagina.

7. The uterus is lined by a mucous membrane, the _____.

8. The routine _____ test can usually detect cervical cancer.

D. The Vagina Functions in Sexual Intercourse, Menstruation, and Birth

Cervix   **Collapsed**   **Endometrium**   **Enlarging**   **Fornices**   **Rugae**   **Vagina**

1. The _____ functions as the sexual organ that receives the penis during sexual intercourse.

2. The vagina serves as an exit through which the discarded _____ is discharged during menstruation.

3. The vagina surrounds the end of the _____.

4. The recesses formed between the vaginal wall and the cervix are called _____.

5. Normally, the vagina is _____ so that its walls touch each other. Two ridges run along the anterior and posterior walls and there are numerous _____, or folds.

6. During sexual intercourse, or during childbirth, the rugae straighten out, greatly _____ the vagina.

E.   The External Genital Structures Are the Vulva

Bartholin's	Clinical perineum	Clitoris	Hymen	Labia majora	Labia minora
Mons pubis	Puberty	Urethra	Vagina	Vestibule	Vulva

1. The term _____ refers to the external female genital structures.

2. The _____ is a mound of fatty tissue that covers the pubic symphysis.

3. At _____, the mons pubis becomes covered by coarse pubic hair.

4. The paired _____ are folds of skin that pass form the mons pubis to the region behind the vaginal opening.

5. Two thin folds of skin, the _____, are located just within the labia majora.

6. The _____ is a small structure that corresponds to the male glans and is a main focus of sexual sensation in the female.

7. The space enclosed by the labia minora is the _____.

8. Two openings can be seen in the vestibule—the opening of the _____ anteriorly, and the opening of the _____ posteriorly.

9. A thin ring of mucous membrane, the _____, surrounds the entrance to the vagina.

10. Two small _____ glands open on each side of the vaginal opening.

11. The region between the vagina and anus is referred to as the _____.

F.   The Breasts Contain the Mammary Glands

Breasts	Colostrum	Lactation	Ligaments of Cooper	Lymphatic
Mammography	Milk	Nipple	Oxytocin	Prolactin

1. The breasts function in _____—production and release of milk for nourishment of the baby.

2. The _____ overlie the pectoral muscles and are attached to them by connective tissue.

3. Fibrous bands of tissue called _____ firmly connect the breasts to the skin.

4. The mammary glands, located within the breasts, produce _____.

5. The _____ consists of smooth muscle that can contract to make it erect in response to sexual stimuli.

6. For the first few days after childbirth, the mammary glands produce a fluid called _____, which contains protein and lactose but little fat.

7. After birth, _____, secreted by the anterior pituitary, stimulates milk production.

8. _____ stimulates ejection of milk from the glands into the ducts.

9. Breast cancer often spreads to the _____ system.

10. _____, a soft-tissue radiologic study of the breast, is helpful in detecting very small lesions that might not be identified by routine examination.

G. Hormones Regulate Female Reproduction

Estrogens   Menarche   Menstrual cycle   Ovulation   Progesterone   Puberty

1. The ovaries secrete estrogens and _____.

2. Like testosterone in the male, _____ are responsible for the growth of sex organs at puberty and for the development of secondary sex characteristics.

3. In girls, _____ typically begins between 10 and 12 years of age and continues until 14 to 16 years of age.

4. _____ is the first menstrual period, and usually occurs between 12 and 14 years of age.

5. During the _____, estrogens stimulate the growth of follicles and stimulate thickening of the endometrium.

6. _____ typically occurs about 14 days before the next menstrual cycle begins.

1. The Preovulatory Phase Consists of the First Two Weeks of the Menstrual Cycle

Estrogen   FSH   LH   Menstruation   Preovulatory   Positive feedback

1. Menstruation occurs during the first 5 or so days of the _____ phase.

2. During _____, the thickened endometrium of the uterus sloughs off.

3. During the early phase of the menstrual cycle, _____ is the principal hormone released by the pituitary gland.

4. During the late preovulatory phase, _____ concentration peaks.

5. The increase in estrogen concentration signals the anterior pituitary to secrete LH. This is a _____ mechanism.

6. The surge of _____ from the anterior pituitary stimulates final maturation of the follicle and ovulation.

2.   *The Corpus Luteum Develops During the Postovulatory Phase*

Corpus luteum   **Endometrium**   **Menstruation**   **Postovulatory**   **Pregnancy**

1.   The _____ phase begins after ovulation.

2.   After ovulation, LH stimulates development of the _____.

3.   Progesterone and estrogen stimulate continued thickening of the _____ in preparation for possible pregnancy.

4.   If _____ does not occur, the corpus luteum begins to degenerate after about eight days.

5.   _____ begins as cells begin to die and damaged arteries rupture and bleed.

3.   *The Menstrual Cycle Stops at Menopause*

Estrogen   **Fertile**   **Hot flashes**   **Menopause**   **Menstrual cycle**   **Progesterone**

1.   At about age 50 years, a woman enters _____—the time when the ovaries become less responsive to gonadotropic hormones and ova are no longer produced.

2.   During menopause, _____ and _____ secretion decreases.

3.   When menopause occurs, the _____ becomes irregular and eventually halts, and the woman is no longer _____.

4.   The decrease in hormones during menopause can cause a variety of symptoms, including a sensation of heat, referred to as _____.

Labeling Exercise

Please fill in the correct labels for Figure 17-3.

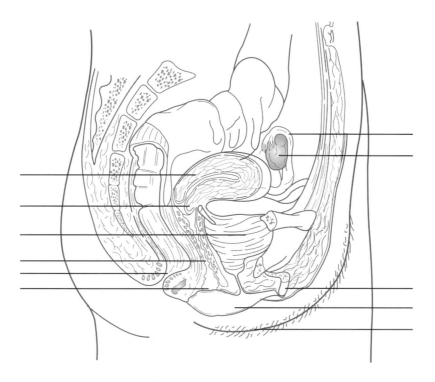

Labeling Exercise

Please fill in the correct labels for Figure 17-4.

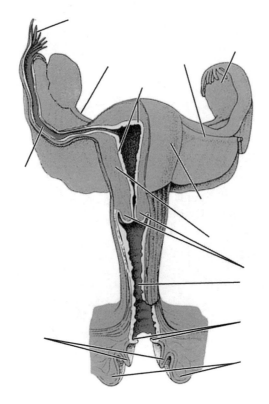

III.   FERTILIZATION IS THE FUSION OF SPERM AND OVUM

Ejaculation   **Fertilization**   **Follicle**   **Ovulation**   **Ovum**   **Uterus**   **Zygote**

1.   When sperm are released in the vagina, some find their way into the _____ and uterine tubes.

2.   _____ is the fusion of the sperm and the egg.

3.   Large numbers of sperm are necessary to penetrate the _____ cells surrounding the ovum (egg).

4.   As soon as one sperm penetrates the _____, no other sperm are able to get into the ovum.

5.   Sperm and ovum fuse to form a fertilized egg, or _____.

6.   After _____, sperm remain viable for only about 48 to 72 hours.

7.   The ovum remains fertile for approximately 12 to 24 hours after _____.

IV.   THE ZYGOTE GIVES RISE TO THE NEW INDIVIDUAL

Cilia   **DNA**   **Embryo**   **Uterine tube**   **Uterus**

1.   The _____ of the zygote contains all of the genetic information needed to produce a complete individual.

2.   The zygote divides to form a(n) _____ composed of two cells.

3.   As the first cell divisions take place, the embryo is slowly moved along the _____ toward the uterus by the action of _____.

4.   By the time the embryo reaches the _____ on the fifth day of development, it is a tiny cluster of about 32 cells.

A.   The Embryo Develops in the Wall of the Uterus

Amnion   **Blood**   **Fetal**   **Human chorionic gonadotropin (hCG)**
Placenta   **Progesterone**   **Umbilical cord**   **Uterus**

1.   On about the seventh day of the development, the embryo begins to implant itself in the wall of the _____.

2.   Several _____ membranes develop around the embryo. They help protect, nourish, and support the developing embryo.

3.   The _____ is a membrane that forms a fluid-filled sac around the embryo.

4.   The _____ is the organ of exchange between the mother and the embryo.

5. Wastes from the embryo move through the placenta and into the mother's _____.

6. During pregnancy, the corpus luteum and the placenta secrete _____.

7. The placenta produces a hormone called _____, which signals the corpus luteum to increase in size and to release large amounts of estrogens and progesterone.

8. The stalk of tissue that connects the embryo with the placenta is the _____.

B. Prenatal Development Requires About 266 Days

Brain	**Cerebrum**	**Fetal movements**	**Fetus**	**Lanugo**
Limb buds	**Menstrual period**	**Premature**	**Spinal cord**	

1. Obstetricians typically count from the onset of the mother's last _____, and consider an average pregnancy 280 days (40 weeks).

2. The _____ and _____ are among the first organs to develop.

3. Small mounds of tissue called _____ can be seen by the end of the first month, and slowly lengthen to form the limbs.

4. After the second month, the embryo is referred to as a(n) _____.

5. The mother usually becomes aware of _____ by about 5 months of development.

6. During the seventh month, the _____ grows rapidly and develops convolutions (folds).

7. Most of the body of the fetus is covered by downy hair called _____.

8. If a baby is born before 37 weeks, it is considered _____.

C. The Birth Process Includes Labor and Delivery

Afterbirth	**Amnion**	**Amniotic**	**Birth canal**	**Delivery**
Dilated	**Effaced**	**Fetus**	**First stage**	**Labor**
Parturition	**Placenta**	**Second stage**	**Third stage**	

1. Several days before birth, the _____ usually assumes an upside-down position, which prepares it to enter the _____ head first.

2. Childbirth, or _____, includes labor and delivery.

3. _____ begins with a long series of involuntary contractions of the uterus.

4. During the _____ of labor, regular uterine contractions become more intense, rhythmic, and frequent.

5. During the first stage of labor, the cervix becomes _____ to about 10 cm, and becomes _____, or continuous with the uterine wall.

6. Rupture of the _____, with the release of the _____ fluid through the vagina may occur during the first stage of labor.

7. The _____ of labor begins when the cervix is fully dilated and ends with the _____ of the baby.

8. When the neonate emerges, it is still connected to the _____ by the umbilical cord.

9. During the _____ of labor, the placenta separates from the uterus and is expelled.

10. After delivery, the placenta is referred to as the _____; it is inspected for abnormalities and then discarded.

D.   Multiple Births May Be Fraternal or Identical

Conjoined	Fertility	Fraternal	Genes	Identical

1. With the use of _____ drugs, multiple births have become much more common.

2. _____ twins develop when a woman ovulates two eggs and each is fertilized by a different sperm.

3. _____ twins develop when the tiny mass of cells that makes up the early embryo divides to form two independent groups of cells, and each develops into a baby.

4. Identical twins, developed from a single fertilized egg, thus have identical _____, and are indeed identical.

5. Rarely, two masses of embryonic cells do not separate completely and give rise to _____ twins.

V.   THE HUMAN LIFE CYCLE EXTENDS FROM FERTILIZATION TO DEATH

Adolescence	Childhood	Development	Infancy
Middle age	Neonatal	Old age	Young adulthood

1. _____ begins at fertilization and continues through the stages of the human life cycle until death.

2. The _____ period extends from birth to the end of the first month of postnatal life.

3. _____ follows the neonatal period and lasts until age 2 years.

4. _____, also a period of rapid growth and development, continues from infancy until adolescence.

5. _____ is the time of development between puberty and adulthood.

6. _____ extends from adolescence until about age 40.

7. _____ is usually considered to be the period between ages 40 and 65.

8. _____ begins after age 65.

CHAPTER TEST

Select the correct response.

1. Reproduction involves several processes, including
   a. formation of gametes.
   b. preparation of the female body for pregnancy.
   c. sexual intercourse.
   d. all of the above.

2. Male reproductive structures include all of the following *except*
   a. testes.
   b. ureters.
   c. urethra.
   d. vas deferens.

3. The sequence of the path that sperm pass through is
   a. tubules in the testis, epididymis, vas deferens, urethra, and ejaculatory duct.
   b. tubules in the testis, vas deferens, epididymis, ejaculatory duct, and urethra.
   c. tubules in the testis, epididymis, vas deferens, ejaculatory duct, and urethra.
   d. epididymis, vas deferens, urethra, ejaculatory duct and tubules in the testes.

4. The _____ is the male copulatory organ.
   a. penis
   b. testis
   c. scrotum
   d. ureter

5. The _____ is removed during circumcision.
   a. shaft
   b. prepuce
   c. glans
   d. vas deferens

6. Primary sex characteristics in the male include
   a. growth of the penis and scrotum.
   b. growth and activity of internal reproductive structures.
   c. muscle development.
   d. both a and b.

7. Secondary sex characteristics in the male include all of the following *except*
   a. muscle development.
   b. growth of the penis and scrotum.
   c. growth of facial, pubic, and underarm hair.
   d. deepening of the voice.

8. A high concentration of _____ in the testes is required for spermatogenesis.
   a. testosterone
   b. estrogen
   c. progesterone
   d. cortisol

9. The organs of the female reproductive system include all of the following *except*
   a. ovaries.
   b. uterine tubes.
   c. urethra.
   d. vagina.

10. The _____ are the female gonads.
    a. uterine tubes
    b. ovaries
    c. breasts
    d. kidneys

11. In a normal pregnancy, the fetus develops in the
    a. ovaries.
    b. scrotum.
    c. uterus.
    d. uterine tubes.

12. The term *vulva* refers to the external female genital structures, which include the
    a. labia.
    b. vestibule.
    c. mons pubis.
    d. all of the above.

13. The mammary glands are located within the
    a. breasts.
    b. vagina.
    c. cervix.
    d. uterus.

14. Female secondary sex characteristics include all of the following *except*
    a. breast development.
    b. broadening of the pelvis.
    c. deepening of the voice.
    d. distribution of fat and muscle that shape the female body.

15. Although there is variation, a "typical" menstrual cycle is _____ days long.
    a. 3
    b. 7
    c. 28
    d. 45

16. During the menstrual cycle, ovulation occurs approximately _____ days before the next cycle begins.
    a. 7
    b. 14
    c. 28
    d. 36

17. By the fourth week of development, many organs in the fetus have begun to develop, including the _____.
    a. brain
    b. hands
    c. feet
    d. sex organs

18. The first stage of labor typically lasts
    a. 4–6 hours.
    b. 8–24 hours.
    c. 1–2 days.
    d. More than 2 days, but less than a week.

19. The umbilical cord connects the neonate to the
    a. mother's umbilicus.
    b. mother's vagina.
    c. placenta.
    d. hospital monitoring equipment.

20. When the cells that make up the early embryo divide completely to form two independent groups of cells, the resulting twins are
    a. fraternal.
    b. identical.
    c. conjoined.
    d. dizygotic.

CROSSWORD PUZZLE FOR CHAPTERS 16 AND 17

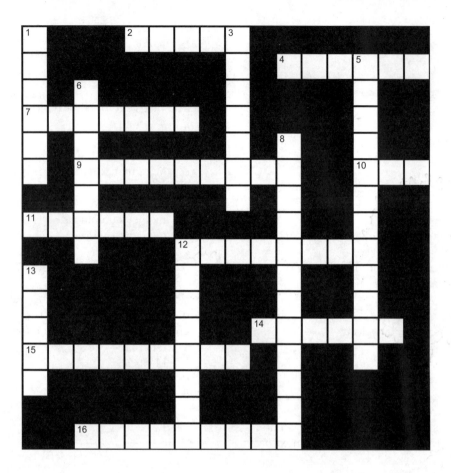

Across

2. Delivers sperm into the vagina
4. Organs that produce sperm
7. Female gonads
9. Stage at which menstrual cycle stops
10. Eggs
11. Portion of the uterus that projects into the vagina
12. Gland that surrounds the male urethra
14. Female sexual organ that receives the penis
15. Female sex hormones
16. Release of ovum from the ovary

Down

1. Fertilized egg
3. Sac that contains the testes
5. Male sex hormone
6. Glands located in the breasts
8. Monthly sloughing of the uterine lining
12. Organ through which the fetus receives nutrients
13. Membrane that partly blocks the entrance to the vagina

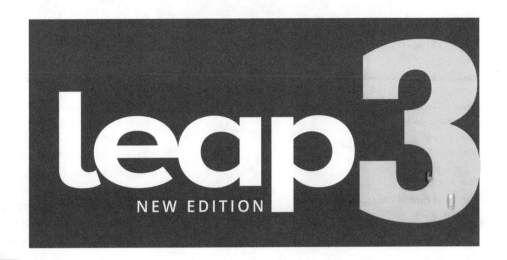

LEAP **3**

NEW EDITION

LISTENING
AND **SPEAKING**

DR. KEN BEATTY

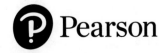

Pearson

Product Owner
Stephan Leduc

Managing Editor
Sharnee Chait

Project Editor
Emily Harrison

Copy Editor
Donna Jensen

Proofreader
Mairi MacKinnon

Rights and Permissions Coordinator
Aude Maggiori

Text Rights and Permissions
Rachel Irwin

Art Director
Hélène Cousineau

Graphic Design Manager
Estelle Cuillerier

Book and Cover Design
Frédérique Bouvier

Book Layout
Marquis Interscript

Cover Photos
Shutterstock © leungchopan
Shutterstock © Rawpixel.com

Dedication

To my MA TESOL and EdD TESOL students; endless thanks
for journeys learning together.

The publisher wishes to thank the following people for their helpful
comments and suggestions:
Janet Baron, Okanagan College
Alex Josef Kasula, Universidad de los Andes
Izabella Kojic-Sabo, University of Windsor
Caitlin May, Universidad de los Andes
Laura Parker, University of Oklahoma
Hélène Prévost, Cégep de l'Outaouais
Jamie Tanzman, Texas A&M International University

INTRODUCTION

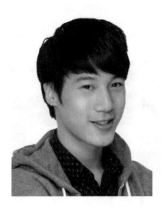

Welcome to *LEAP 3: Listening and Speaking*. This new edition builds on the work of the previous edition and incorporates feedback from teachers in Canada, the USA, and around the world. Changes include new focuses on critical thinking and accuracy, as well as new listenings and videos in each chapter. Updated science, technology, engineering, and mathematics (STEM) topics include economics, secret codes, and statistics. A Critical Connections task at the end of each chapter allows students to build on what they have learned and apply it to new ideas.

Traditional English programs don't always develop students' thinking and language skills that are so necessary for college and university. *LEAP 3*'s cross-curricular approach focuses on developing critical thinking skills, while giving students opportunities to explore content from a range of subject areas.

Students use *LEAP 3: Listening and Speaking* to study and engage in discussions of open-ended questions. Students work on their own, in pairs, or in small groups, exploring a variety of perspectives and listening genres in each chapter. This work leads students toward structured speaking assignments such as panel discussions, presentations, and informal debates. Along the way, students build their comprehension of concepts and vocabulary including key words from the Academic Word List.

In an ever-changing world, students need critical thinking and interaction skills. They need to know how to engage in active listening, understand the subtexts of the messages they hear, and fashion their own spoken responses using informative, compelling, and persuasive language in formal and informal settings. *LEAP 3: Listening and Speaking* helps students meet these and other challenges.

ACKNOWLEDGEMENTS

Any book of this scope requires the help of many heroes—thanks to all the teachers in Canada and around the world who give their time and ideas to help shape the materials that they and others will use. Thanks also to Pearson ELT Product Owner Stephan Leduc and my creative and vigilant editor, Sharnee Chait, and others who promote the *LEAP* series. Finally, thanks to Julia Williams, who wrote the companion volume to this book, *LEAP 3: Reading and Writing*.

Dr. Ken Beatty, Bowen Island, Canada

HIGHLIGHTS

Gearing Up uses diagrams to spark critical thinking, reflection, and discussion about the chapter topic.

The **overview** outlines the chapter's objectives and features.

Vocabulary Build strengthens comprehension of key vocabulary words and reinforces them through tasks.

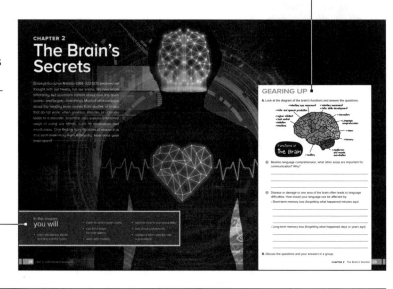

Focus on Critical Thinking helps you learn strategies to think critically about what you hear and how to apply these strategies to listening and speaking tasks.

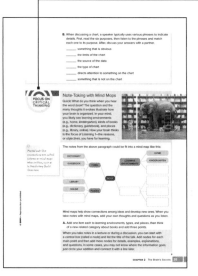

The **listenings**, including one video per chapter, come from various sources: lectures, debates, interviews, and podcasts.

Focus on Listening develops specific strategies you need to fully understand the content and structure of different listening genres.

Before You Listen activities elicit your prior knowledge of a subject and stimulate interest.

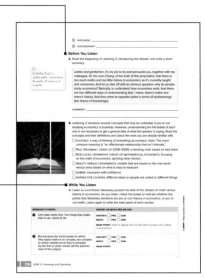

After You Listen activities give you an opportunity to show your comprehension and reflect on personal or larger issues related to what you have heard.

While You Listen activities engage you in a variety of active listening strategies, including taking notes.

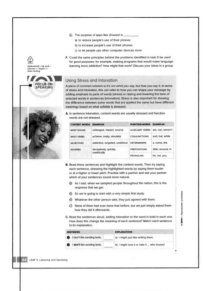

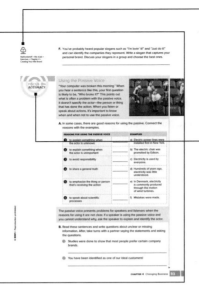

My eLab provides practice and additional content.

Focus on Accuracy reviews important grammar features that you can apply when listening to and speaking academic English.

Academic Survival Skill helps you develop essential skills for academic coursework.

Focus on Speaking develops the skills you need to effectively discuss issues and express opinions.

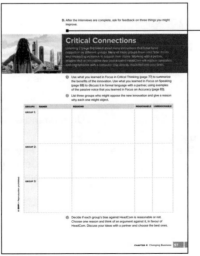

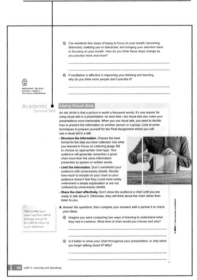

The **Warm-Up Assignment** prepares you for the Final Assignment.

The **Final Assignment** synthesizes the chapter content and theme into an in-depth speaking task. Each chapter focuses on a different type of assignment.

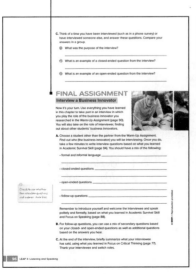

Critical Connections allows you to reinvest what you learned in the chapter while applying critical thinking.

SCOPE AND SEQUENCE

CHAPTER	LISTENING	CRITICAL THINKING	SPEAKING
CHAPTER 1 **ENGINEERING LIFE** SUBJECT AREAS: education, engineering, robotics	• Listen to infer attitudes, emotions, and intentions - Pay attention to word choice and sentence structure	• Think about hypothetical situations - Explore positive and negative consequences	• Give presentations - Structure your presentation with a template and key phrases
CHAPTER 2 **THE BRAIN'S SECRETS** SUBJECT AREAS: education, neuroscience, psychology	• Listen to understand charts - Recognize the differences among charts	• Use mind maps for note-taking - Show connections among ideas and develop new ones	• Talk about procedures - Use linking words
CHAPTER 3 **SELLING DREAMS** SUBJECT AREAS: computer science, marketing, political science	• Listen for how speakers organize ideas - Recognize organization types using signal words	• Use strategies to propose solutions - Identify the consequences of a solution	• Use stress and intonation to enhance meaning - Learn the difference between content and function words
CHAPTER 4 **CHANGING BUSINESS** SUBJECT AREAS: history, marketing, psychology	• Listen to identify bias - Identify biased strategies and the speaker's purpose	• Summarize key information - Identify main ideas, answer the 5-W questions, and keep opinions separate	• Use formal and informal language - Recognize the differences between formal and informal language
CHAPTER 5 **APPLYING SCIENCE** SUBJECT AREAS: biology, ecology, history	• Listen for cause and effect - Identify words and phrases showing cause and effect	• Evaluate a presentation - Learn key evaluation factors	• Develop an argument - Learn techniques to follow
CHAPTER 6 **FROM NUMBERS TO IDEAS** SUBJECT AREAS: mathematics, statistics, economics	• Listen to recognize certainty - Identify key words and expressions	• Identify logical fallacies - Recognize argument techniques	• Discuss pros and cons - Use pro and con points to build arguments
CHAPTER 7 **THINKING MACHINES** SUBJECT AREAS: computer science, innovation, psychology	• Listen to recognize paraphrases - Identify signal words	• Play the devil's advocate - Challenge others' thinking using strategies	• Apply turn-taking to conversations - Recognize signalling strategies
CHAPTER 8 **OUR HUNGRY PLANET** SUBJECT AREAS: agriculture, political science	• Listen for clarification - Recognize clarification strategies	• Understand complex ideas - Use the Feynman Technique to break down complex ideas	• Discuss problems and solutions - Follow logical steps to provide solutions

ACCURACY	ACADEMIC SURVIVAL SKILL	ASSIGNMENTS	My eLab

• Talk about *if*
  - Use the first, second, and third conditional forms
	• Learn note-taking skills
	  - Use the Cornell Note-taking System
		• Develop a hypothetical situation
		• Present, discuss, and take notes on a hypothetical situation	

• Work with modals
  - Understand which modals are more polite
	• Use visual aids
	  - Understand how to structure and limit the information
		• Explain a chart
		• Present and discuss a procedure	

• Talk about the past
  - Use the simple past, past progressive, and present perfect tenses
	• Answer questions in a presentation
	  - Recognize key question types and when and how to answer them
		• Discuss ideas about how to create a marketing campaign
		• Present a marketing campaign to a group
			• Online practice for each chapter:
			  - More comprehension exercises for the listenings
			  - Vocabulary review
			  - Accuracy practice
			  - Speaking focus review
			  - Chapter test

• Use the passive voice
  - Understand the reasons for using the passive voice
	• Develop interview skills
	  - Learn tips to conduct an effective interview
		• Profile a business innovator
		• Conduct an interview	

• Use linking words to talk about cause and effect	• Cite sources in a discussion
	  - Learn about spoken citations
		• Explore a scientific issue
		• Discuss cause and effect in a group
			• Additional online listening texts:
			  - Extra listening with comprehension and critical thinking questions
			• Study resources in Documents including:
			  - All audio and video clips from the coursebook
			  - Irregular Verbs List

• Create cohesion for communicating
  - Use pronouns and conjunctions to connect clauses
	• Learn informal debating strategies
	  - Develop ideas using a debate structure
		• Prepare for a debate
		• Participate in an informal debate	

• Make and understand comparisons
  - Use words to connect clauses
	• Brainstorm in a group
	  - Learn brainstorming techniques
		• Brainstorm intelligences
		• Discuss brainstormed ideas in a group	

• Review gerunds and infinitives	• Take part in discussions - Learn about the role of a moderator	• Develop a topic for discussion • Contribute to a panel discussion	

TABLE OF CONTENTS

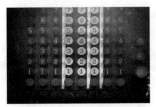

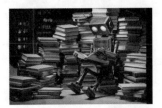
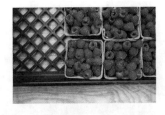

CHAPTER 1
Engineering Life

If you were asked to gather a team to go to Mars, what professionals would you call on to help get you there? Your answer would likely include an engineer. Many people think of engineers as people who work with big machines and, until recently, the profession was narrowly divided into *chemical, civil, electrical* and *mechanical* engineers. But today, there are about 200 engineering degrees as society demands educated workers with specialized skills in many fields. All engineers typically have an interest in analyzing processes and solving problems. **How are process analysis and problem solving part of your education and career interests?**

In this chapter,
you will

- learn vocabulary related to analysis and problem solving;

- listen to infer attitudes, emotions, and intentions;

- think about hypothetical situations;

- talk about possibilities with conditional tenses;

- learn about note-taking;

- learn how to give presentations;

- present and discuss a hypothetical situation about the automation of a career.

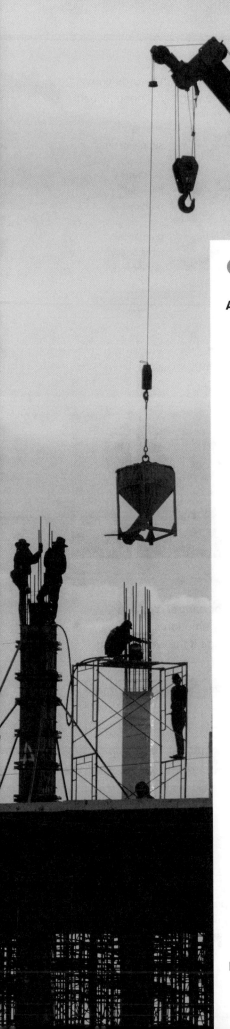

GEARING UP

A. Designing products, ideas, and solutions is a common process. Look at the flow chart and answer the questions.

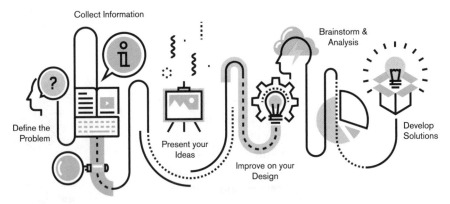

Collect Information

Brainstorm & Analysis

Define the Problem

Present your Ideas

Improve on your Design

Develop Solutions

1. Why is it important to define the problem at the beginning of a process?

_____

_____

2. What are three ways you might collect information about a large real-world problem?

_____

_____

3. After presenting your ideas, why is a common next step "improve on your design"?

_____

_____

4. Is brainstorming and analysis best left to the end of the process, or should it occur at different times? Why?

_____

_____

_____

B. Work in groups. Compare your answers with those of other students.

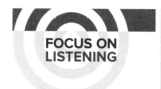
Below are the key words you will practise in this chapter. Check the words you understand, then underline the words you use. Highlight the words you need to learn.

adoption	foundation*	parameters*
automation*	implications*	persistence*
awareness*	inspiration	perspective*
communities*	internship	policy*
consulting*	investors*	sectors*
cycle*	mentality*	transition*
feasibility	paradigm*	

nouns → analysis and problem solving

verbs → affected*, supplemented*

adjectives → aesthetic, financial*, predictable*

adverbs → dramatically*, functionally*, significantly*

* Appears on the Academic Word List.

FOCUS ON LISTENING

Inferring Attitudes, Emotions, and Intentions

"What did he mean when he said *no*?" It seems like the answer to such a question should be obvious, but people do not always say exactly what they mean. It is necessary to listen beyond the words to infer—or understand the true meaning—based on clues about their attitudes, emotions, and intentions. Understanding each clue means paying attention to word choice and sentence structure.

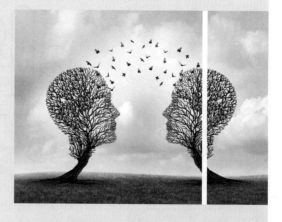

A. A speaker's attitudes are seen as *positive*, *negative*, or *neutral*. You can identify attitudes from the choice of words, particularly emotional verbs, adjectives, and adverbs. Read the sentences and decide if the word in bold in each one is positive, negative, or neutral.

ADJECTIVES AND ADVERBS	POSITIVE	NEGATIVE	NEUTRAL
❶ The new electric motorcycle is **amazingly** fast.	✓		
❷ He presented a long argument why we all **supposedly** need new headphones.			
❸ He puts a lot of **hard** work into developing robotic friends for autistic children.			
❹ She **explained** that buildings are similar to human bodies.			
❺ It's **questionable** whether she'll discover anything in the Antarctic.			
❻ The software is always based on the **current** needs of customers.			

One way speakers convey their intentions while they speak is by introducing new topics with rhetorical questions. Rhetorical questions are questions for which the answer is obvious; they help develop the speaker's argument.

B. Read the following rhetorical questions. Explain what the speaker's intention is in using each question. For example, is the speaker sharing an attitude or trying to make you think something in particular?

1 No one really wants to work on a construction site for an hourly rate, do they?

SPEAKER'S INTENTION: *to make you feel that working for an hourly rate is not*

a good idea

2 You don't believe in ghosts or that people have equal opportunities, do you?

SPEAKER'S INTENTION: _____

3 Who doesn't think that taller buildings are the way of the future?

SPEAKER'S INTENTION: _____

4 Would any of us be successful if we hadn't learned how to study properly?

SPEAKER'S INTENTION: _____

5 Can you be a famous architect without studying engineering? Of course not!

SPEAKER'S INTENTION: _____

_____

C. With a partner, look at task B's questions and your ideas about the speakers' intentions. Think of opposing arguments for each one.

1 _____

_____

2 _____

_____

3 _____

_____

4 _____

_____

5 _____

_____

D. A speaker's attitudes, emotions, and intentions are often expressed in several ways. Read the questions below. Listen to the paragraph two or three times to answer the questions.

1 What is the speaker's attitude toward students taking a gap year?

_____

2 What is an example of a rhetorical question he uses to make his point?

_____

_____

③ What is an emotional expression the speaker uses to indicate his personal preference?

_____

_____

④ What are three words or expressions the speaker uses to show his attitude?

_____

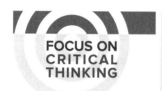

Thinking about Hypothetical Situations

Are you a dreamer? Dreamers are people who think hypothetically, imagining what might happen in the future and what the consequences would be. Listening 1 is about a hypothetical situation, imagining a world without bridges. Hypothetical situations help us to explore ideas through *if* questions. How would the world be different if there were no bridges? What would be the consequences? Exploring hypothetical scenarios leads to insights about underlying ideas and principles.

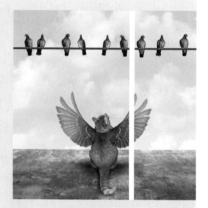

A. You can recognize a hypothetical situation when someone uses the word *hypothetical* or *imagine*. Other common expressions are *it's time*, *perhaps*, *wishes*, and *would rather*. Match the following hypothetical situations to their possible consequences.

HYPOTHETICAL SITUATIONS		CONSEQUENCES
❶ Perhaps it's time to consider offering free university education to medical students.	*d*	a) There would be more social support in communities.
❷ Imagine if every student had to take a year out to volunteer.	_____	b) They would bring real-world expertise to the classroom.
❸ I wish that everyone would wear school uniforms, even at university.	_____	c) Classes would be less crowded.
❹ Hypothetically, what if all teachers also had to work in their field?	_____	d) The number of doctors would increase.
❺ I'd rather see universities offer courses in the evening and seven days a week.	_____	e) Less paper would be used.
❻ Could you see a way that we might replace all textbooks with computer tablets?	_____	f) Students would save money on clothing.

© ERPI • Reproduction prohibited

B. Consider the following hypothetical situations and imagine what the positive and negative consequences might be. These consequences should be based on realistic ideas, even if the hypothetical situation is not realistic. Write brief points, then discuss your answers in a group to choose the best ones.

1 Everyone could afford a personal robot to do jobs around the home.

POSITIVE CONSEQUENCE: _____

_____

NEGATIVE CONSEQUENCE: _____

_____

2 The cost of fossil fuels suddenly rises, making gasoline (for cars) too expensive for most people.

POSITIVE CONSEQUENCE: _____

_____

NEGATIVE CONSEQUENCE: _____

_____

3 Laws were passed making four years of university a requirement for all young adults.

POSITIVE CONSEQUENCE: _____

_____

NEGATIVE CONSEQUENCE: _____

_____

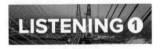 **LISTENING ❶**   **Choosing the Right Path**

Listening 1 sets out a hypothetical situation of a world without bridges. The point is not to stop building bridges, but rather to reflect on a hypothetical situation and ways you should prepare yourself to think about the future.

VOCABULARY BUILD

In the following exercises, explore key words from Listening 1. Look up any words you don't know.

A. Collocations are words that are commonly found in combination, such as *salt and pepper*. Complete the sentences by using the words in the box to fill in the blanks. Then highlight the other term of the collocation for each of the key words.

awareness	financial	foundation	~~paradigm~~	perspective	significantly

1 A changing _____*paradigm*_____ in work is the idea of the home office.

2 The number of jobs in computing is _____ higher.

3 We're facing a _____ crisis because of the loss of jobs.

④ Looking for jobs after university gives you a new _____.

⑤ We are hoping to raise _____ of the key issues.

⑥ We need a strong _____ to make a company work.

B. Use the words in the box to complete the paragraph. Then highlight the other term of the collocation for each of the key words.

communities inspiration investors paradigm perspectives

Traditionally, wise _____ have been the ones who have
spent money in new construction that leads to the growth of cities. But now,
local _____ are creating this new _____
and putting control back into the hands of people who live and work in
neighbourhoods. These shifting _____ have happened
because people are becoming more vocal about engaging in political
processes. Many draw _____ from various human rights
protests where people have stood up for themselves and the interests
of those around them.

C. Write sentences using the pairs of words in parentheses. Share your sentences
with a partner and practise saying them to check if they make sense and for
speaking practice.

① (paradigm / perspective) _____

_____

② (financial / investors) _____

_____

③ (awareness / communities) _____

_____

Before You Listen

A. Whenever you look at a problem and a
hypothetical solution, you need to consider
what happens next, or the positive and
negative *effects* of any solution. What would
be the effects of *not* repairing or replacing
old bridges and *not* building new ones?
Compare your answers with a partner's
to check that your ideas are realistic.

① If we didn't *repair* bridges, the positive
effects might be ...

_____

② If we didn't *repair* bridges, the negative effects might be ...

_____

③ If we didn't *build* bridges, the positive effects might be …

_____

④ If we didn't *build* bridges, the negative effects might be …

_____

B. In Listening 1, lecturer Dr. Quinn puts forward the hypothetical idea of no longer building bridges and getting rid of old ones. This is a hypothetical situation that is highly unlikely to happen. Choose the point that is most likely Quinn's intention for discussing the idea with her students.

  a) She would like to propose destroying all the bridges in a city where she lives, and she is looking for support.

  b) She wants them to explore consequences of a hypothetical situation and develop their thinking.

  c) She wants to use the ideas to develop ways to build new bridges in the place where she lives.

While You Listen

C. The first time you listen, consider what Dr. Quinn and Max are saying. Listen a second time to complete your notes and add details.

DR. QUINN AND MAX	NOTES
❶ Welcome to this week's lecture. Throughout your different fields you study, …	You are not prepared *for the future.*
❷ When you talk about the future, you cannot know exactly what will happen, so …	Going to Mars is hypothetical and won't happen unless
❸ For inspiration, let's start with a topic that's familiar to you: bridges.	Bridges is a topic that
❹ Can someone give me the opposite argument?	There is more than one
❺ I'd say that bridges are necessary because …	There are multiple reasons for building bridges.
❻ Great answer, Max. If I can summarize your ideas, you're mostly concerned about …	Max's points are all about
❼ Okay, it's important to have an awareness of the opposite point of view.	Knowing another point of view helps you
❽ I don't think that anyone would disagree that bridges are expensive to build, but …	Quinn thinks cost
❾ For the second premise from the planning perspective, …	Words like *likely* and *often* mean
❿ The third premise is the most serious one. From the engineering perspective, …	Even if you don't agree with the other points,
⓫ Okay, so that's the foundation of my argument, but let's take it to the next level.	If you agree with the first points,
⓬ Can anyone tell me what is meant by paradigm shift?	Computer usage today can be compared to

DR. QUINN AND MAX	NOTES
⑬ What are some hypothetical paradigm shifts you might consider? What if ... in thirty years,	One change would lead to
⑭ As you can probably guess, I am not telling you all this because ...	Bridges are just an example
⑮ Besides exploring hypothetical situations, what else can you do?	Study outside
⑯ Really? Why biology? Max: Well, I've always been interested in ...	Growing up on a farm made Max
⑰ Let me push you a little further on this. Can you relate ...	Quinn sees a relationship between
⑱ Yes, bees live together but when a hive gets too big, some [bees] leave and ...	Bees and humans are similar
⑲ Wow! If only we could think like bees! So let's build a hypothetical situation ...	Money not spent on bridges might be spent on
⑳ Of course all of this is hypothetical, but at least it is a first step in ...	Hypothetical situations help improve

After You Listen

D. Review your notes from task C and use what you learned in Focus on Listening (page 4) to answer the following two questions.

① What can you infer about Dr. Quinn's attitudes toward her students?

_____

_____

② What can you infer about Max's attitudes from his time growing up on a farm?

_____

_____

E. Read the following statements and indicate whether you think each one is true or false. For each false statement, write the true statement.

STATEMENTS	TRUE	FALSE
① Quinn suggests that the idea of humans going to Mars is hypothetical. _____ _____		
② The topic of bridges was suggested because it mainly interests engineers. _____ _____		
③ Quinn's point about convenience is a summary of what Max said about bridges. _____ _____		

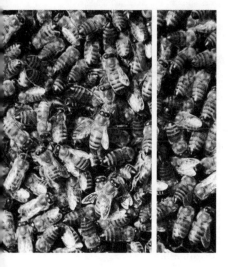

STATEMENTS		TRUE	FALSE
④	Quinn talks about point of view to suggest that you only need to understand one side of an argument.		
⑤	A paradigm shift is the idea that your view of the world should never change.		
⑥	One paradigm shift can result in multiple side effects, some of which are unexpected.		
⑦	The example of bees is meant to model how groups organize their society based on resources.		
⑧	The importance of hypothetical situations is that they help us think about the past.		

F. Max's study of biology will probably impact on his work as an engineer. Think of a career you are interested in. Then choose another subject area from the list below. How might you use the combination for a new job?

Psychology Robotics Engineering
Geography Literature Business
Languages Music History Theater
Law Medicine Education
Mathematics Astronomy

MyBookshelf > My eLab > Exercises > Chapter 1 > Choosing the Right Path

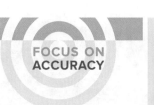

FOCUS ON ACCURACY

Talking about *If*

What would you do if you were given a million dollars? Questions that begin with "What would you do if ..." and "What will you do if ..." are two common ways to start hypothetical questions. To answer, you need to think about whether or not something is or was possible and then what you would do about it.

These are the three conditional tenses. Compare these tenses.

SITUATION	IF CLAUSE	RESULT CLAUSE	EXAMPLE SENTENCE
First conditional: true in the present or future	simple present	*will* + base form	If I have time, I will study.
Second conditional: untrue in the present or future	simple past	*would* + base form	If I had time, I would study.
Third conditional: untrue in the past	past perfect	*would have* + past participle	If I had had time, I would have studied.

The example sentences are made of clauses. The *if* clause is the condition; the other clause is the result or consequence of the condition. However, the order of the clauses can be switched (for example, *I will study if I have time).* When the *if* clause comes second, a comma between the clauses is not necessary.

A. Read the conditional sentences and choose the correct meaning of each one.

① However, if your dreams begin with sound premises, you will be in a better position to achieve them.

    a) Your dreams may sound good but they won't help your position.

    b) Base your dreams on facts and you will likely act on them.

    c) Position your dreams to get yourself into better premises.

② If we built communities that had everything they needed, we wouldn't need bridges.

    a) Our communities don't have everything so we still need bridges.

    b) The main thing we need in our communities are better bridges.

    c) We can still build communities with the bridges that we all need.

③ I wouldn't have gotten a better job if I hadn't worked hard at school.

    a) I got a job at school because I worked harder.

    b) I didn't work hard so I don't have the job I want.

    c) I worked hard and it led to getting the job I wanted.

④ If you had woken up earlier, you wouldn't have missed today's test.

    a) Today's test was too late for you.

    b) You overslept and missed the test.

    c) Getting to sleep earlier affects your tests.

⑤ If she hadn't forgotten, she would have visited the exhibition.

    a) She did forget and regrets missing the exhibition.

    b) She forgot but did not intend on attending the exhibition.

    c) Forgetting the time is a good reason to miss something.

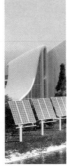
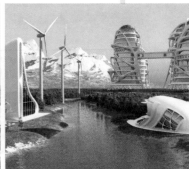

⑥ If that had happened fifty years ago, what would our cities have looked like?

    a) Cities will continue to change in future.

    b) It didn't happen so we can only guess.

    c) Cities fifty years ago were far different.

B. Use the words in parentheses to write sentences about hypothetical situations using the first, second, and third conditional forms. After, practise your sentences with a partner and make sure each of you has used the correct conditional form.

1 first conditional (everyone / show respect / get along)

If everyone shows respect, we will get along.

2 first conditional (you / learn from mistakes / make a better person)

_____

3 second conditional (they / study / urban geography, engineering, or business / understand the urban landscape)

_____

_____

4 third conditional (we / complete / engineering degrees / opportunity to work on bridges)

_____

_____

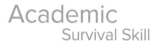

MyBookshelf > My eLab >
Exercises > Chapter 1 >
Focus on Accuracy

Academic
Survival Skill

Note-Taking

When you listen and take notes, you need a method that helps you capture important information for later study. The widely used Cornell Note-taking System was developed in the 1950s at Cornell University. To begin, divide your page of notes into four sections.

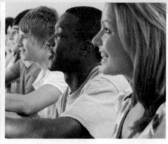

List information that identifies the talk.

TOPIC *Vanishing Trades in the Digital Age* _____

COURSE/CLASS _____

DATE _____

Fill in the main ideas and questions while you listen and after.

• MAIN IDEAS	• KEY WORDS AND IDEAS
_____	_____
_____	_____
_____	• IMPORTANT NUMBERS (INCLUDING DATES)
• KEY QUESTIONS	_____
_____	• REPEATED / STRESSED INFORMATION
_____	_____
_____	• NOTES ON ANY VISUALS *no visuals in this talk*

Write your notes about the talk.

SUMMARY	
_____	

Write a short summary.

© **ERPI** • Reproduction prohibited

A. Read the following paragraph from Listening 2 with a partner. In the above table, first fill in the *key words and ideas* box (including important numbers and key/stressed information).

> We have, first of all, defined automation pretty broadly, so we have included robotics, but also artificial intelligence and machine learning, and we've been looking at how those different technology areas will impact both the jobs that we all do, but also the tasks that are done within jobs. And what we are learning is that 50 percent of the activities that people currently get paid for can be automated by some of those technologies by 2055.

B. Look at your notes in the key words and ideas box and write down the main idea; the longer a talk, the more main ideas you will have. Write one question about it. In a lecture, key questions are ones you would research on your own or ask the speaker about later. Then write a short summary of the talk.

C. In the summary, *artificial intelligence* is abbreviated to *AI*. Use short forms like *AI* for *artificial intelligence* so you can write more quickly as you listen. Write five abbreviations for words or terms that are common in your field.

ABBREVIATIONS				
_____	_____	_____	_____	_____

D. Write five symbols that can help you write faster notes. Compare your abbreviations and symbols in a group to get new ideas about how you can take notes more efficiently.

SYMBOLS				
_____	_____	_____	_____	_____

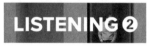 **LISTENING ②**

Vanishing Trades in the Digital Age

How many jobs have completely disappeared because of technology? In the past sixty years, perhaps only the job of elevator operator is completely gone. However, many other jobs are likely to vanish in the coming decades. In other cases, technology will make some jobs more efficient and effective so one person can do the work of many.

VOCABULARY BUILD

In the following exercises, explore key words from Listening 2.

A. Choose the word that best completes each of the sentences adapted from Listening 2.

dramatically	affected	sectors	supplemented	transition

❶ The year 2055 is when we would see most of the activities we've projected

that could be automated—when that _____ will be complete.

2 Are some areas of the world going to be _____ in greater ways than others?

3 But almost every job will change form quite _____.

4 So doctors, lawyers, all sorts of professions will have parts of their current jobs replaced by automation, and frankly _____ by automation.

5 We're not looking at a world where entire _____ of the workforce are going to vanish as jobs are completely automated.

B. It's often easier to understand new words if you understand the root words within them. First, write the root word for each of the following and then write a synonym or definition for the key word.

Learn root words to expand your vocabulary.

KEY WORD	ROOT WORD	DEFINITION
1 adoption	*adopt*	
2 automation		
3 feasibility		
4 implications		
5 predictable		

Before You Listen

A. Machine learning is part of artificial intelligence and refers to how a computer can look at large amounts of data and learn to recognize patterns. An example is looking at test results from millions of patients so it can identify problems more quickly and accurately than a human doctor. Read an excerpt from Listening 2. Then answer the questions and compare your ideas with a partner.

> We have first of all defined automation pretty broadly, so we have included robotics, but also artificial intelligence and machine learning, and we've been looking at how those different technology areas will impact both the jobs that we all do, but also the tasks that are done within jobs. And what we are learning is that 50 percent of the activities that people currently get paid for can be automated by some of those technologies by 2055.

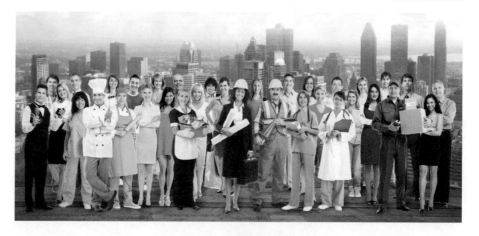

1 What human jobs might be replaced by robotics?

_____

② What human jobs might be replaced by machine learning and artificial intelligence?

_____

③ What jobs are unlikely to be completely replaced by robotics, artificial intelligence, and machine learning?

_____

B. An outcome of increased automation is likely to be higher unemployment, even if companies save money and make greater profits. High unemployment often leads to social unrest. Governments in Sweden and Canada are experimenting with guaranteed incomes—paying everyone in a community enough to live, whether or not they are working. If you lost your job to automation but didn't have to work to support yourself, would you still want to work? Why or why not? Discuss in a group.

While You Listen

C. The Cornell System encourages you to listen for significant numbers and dates. Listening 2 features many number and time expressions. The first time you listen, consider what interviewer Nora Young and think-tank researcher Katy George have to say about automation, and make notes on their number and time expressions. Listen again and add details to your notes.

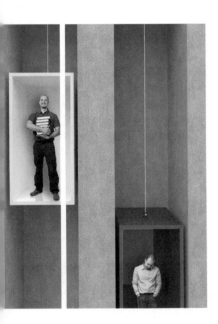

NUMBER AND TIME EXPRESSIONS	NOTES
❶ At least according to one source, in the past **sixty years**,	_elevator operator is the only career that's been completely automated_
❷ There are less than **5 percent** of today's occupations ...	
❸ And what we are learning is that **50 percent** of the activities that people currently get paid for ... by **2055.**	
❹ Almost **60 percent** of the occupations that exist today have tasks like ...	
❺ I read that about **60 percent** of all jobs are ...	_something like 30% automatable_
❻ So, think about **a third** of everybody's, almost everybody's, jobs will be ...	

NUMBER AND TIME EXPRESSIONS	NOTES
7 The **top three** are **first** of all …	
8 **Second,** tasks that are …	
9 and, **third**, tasks that are collecting data. The sectors that will be most affected are …	
10 but we actually see that these tasks that can be automated cut across **all** industries and all different wage levels. So …	*Doctors, lawyers, will have parts of their current jobs replaced and supplemented by automation.*
11 There are **several different factors** that are quite important in …	
12 But at the macro level, we believe that it's gonna [going to] take **decades** to play out, and there are …	
13 **Every** part of the world as we evaluated this will be affected, so there's really **no part** of the world that …	
14 But **the Big Five** in Europe, the United States, Japan … **all** countries have very significant amounts of …	
15 At one level, countries with **lower wages** have some roles that are …	
16 Although, as I said, we also see the same kind of susceptibility to automation in very **high-** …	
17 And so in that sense, you would expect **faster**-paced technology adoption in some of those industries. On the other hand, there's **less** of an economic imperative in place where …	

NUMBER AND TIME EXPRESSIONS	NOTES
⑱ I think the **two messages** that I hope policy makers take away to the highest level would be, **number one**, that ...	• *automation and new technology are very important*
⑲ But the **second takeaway** is that, in order to manage this in a way that does not drive even greater income inequality and disruption to communities and to parts of our workforce, we really need to ...	
⑳ **2055** is kind of our baseline projection as to when we would see most of the activities that we've projected ...	
㉑ But we think that that could happen **twenty years earlier**, or ...	
㉒ Well, **two pieces of advice. One** is to really become a confident and skilled user of ...	
㉓ But **secondly**, the kinds of tasks that are not susceptible to automation are things like ...	• *interfacing and facilitating relationships* • *applying expertise in decision making or planning*

After You Listen

D. Use your notes from task C and what you learned about the Cornell System (page 13) to write one main idea and one key question about Listening 2, and then write a summary.

① MAIN IDEA: _____

② KEY QUESTION: _____

_____

③ SUMMARY: _____

_____

_____

E. Read questions and statements from Listening 2 and choose the best explanation for each one.

① "Eventually, everything will be so automated that we'll just sit on our *Jetsons*' (a cartoon series about the future) couch and live a life of leisure."

    a) In the future, all work will be done by computers, robots, and other machines.

    b) Most people in the future will work on their couches, not at desks.

    c) We will have lives of leisure and sleep far more on couches than in beds.

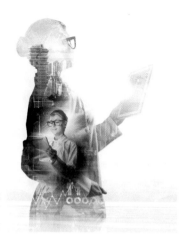

2 "So doctors, lawyers, all sorts of professions will have parts of their current jobs ... supplemented by automation, in a way that should make all of those occupations even more productive."

  a) Technology will train us to be both doctors and lawyers.

  b) Doctors and lawyers will help others become more productive at work.

  c) More professionals will use technological tools to help them do their jobs.

3 "And then there are a bunch of other factors, things like regulatory factors, as well as other social factors, that will determine the pace of adoption."

  a) Regulatory and social factors will slow the pace of automation.

  b) We will only understand factors when they are being adopted.

  c) Few regulatory factors will involve social factors as well.

4 "We actually have labour shortages in some of those same industries because we don't have people who are in the right location or with the right skills."

  a) Labour shortages will likely change the ways we look for work.

  b) We'll all look for jobs online without worrying about skills.

  c) People with the right skills will travel farther to find work.

5 "On the other hand, there's less of an economic imperative in place—where labour costs are really low—to automate those roles."

  a) We will have to invest in automation in poorer areas.

  b) There will be little investment in automation in poorer areas.

  c) Richer areas will eventually invest in even the poorest areas.

6 "In the long run it will work out, but in the short run there could be some painful disruptions."

  a) Almost everyone will go for longer runs, not shorter runs.

  b) Automation may lead to many people suffering if they can't find work.

  c) We will create disruptions that may or may not be painful to others.

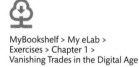

MyBookshelf > My eLab >
Exercises > Chapter 1 >
Vanishing Trades in the Digital Age

F. In a group, look at the key questions you and others wrote in task D. Share the questions and discuss your answers.

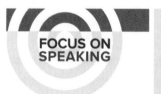

FOCUS ON SPEAKING

Giving Presentations

Giving presentations is a long-term skill that you will use in many contexts. For example, you will likely give presentations in university as well as throughout your future career. Sometimes presentations will be to a single person; in other cases, to small groups or to large crowds. In each case, you need to organize your ideas so they are easy to follow and remember. The following tasks will help you prepare a hypothetical situation in the Warm-Up Assignment and to make a presentation in the Final Assignment.

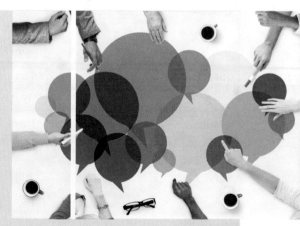

A. Think about a speaker or presenter you have heard who impressed you. Why did the presentation stand out? Was it the content (what was said), the structure (how the ideas were organized and the visual aids were used), or the presentation (the speaker's style and delivery)? Make notes, then compare your ideas in a group.

1 THE SPEAKER: _____

_____

2 THE TOPIC: _____

_____

3 WHY THE PRESENTATION STOOD OUT: _____

_____

B. On a separate page, use these phrases to help you structure your presentation. Where you see an ellipsis (...), insert information about the presentation you described in task A. After, practise the sentences with a partner.

STRUCTURE	SENTENCES
GREETING AND INTRODUCTION (introduce yourself and your topic)	"Hello, my name is ... and I'd like to give you a brief presentation on ..." Or, "In this presentation, I'd like to describe/analyze/discuss ..." Or, you might want to use a rhetorical question (a question for which the answer is already understood by the audience): "Have you ever thought about ...?"
OBJECTIVE (explain your problem)	"The purpose of this presentation is to ... It is important to you because ..."
ORGANIZATION (explain what you will talk about)	"First, I'll explain the causes of ... Then, I will talk about the effects ... Finally, I'll conclude with a suggestion ..."
MAIN POINTS (your examples and explanations)	Add transitions between points to let your audience know that you are finishing one idea and going on to the next one. "Next, I'd like to turn to ..." "I've discussed ... now I'd like to talk about ..." Add examples and explanations.
CONCLUSION (a summary, solution, or request for action)	End with a clear and final message. "I'd like to conclude by saying ..." "To sum up, I'd like to say ..." "Now, it's your turn to ..."
QUESTIONS	"If anyone has any questions, I'd be happy to answer them." "We have time for a few questions."
THANKS	"Thanks for listening, and if you have any more questions, you can always contact me later / after the presentation."

MyBookshelf > My eLab > Exercises > Chapter 1 > Focus on Speaking

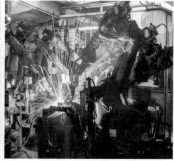

WARM-UP ASSIGNMENT
Develop a Hypothetical Situation

Now it's time to develop a hypothetical situation related to the automation of a career and to consider the consequences.

A. Working with a partner, choose one career that requires a university education. You might choose a career that one or both of you are interested in pursuing. In your hypothetical situation, imagine that your chosen career is replaced by automation.

The career: _____

B. Brainstorm (think of different ideas) by discussing the possible consequences of your career no longer being done by humans. For example, imagine if doctors were automated—replaced by robots. Perhaps a consequence would be that robot doctors would visit patients at home more often. List your three best ideas about what the consequences would be of the career being automated.

CONSEQUENCE 1: _____

CONSEQUENCE 2: _____

CONSEQUENCE 3: _____

C. Consider the follow-up consequences that might occur as a result of your initial consequences (task B). For example, if robot doctors visited people at their homes more often, the idea of the emergency room might disappear and instead, every neighbourhood would have a robot doctor who worked twenty-four hours a day, seven days a week. Or perhaps robot doctors would be in the form of drones that could travel to your home at a moment's notice.

FOLLOW-UP CONSEQUENCE 1: _____

FOLLOW-UP CONSEQUENCE 2: _____

FOLLOW-UP CONSEQUENCE 3: _____

D. Make notes about your ideas. You will expand on your points and discuss them in your Final Assignment.

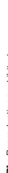

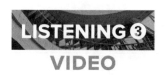
LISTENING ③
VIDEO

One Day in the Life: Six Jobs

What do these occupations have in common: architect, electric motorcycle engineer, mechanical engineer, planetary research scientist, roboticist, and software engineer? All of them are involved in solving problems in unusual ways. Which occupation might you be interested in doing?

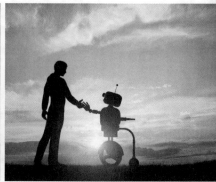

In the following exercises, explore key words from Listening 3.

A. Reading words in context can help give an idea as to their meaning. Read the sentences adapted from Listening 3 and fill in the blanks.

functionally	internships	mentality	parameters	policy

1. It requires the scientist; it requires the engineers, the people who come up with _____, the people who come up with the money.

2. We've left instruments out in the field for years at a time so that we can really look at what the different environmental _____ are, how does the light vary?

3. As a start-up, our _____ really is to work fast and fail fast.

4. The experiences at my previous _____ taught me a lot about this career and just exposed me to a lot of things in the software universe.

5. You then start to test those concepts either by building them out and _____ using them and seeing if they perform the way you want them to, or by building them out virtually.

B. Complete each sentence with a phrase that helps to explain the key word in bold. After, practise your sentences with a partner to decide if each makes sense.

1. Architecture is all about being **aesthetic**, which means that _____
_____

2. Often in the classroom, we were too focused on the very **specific** rules such as _____
_____

3. At university and in your career, you have to show **persistence** by _____
_____

4. One step in the **cycle** of project development is _____
_____

5. As a **consulting** firm, most of our work involves _____
_____

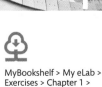

MyBookshelf > My eLab >
Exercises > Chapter 1 >
Vocabulary Review

CEO = Chief
Executive Officer

Before You Listen

A. Marc Fenigstein is the CEO of an electric motorcycle company. Read about his company and his responsibilities, and then list three skills that might be important in his job.

Our first product is a race-level electric motocross bike. And because it's electric, there's also a street-legal version of it that is potentially the fastest urban vehicle on the planet. As CEO, ultimately I'm responsible for everything that happens under our roof, but my day-to-day [job] is primarily running the business side and keeping everything out of the way of our design and engineering team to let them do what they do best.

_____ _____ _____

B. As you watch the video in Listening 3, you will focus on the main jobs, education, and advice or lessons of six professionals. Think about a career you would like to have some day and answer the questions. Share your answers with a partner to see if you both can find additional points to include.

1 What is the main job or work of a person in this position?

_____

2 What education is required to work in this position?

_____

3 What are the advantages and disadvantages of this position?

_____

While You Listen

See what you can understand from the speakers' facial expressions, gestures, and body language.

C. Use what you learned about the Cornell System (page 13) to take notes as you listen to six people talk about their jobs. For each one, take notes about what their main job is (beyond each one's job title), the education they received (both at university and informally), and the advice they have or lesson they have learned in their professions. Listen again and fill in details.

JOBS	DETAILS
ELECTRIC MOTORCYCLE ENGINEER: MARC FENIGSTEIN	MAIN JOBS: *running the business side so the design and engineering teams can work*
	EDUCATION:
	ADVICE/LESSONS: *Don't be afraid to …*
SOFTWARE ENGINEER: VICTORIA SUN	MAIN JOBS:
	EDUCATION: *her engineer*
	ADVICE/LESSONS:
ROBOTICIST: MAREK MICHALOWSKI	MAIN JOBS:
	EDUCATION:
	ADVICE/LESSONS:

JOBS	DETAILS	
PLANETARY RESEARCH SCIENTIST: MARGARITA MARINOVA	MAIN JOBS:	
	EDUCATION: *engineering*	
	ADVICE/LESSONS:	
MECHANICAL ENGINEER: NIVAY ANANDA-RAJAH	MAIN JOBS:	
	EDUCATION:	
	ADVICE/LESSONS:	
ARCHITECT: RACHELE LOUIS	MAIN JOBS:	
	EDUCATION:	
	ADVICE/LESSONS: *She loves how her career integrates so many different aspects of the human spirit.*	

After You Listen

D. Review your notes from task C. Continue with the format of the Cornell System and work with a partner to write a main idea, key question, and summary for each of the six professions.

JOBS	NOTES
ELECTRIC MOTORCYCLE ENGINEER	MAIN IDEA: *His job is about making it easy for others in his company to work.* KEY QUESTION: SUMMARY:
SOFTWARE ENGINEER	MAIN IDEA: KEY QUESTION: SUMMARY:
ROBOTICIST	MAIN IDEA: KEY QUESTION: SUMMARY:

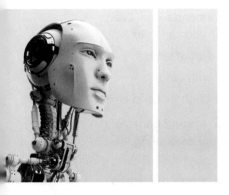

JOBS	NOTES
PLANETARY RESEARCH SCIENTIST	MAIN IDEA: KEY QUESTION: SUMMARY:
MECHANICAL ENGINEER	MAIN IDEA: KEY QUESTION: SUMMARY:
ARCHITECT	MAIN IDEA: KEY QUESTION: SUMMARY:

E. Read the statements and choose the best inferences.

1 When the electric motorcycle engineer says, "Managing an operation like this is not easy and it requires a lot of multidisciplinary thinking," you can infer:

a) Most jobs require many people to work with every possible tool.

b) No one is likely to have enough skills to do the jobs of the future.

c) Multidisciplinary thinking means that you have to have lots of skills.

2 When the software engineer says, "I really ... dreamed about being a games developer when I was in high school and I thought building video games was so much fun," you can infer:

a) All video game players should dream about doing her same job.

b) She enjoys her job because it relates directly to her passions.

c) If you don't start young, you will never learn about the job of your dreams.

3 When the roboticist says, "As an undergraduate, I studied computer science and psychology," you can infer:

a) Creating robots for autistic children combined his interests.

b) Autism is a topic that is commonly considered in computer science.

c) Sometimes things you study have no relationship to your future job.

4 When the planetary research scientist says, "I think the biggest key to success is being passionate about something and allowing yourself to be passionate about something," you can infer:

a) She is passionate about her job.

b) Success is the most important thing to her.

c) She works with passionate people.

⑤ When the mechanical engineer says, "With this headband alone, I've probably made thirty different prototypes (models)," you can infer:

a) If you don't know what you're doing, you waste a lot of time.

b) He only works on his own when he should work with others.

c) Much of his work involves getting things right through trial and error.

⑥ When the architect says, "The core and shell is the skin and bones of the building, the shell being the skin, the outside, and the core being the inside," you can infer:

a) Her building designs will tend to have faces like people or animals.

b) She likely has a background in a medical field such as nursing.

c) She has a strong interest in relating biology to architecture.

F. Based on what you now understand about each of the six occupations, which would be most interesting to you? Why? Compare your choices in a group and explain your reasons.

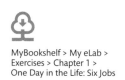

MyBookshelf > My eLab > Exercises > Chapter 1 > One Day in the Life: Six Jobs

FINAL ASSIGNMENT

Present, Discuss, and Take Notes on a Hypothetical Situation

Now it's your turn. Use everything you have learned in this chapter to present the ideas you developed in the Warm-Up Assignment and then discuss them in a group.

A. Review your notes from the Warm-Up Assignment (page 21) and prepare them for your presentation. Use what you learned in Focus on Speaking (page 19) to write brief cue-card notes for your key points about consequences and follow-up consequences. Divide up the tasks with your partner.

cue cards

STEPS IN YOUR PRESENTATION	BRIEF CUE-CARD NOTES
GREETING AND INTRODUCTION (explain the profession)	
OBJECTIVE (explain that you will explore the consequences of automation)	It's possible that careers in _____ could disappear with automation and it's important to consider the consequences if they do.
ORGANIZATION (explain your talk)	First, we will explain (the profession _____), then we will talk about how automation might cause it to disappear, and then we'll discuss possible consequences.
MAIN POINTS (consequences and explanations)	**CONSEQUENCE 1 + FOLLOW-UP:**
	CONSEQUENCE 2 + FOLLOW-UP:
	CONSEQUENCE 3 + FOLLOW-UP:
CONCLUSION	

STEPS IN YOUR PRESENTATION	BRIEF CUE-CARD NOTES
QUESTIONS (ask if there are any questions)	
THANK THE AUDIENCE	

B. As others present, use what you learned in Academic Survival Skill (page 13) to take notes. Build on what you learned in Focus on Listening (page 4) to see what you can infer about each speaker's attitudes, emotions, and intentions. Use these inferences to ask questions.

C. When everyone has presented, look for connections between the consequences of different careers being automated. For example, if we have robot doctors and robot police officers, could the two robots be combined into one?

D. When everyone has finished presenting, ask your teacher and other students for feedback so you can improve your presentation and discussion skills.

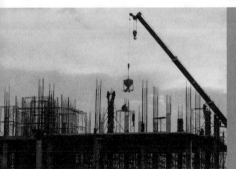

Critical Connections

In today's homes and factories, automation increasingly relies on software to run computers, robots, and other machines. A threat to automation is malware: computer viruses aimed at disabling or destroying machines. In some cases, individual hackers spread malware to get money from victims. In other cases, governments use malware to attack their enemies. For example, a virus called Stuxnet was used to disable part of one country's nuclear weapons program.

A. Imagine yourself in ten years. What will you be doing in terms of a job?

I will be working as a _____.

B. Imagine yourself in this hypothetical situation: A malware virus similar to Stuxnet has spread and evolved to destroy every automated machine in the world. As you walk outside your suddenly dark home, you find a much quieter world. Dams and power plants that produce electricity have stopped working. Newer cars are still in the middle of the roads, and there are no airplanes in the sky. Many people are trapped in buildings where automatic doors will not open. Hardest hit are hospitals. The computers that could be used to battle the malware are largely disabled.

On a separate page, answer these questions using the conditional tenses you learned in Focus on Accuracy (page 11):

1 How will the loss of automation affect the job you identified in task A?

2 What do you think you will be doing from day to day if you can't do your chosen job?

3 What do you think you will try to do to help yourself and others?

C. Discuss the effects of the hypothetical situation in a small group. As others talk about their lives in the future, use what you learned in Focus on Listening (page 4) to infer their attitudes, emotions, and intentions.

CHAPTER 2

The Brain's Secrets

Greek philosopher Aristotle (384–322 BCE) believed we thought with our hearts, not our brains. We now know differently, but questions remain about how the brain learns—and forgets—new things. Much of what we know about the healthy brain comes from studies of brains that do not work: when genetics, disease, or damage leads to a disorder. Scientists also explore traditional ways of using our minds, such as meditation and mindfulness. One finding from decades of research is that each brain may learn differently. How does your brain learn?

In this chapter, you will

- learn vocabulary about learning and the brain;

- listen to understand charts;
- use mind maps for note-taking;
- work with modals;

- explore how to use visual aids;
- talk about procedures;
- explain a chart and discuss a procedure.

GEARING UP

A. Look at the diagram of the brain's functions and answer the questions.

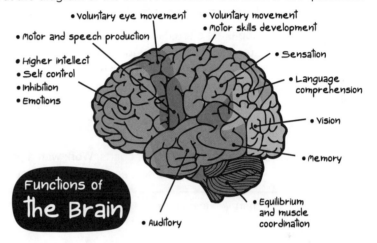

- Voluntary eye movement
- Voluntary movement
- Motor skills development
- Motor and speech production
- Sensation
- Higher intellect
- Self control
- Inhibition
- Emotions
- Language comprehension
- Vision
- Memory
- Equilibrium and muscle coordination
- Auditory

Functions of the Brain

① Besides language comprehension, what other areas are important for communication? Why?

_____

_____

_____

② Disease or damage to one area of the brain often leads to language difficulties. How would your language use be affected by:

• Short-term memory loss (forgetting what happened minutes ago)

_____

_____

_____

• Long-term memory loss (forgetting what happened days or years ago)

_____

_____

_____

B. Discuss the questions and your answers in a group.

Below are the key words you will practise in this chapter. Check the words you understand, then underline the words you use. Highlight the words you need to learn.

nouns
chemical*
conjecture
criteria*
formula*
insight*
mobility
participants*
psychology*
symptoms
synchronization
technique*
variation*

adverb
presumably*

learning and the brain

verbs
alter*
analyzing*
categorize*
distracted
distributed*
encounter*
evaluating*
inhibit*
modified*
resolve*
ruminate

adjectives
abstract*
conscious
enhanced*
philosophical*
radical*
rational*

* Appears on the Academic Word List.

FOCUS ON LISTENING

Understanding Charts

Speakers often use charts to help explain their ideas. A chart is usually a summary of a large amount of data that has more details than speakers would want to explain or listeners would want to hear about. Instead, charts present information in ways that are easy to understand and compare. But you need to recognize the differences among charts so you can predict what types of information they typically display.

A. Look at six types of charts. Work with a partner to name each chart, using the types in the box, and then write what each is used for.

| column chart | flow chart | line chart | organizational chart | pie chart | Venn diagram |

❶
Venn diagram; shows what two
or more things have in common

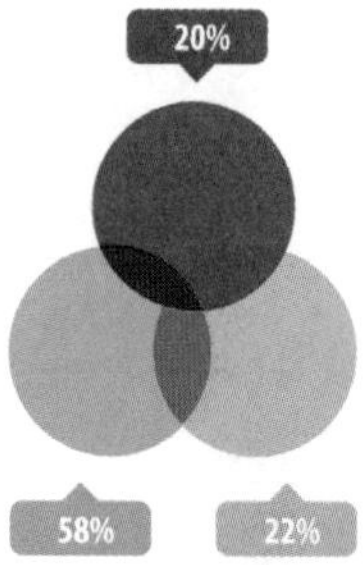

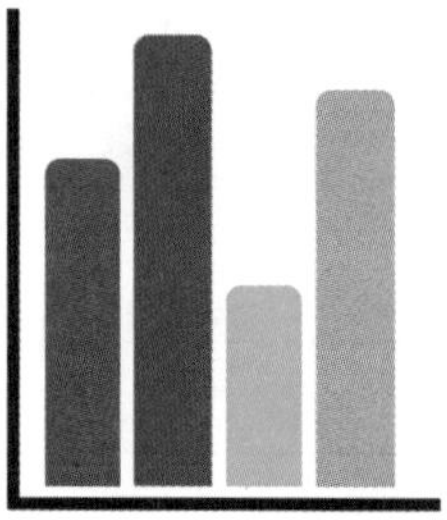

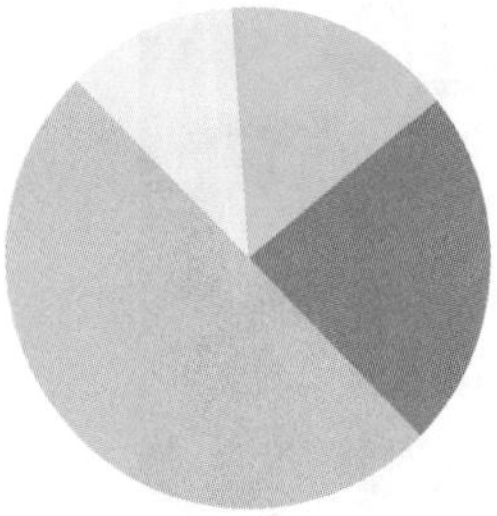

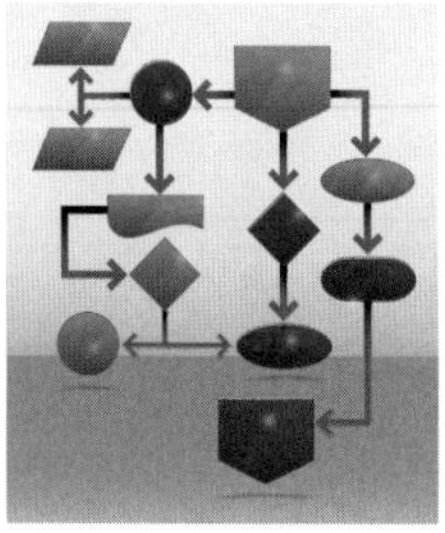

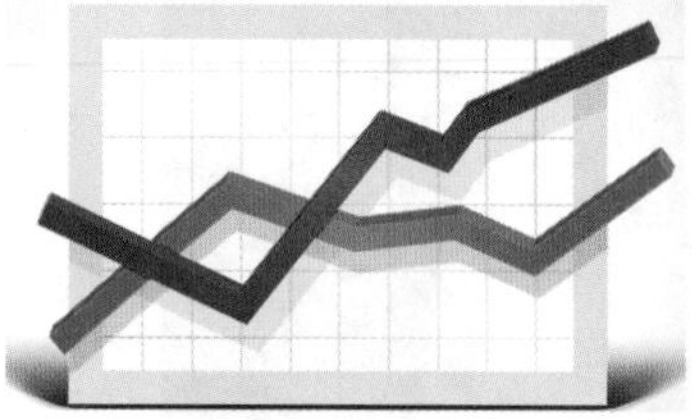

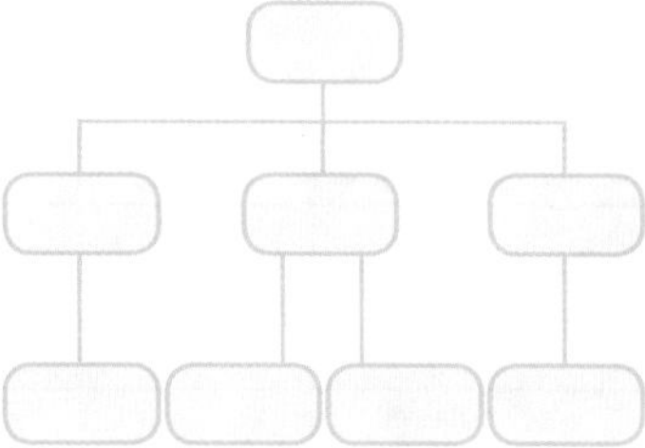

❷
_____

❸
_____

❹
_____

❺
_____

❻
_____

B. When discussing a chart, a speaker typically uses various phrases to indicate details. First, read the six purposes, then listen to the phrases and match each one to its purpose. After, discuss your answers with a partner.

_____ something that is obvious

_____ the limits of the chart

_____ the source of the data

_____ the type of chart

_____ directs attention to something on the chart

_____ something that is not on the chart

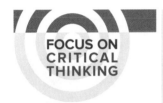

FOCUS ON CRITICAL THINKING

Note-Taking with Mind Maps

Quick! What do you think when you hear the word _book_? The question and the many thoughts it evokes illustrate how your brain is organized. In your mind, you likely see learning environments (e.g., home, kindergarten), kinds of books (e.g., dictionary, guidebook), and places (e.g., library, online). How your brain thinks is the focus of Listening 1—the reasons, or _objectives_, you have for learning.

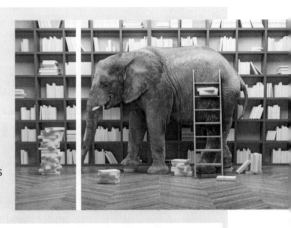

> Mental web-like connections are called schema or mind maps when written, such as in Vocabulary Build Overview.

The notes from the above paragraph could be fit into a mind map like this:

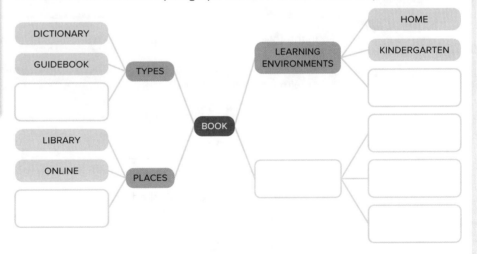

Mind maps help show connections among ideas and develop new ones. When you take notes with mind maps, add your own thoughts and questions as you listen.

A. Add one item each to _learning environments_, _types_, and _places_, then think of a new related category about books and add three points.

When you take notes in a lecture or during a discussion, you can start with a central box (called a _node_) and list the title of the talk. Add nodes for each main point and then add more nodes for details, examples, explanations, and questions. In some cases, you may not know where the information goes; just circle your addition and connect it with a line later.

B. Here is some information about Benjamin Bloom (1913–1999), who created a taxonomy, or classification, of learning objectives. Some key words are indicated in bold. On a separate sheet, start with *taxonomy* as the central node and add the other words into a mind map. Remember to connect key word nodes that belong together.

> In the 1950s, **Bloom** was working at the University of Chicago (**U of C**) and was involved in evaluating examinations. He looked at the **exams** being developed by university professors at the time and tried to see general **patterns** in the kinds of questions that students were being asked. He thought that if he could organize the **questions** in a logical way, then professors could write better exams with **clearer objectives** for what was expected from students. What he ended up with was a set of **six levels** of questioning.

LISTENING ❶   The Best Way to Learn

Why do some things seem easy to learn while others are a struggle? How do you learn? Is there a best way to learn? Does everyone learn differently? Bloom and his colleagues considered these and other questions and produced a taxonomy of learning objectives to help understand how learners process knowledge.

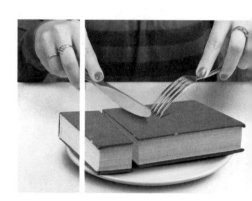

VOCABULARY BUILD

In the following exercises, explore key words from Listening 1.

A. Consider the context of these sentences from Listening 1 to fill in the blanks with words from the box.

analyzing	chemical	evaluating	categorize	psychology

❶ In educational _____, Bloom's interest was with the *cognitive*, and *cognition*—both of which refer to how we learn.

❷ In this case, you are asked to simply repeat something you have memorized, such as a list of dates or _____ formulae.

❸ In biology, for instance, taxonomies group and _____ plants and animals based on similarities and differences and on relationships.

❹ Often this process of _____ includes deciding what is important and what is not important.

❺ Bloom was working at the University of Chicago and was involved in _____ examinations.

B. Match each word from the box with its three synonyms.

conjecture	criteria	encounter	formula	insight

1 vision, understanding, awareness _____

2 standards, principles, measures _____

3 method, recipe, procedure _____

4 guesswork, estimation, inference _____

5 meet, face, confront _____

Before You Listen

A. Bloom's Taxonomy is most often represented as a pyramid. Review the chart, answer the questions, and discuss your answers with a partner.

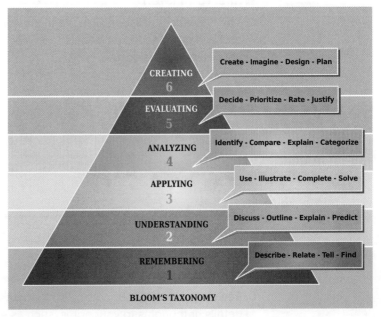

1 Review the chart types in Focus on Listening (page 30). What type of chart is this?

_____

2 Why do you think that *remembering* is indicated as the biggest section and *creating* as the smallest section?

_____

_____

_____

3 Consider the topic of *how the brain works*. What might be an *evaluating* task that students could do to better understand the topic?

_____

_____

B. Look at the Bloom's Taxonomy again and write one thing you learn each way. For example, you may learn an address and only have to remember it, not understand or analyze it. Discuss your answers with a partner.

SKILLS	EXAMPLES
❶ creating	
❷ evaluating	
❸ analyzing	
❹ applying	
❺ understanding	
❻ remembering	

While You Listen

C. The first time you listen, fill in the blank nodes to explain the skills (in yellow) and add other nodes for details. Listen again to add questions and check your comprehension.

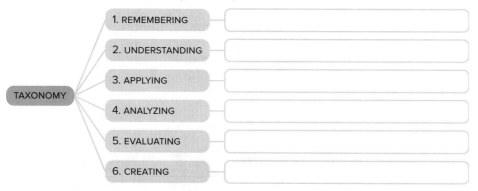

After You Listen

D. Review your mind-map notes. Think about what you've written. Add other details or thoughts to your notes, such as examples that help you understand. Compare mind maps with a partner.

E. Read the following statements and indicate whether you think each one is true or false. For each false statement, write the true statement.

STATEMENTS	TRUE	FALSE
❶ Remembering is Bloom's highest cognitive skill. _____ _____		
❷ Understanding is about constructing meaning from something that you've learned. _____ _____		
❸ A typical *apply* question would be to think about something you've read. _____ _____		

STATEMENTS		TRUE	FALSE
❹ You need to *remember*, *understand* and be able to *apply* what you've learned. _____ _____			
❺ Evaluating is often based on criteria or a set of standards. _____ _____			
❻ The cognitive skill of creating is seldom about producing something new. _____ _____			

F. Use what you learned about the taxonomy of learning to match the skills to the statements. Check your answers with a partner's.

SKILLS		STATEMENTS
❶ remembering	_____	a) After a whole summer of sitting in a chair, the lifeguard had to use her skills.
❷ understanding	_____	b) There are courses I could take and I'm trying to choose the best ones.
❸ applying	_____	c) Look at the two pictures and tell me if you can see a difference.
❹ analyzing	_____	d) The book is in the library, isn't it?
❺ evaluating	_____	e) I started a business selling something new.
❻ creating	_____	f) I know how an engine works. I just can't fix one.

MyBookshelf > My eLab > Exercises > Chapter 2 > The Best Way to Learn

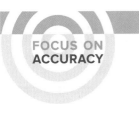
FOCUS ON
ACCURACY

Working with Modals

"Can you help me? Could you help me? Will you help me?" These three questions look like they are asking the same thing, but subtle differences among modals change the meaning. Modals help a speaker introduce an attitude on a topic; for example, suggesting something is a possibility, a probability, a necessity, or something just to be taken as advice. In Listening 2, you will use this information to better understand the speakers.

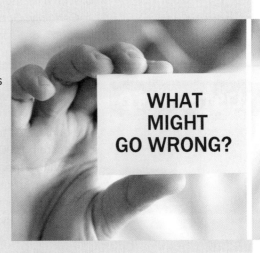

WHAT MIGHT GO WRONG?

A. Look at the modals and their functions and write sentences about the theme of this chapter (the learning brain) using each vocabulary word (in parentheses) from Listening 1.

MODALS	FUNCTIONS	SENTENCES
❶ can	ability or permission	(analyze) *You can analyze the mistakes you made in order to improve.*
❷ could	possibility/ability	(psychological)
❸ have to / had to	obligation/necessity	(formula)
❹ may	possibility or permission	(insight)
❺ might	possibility	(encounter)
❻ must	obligation or logical conclusion	(evaluate)
❼ should	suggestion or advice	(analyze)
❽ would	desire or request	(categorize)

When you use modals for requests, it's important to understand that some are more polite than others. In particular, the phrase *would you mind* is used for polite requests. Compare these two sentences:

- Can you help me with my homework?
- *Would you mind helping me with my homework?*

B. Choose the more polite word or phrase in parentheses for each sentence.

❶ (Can / Could) you teach me how to use this computer program?

❷ (May / Might) I borrow your extra pencil during this test?

❸ (Could you / Will you) turn your phone off while the teacher is speaking?

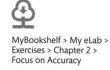

MyBookshelf > My eLab > Exercises > Chapter 2 > Focus on Accuracy

C. With a partner, practise responding positively to the questions in task B with *Certainly, Of course,* or less formally, *Sure.* Reply negatively with *Sorry, I can't,* or *Sorry, I'm afraid not.*

LISTENING ❷ ## The Science of Mindfulness

The earliest written mention of meditation comes from 1500 BCE, but the practice of meditating—spending quiet time in thought for religious or other reasons—probably began much earlier. Today, scientists are examining the health and learning benefits of taking time from your schedule to think deeply and relax. Do you think meditating and mindfulness can improve your thinking?

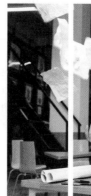
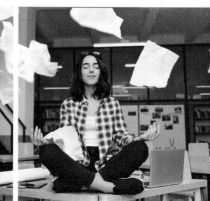

In the following exercises, explore key words from Listening 2.

A. Read the sentences and match each word in bold to its antonym—a word with the opposite meaning. Look up words you don't know. Practise reading each sentence once, then a second time using the antonym.

SENTENCES		ANTONYMS
❶ It's easy to be **distracted** when you study.	_____	a) reduced
❷ A large crowd can **inhibit** interest in asking questions.	_____	b) forget
❸ Do you make **rational** choices to balance work and fun?	_____	c) help
❹ The quiet let him **ruminate** about his past mistakes.	_____	d) focused
❺ The **enhanced** textbook has computer resources.	_____	e) unreasonable

B. Use the words in the box to complete the sentences.

participants	presumably	synchronization	technique	variation

❶ He said he lost his money but _____ he had other money in his pocket.

❷ It wasn't exactly the same class she held last year; rather, it was a

_____.

❸ A simple _____ for relaxation is simply to close your eyes.

❹ Although only thirty people had signed up, seventy-seven _____ came to the class.

❺ We insist on the _____ of everyone's watches to time the race.

Before You Listen

A. Two key concepts in Listening 2 are *meditation* and *mindfulness*. Read the definitions and write reasons why you might do each one.

TERMS	DEFINITIONS	REASONS FOR DOING IT
❶ meditation	spending quiet time in thought for religious or other reasons	
❷ mindfulness	focusing on the moment using all of your senses	

B. Read a paragraph from Listening 2. Why might some people prefer learning from a phone app rather than from a human teacher? Discuss your answers with a partner to choose the best ideas.

> Basically, the app on your phone reminds you to meditate, guides you through the process, and provides videos to help out. The meditation programs offered range from relationships to sports to happiness, dealing with cancer, even mini-meditations on mindful cooking. And at the root of all these programs are scientific claims about what meditation can offer you.

While You Listen

C. Read the key sentences below and highlight the modals to better understand each sentence. Listen to McDonald interview Krigolson and Cox to get a general idea about the context of each sentence, then listen again to add explanations. Listen a third time to add details to your answers.

KEY SENTENCES	EXPLANATIONS
1 What are some of the telltale signs you might be able to pick up from a person's brain while they're meditating?	*If the technology works, brainwaves can indicate your level of relaxation.*
2 So you should get more alpha activity during a meditation because you're a bit more relaxed.	
3 So more gamma would basically mean your brain is working; the different parts of your brain are working more effectively.	
4 In terms of the game and the game response, assuming that everything's in line with what's been done before, we should actually see some enhanced brain function in you, Bob.	
5 So, you know, just like you might want to play tennis and you need to get stronger to be better at tennis.	
6 It could be, you know, a memory. It could be your shopping list. It could be anything, but you get distracted.	
7 And frequently the thing that you focus on is your breath, but it doesn't have to be.	
8 I would say you probably have to do it at least three or four times a week for up to four to six months or so to start feeling the level two benefits.	*level one benefits of meditation:* *level two benefits of meditation:*

KEY SENTENCES	EXPLANATIONS
9 It can be something in the past, an argument you had or something that you said and you wish you hadn't or it might be something you're worried about happening in the future.	

After You Listen

D. Use your notes to complete the mind map and summarize Listening 2. Add questions you have about the ideas and then compare your mind map with a partner's.

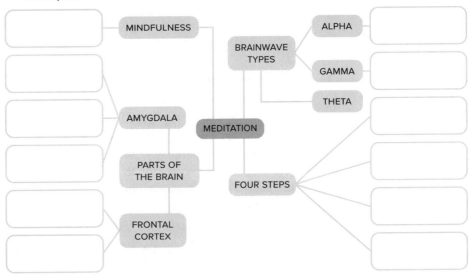

E. Write a response to each of the following questions. Practise the questions and answers with a partner to check your answers.

1 What's the difference between *relaxing* and *meditating*?

_____

2 What's the difference in the relaxation of novices versus people like monks who meditate long-term?

_____

3 What does *cortical synchronization* mean?

_____

4 How does meditation affect your cognitive abilities?

_____

5 What should one expect after ten sessions of ten-minute meditations?

_____

F. Write answers to the three questions and then, in a group, discuss them to compare your answers and choose the best ones.

1 If you don't practise meditation now, does Listening 2 make you want to start doing it? Why or why not?

_____

_____

② Cox mentions four steps of trying to focus on your breath, becoming distracted, realizing you're distracted, and bringing your attention back to focusing on your breath. How do you think these steps change as you practise more and more?

_____

_____

③ If meditation is effective in improving your thinking and learning, why do you think more people don't practise it?

_____

_____

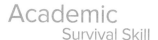

MyBookshelf > My eLab >
Exercises > Chapter 2 >
The Science of Mindfulness

Academic
Survival Skill

Using Visual Aids

An old cliché is that a picture is worth a thousand words. It's one reason for using visual aids in a presentation—to save time—but visual aids also make your presentations more memorable. When you use visual aids, you need to decide how to present the information to another person or a group. Look at some techniques to prepare yourself for the Final Assignment where you will use a visual aid in a talk.

- **Structure the information.** Choose the best format for the data you have collected. Use what you learned in Focus on Listening (page 30) to choose an appropriate chart type. Your audience will generally remember a good chart more than the same information presented as spoken or written words.

- **Limit the information.** Don't overwhelm your audience with unnecessary details. Decide how much to include on your chart so your audience doesn't feel they could more easily understand a simple explanation or are not confused by unnecessary details.

- **Share the chart effectively.** Don't show the audience a chart until you are ready to talk about it. Otherwise, they will think about the chart rather than listen to you.

A. Answer the questions, then compare your answers with a partner's to check your ideas.

① Imagine you were comparing two ways of learning to understand what they had in common. What kind of chart would you choose and why?

_____

_____

② Is it better to show your chart throughout your presentation, or only when you begin talking about it? Why?

_____

_____

Make certain your charts and their details are large enough to be visible to everyone in your audience.

3 Is it better to include all your data on a chart or only those portions you intend to talk about? Why?

_____

_____

B. Autism, a topic in Listening 3, is a mental condition that makes it difficult for some people to communicate and form relationships. It is a spectrum disorder, which means it can be easy or extremely difficult for autistic individuals to fit into society. The two charts below show the ratio of autistic people in the general population. Look at the charts, answer the questions, and compare your answers with a partner's.

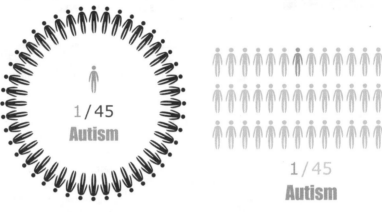

1 Based on what you learned in Focus on Listening (page 30), what is another way you could present this information?

_____

_____

_____

2 Why would you use a chart rather than just saying, "One in forty-five people is autistic"?

_____

_____

_____

3 How might the organization of each of the two charts change what you think about autism? That is, what message or point of view might you understand from each chart?

_____

_____

_____

C. Work with a partner and use what you learned about autism in task A to talk about one of the two charts. Your partner then talks about the other. After you both present, discuss what you can do to improve your presentation skills when you explain a chart in the Warm-Up Assignment.

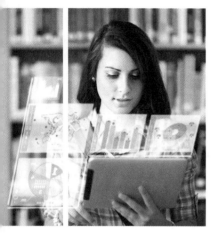

WARM-UP ASSIGNMENT
Explain a Chart

Now it's your turn to research and present a short talk on one of the types of charts you learned about in Focus on Listening.

A. Consider the themes of this chapter: education, neuroscience, and psychology. Use key words to search online. Key words might include *chart + brain, meditation, learning, remembering, understanding, applying, analyzing, evaluating,* and *creating.* Be prepared to share a copy of your chart on screen or on paper.

B. Review the information on your chart. Write answers to these questions to structure your presentation based on what you learned in Academic Survival Skill (page 40).

QUESTIONS	YOUR ANSWERS
❶ What is the title of your chart?	*The title of the chart is …*
❷ What kind of chart is it?	*This is a …*
❸ Who or what organization created the chart?	*The chart was created by …*
❹ What kind of data does it share?	*The chart displays data on …*
❺ What is significant in the chart; that is, what is unusual or important?	*An important/unusual feature of the chart is …*
❻ What is another way to present the chart's data?	*The data could also have been presented …*
❼ What would improve the chart (e.g., limit unnecessary details)?	*The chart could be improved by …*
❽ How can you summarize the chart?	*Overall, this chart …*

C. Practise your presentation with a partner or in a small group, using your notes to guide you. After, ask for feedback so you can improve your presentation.

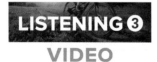

LISTENING ❸
VIDEO

Harnessing the Power of Brain Plasticity

A stroke happens when your brain loses control over part of your body, usually on one side and in one or more limbs. Most stroke patients end up using their other arm more and the affected one does not improve. But a new treatment restrains the good arm and forces the patient's brain to rewire the damaged arm. It's an example of how plastic—or flexible—the brain is in terms of new learning.

In the following exercises, explore key words from Listening 3.

A. The following sentences feature synonyms of the words in the box. Highlight the synonyms and write in the correct key word in each blank from the choices in the box.

alter	distributed	philosophical	radical	resolve

1 The doctors decided to modify the brain patients' treatment.

_____

2 She had theoretical concerns about the future.

_____

3 A new idea was looking at the patients' hearing.

_____

4 The results were spread by the doctors and the nurses.

_____

5 It was felt by some that the treatment would fix the problem.

_____

B. Fill in the blanks with words from the box to form common collocations (words that naturally fit together).

abstract	conscious	mobility	modified	symptoms

1 major _____

2 losing _____

3 _____ concepts

4 _____ decision

5 genetically _____

C. Write sentences using the pairs of words below.

1 collected / philosophical

_____

2 ignore / symptoms

_____

3 ignorant / unimportant

_____

Before You Listen

A. What do you know about the brain? The introduction to Listening 3 mentions strokes. Other common brain disorders are *attention deficit hyperactivity disorder* (*ADHD*) and Parkinson's, a disease that makes victims shake and affects their balance. What other disorders affect the brain?

_____

MyBookshelf > My eLab >
Exercises > Chapter 2 >
Vocabulary Review

B. Read part of the introduction to Listening 3. It contrasts the theory of neuroplasticity with the theory that the brain is a machine. Why might these two theories have opposite views of learning? Discuss the question with a partner.

> Dr. Norman Doidge [is] making waves again. His first book explained the theory of neuroplasticity, the discovery that the brain can change. Now, in a new book, he says he's found evidence the brain can be rewired to help treat people with everything from Parkinson's disease to autism, and he's challenging the medical community to be more supportive of these new approaches. I sat down with him earlier this week. But first, some background. For years, the brain has been described as a machine.

While You Listen

C. First read the questions and, as you listen to Dr. Doidge's responses, add details to fill out his points. Listen again to add more details and examples, and to check your answers.

INTERVIEWER	DR. DOIDGE
❶ You talk about one case: another doctor who had experienced many years of chronic neck pain, and he was able to cure himself by flooding his brain. Explain that.	• *Dr. Michael Moscowitz, psychiatrist /* • *switches in the brain that can*
❷ So it's not the neck that actually hurts, it's the brain sending a signal that your neck hurts.	• *a whole system, but "gates" go*
❸ And if you can stop the signal, then ...	• *anaesthetic drugs also*
❹ And you can do that through a thought process.	• *a lot of patients went completely off* • *some patients have damaged body parts, but*
❺ The next chapter is about a fellow in South Africa with Parkinson's who walked off some of his symptoms.	• *John Pepper got Parkinson's*
❻ Instead of losing mobility, he became more mobile. He taught himself.	• *more mobile with what he called his*
❼ What is "conscious walking"?	• *aware of details*
❽ So in doing that, he was creating ... developing a different part of his brain?	• *using his brain to* • *walking is important* • *brain is connected to* • *brain growth between nerve cells when* • *generate new* • *helps Parkinson's patients and*
❾ And yet, he was a big deal in the Parkinson's community, and he was kind of kicked out for giving people false hopes.	• *people had difficulty accepting that activity of various kinds, mental and physical, might actually*
❿ A lot of people suffer from autism, ADHD ... it's pretty common these days. You say that this theory can be applied there as well. How?	• *research shows children with autism have inflammation* • *autism is a whole-body disease that*

© ERPI • Reproduction prohibited

INTERVIEWER	DR. DOIDGE
⑪ So how do you help that, then?	• *inflamed brains are* • *autistic children often cover their ears because of* • *among autistic children, auditory zoom* • *they hear low sounds, not* • *music can train*
⑫ You've seen kids helped with this?	• *yes*
⑬ What kind of difference does it make?	• *example: child with severe autism:* • *parents told he'd be institutionalized* • *After treatment, the child*
⑭ But why aren't all the doctors recommending this, then?	• *1. People think autism is* • *2. studies are* • *3. this idea of talking to the brain in its own language is*
⑮ You say that the mind can alter the brain. Where is the mind? It's not in the brain?	
⑯ People say that to me all the time. (laughs)	• *brain = your thoughts, your feelings are in your neurons but perhaps not*
⑰ That is not true?	• *most neuroscientists believe that mind is very diffusely distributed* • *perhaps neurons in the gut (stomach)*
⑱ So your mind could be down here?	• *We can show mental activity when people listen to music but perhaps the whole body*

After You Listen

D. Use your notes from task C and what you learned in Focus on Critical Thinking (page 31) to explain what links these ideas.

IDEAS	LINKS
❶ brain flooding / pain	*Flooding the brain with new messages can help control pain.*
❷ physical activity / brain structure	
❸ autism / inflammation	
❹ autism / hearing	
❺ genetics / environment	
❻ mind / the body	

E. Choose the word or phrase that best completes each sentence.

1. Chronic pain is _____.
   a) ever-changing
   b) always present
   c) hard to identify

2. The idea of "gates" in the body is about _____.
   a) opening and closing your thoughts
   b) dividing your arms and your legs
   c) points where pain can be stopped

3. The purpose of anaesthetics is _____.
   a) to cure illnesses
   b) to stop pain signals
   c) to make the brain think

4. John Pepper was able to deal with Parkinson's disease by _____.
   a) walking
   b) talking
   c) singing

5. The interview suggests cutting-edge treatments are not translated (adapted to other uses) because _____.
   a) doctors cannot accept new ideas
   b) few people can translate medical terms
   c) cutting involves unnecessary surgery

6. Dr. Doidge discusses a child who avoids eye contact and cannot communicate because _____.
   a) of his fear of doctors
   b) he has Parkinson's
   c) he has autism

MyBookshelf > My eLab >
Exercises > Chapter 2 >
Harnessing the Power
of Brain Plasticity

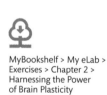

**FOCUS ON
SPEAKING**

Talking about Procedures

You often have to describe a *procedure* or the steps you need to do something, such as learning to ride a bicycle. Unlike processes (explanations of how things work), procedures often use the active voice with the imperative and don't include a subject; listeners or readers understand they are the subjects. In Final Assignment, you will use the ideas in this focus to talk about a procedure.

Compare these two sentences:

- **Passive voice process:** A mindfulness app is used to help people concentrate.

- **Active voice procedure with the imperative *use*:** Use a mindfulness app to help you concentrate.

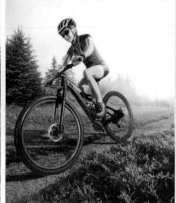

A. Read the following dialogue and rewrite it as a procedure in point form; that is, one point for each action in the procedure.

> **Host**: What is "conscious walking"?
>
> **Dr. Doidge**: Well, just being aware that you're not going to just start to walk, but you're going to lift your right leg, swing it forward at the knee, shift your weight down to your right foot, pay attention ...
>
> **Host**: So in doing that, he was creating ... developing a different part of his brain?

_____

_____

_____

_____

_____

_____

Written in point form, procedures are efficient because they are easy to _read_ and follow. However, when you _talk_ about a procedure, it's necessary to use linking words such as ordinal numbers (first, second, third) and words like _after, and, before, finally, next, then,_ and _while._

B. Rewrite your points from task A into a paragraph, using one linking word for each point and adding extra words as necessary. To check your answer, take turns reading your paragraph to a partner.

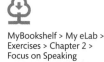

MyBookshelf > My eLab >
Exercises > Chapter 2 >
Focus on Speaking

_____

_____

_____

FINAL ASSIGNMENT
Present a Procedure and Discuss

Now it's your turn. Use everything you have learned in this chapter to prepare for and give a presentation on a procedure related to learning a new skill. For your presentation, you will build on what you did in the Warm-Up Assignment (page 42) and use what you learned in Focus on Listening (page 30) and Academic Survival Skill (page 40) to create a bar chart related to your topic.

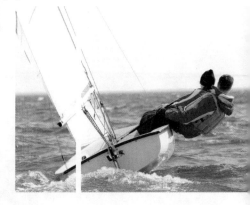

A. Choose something you are familiar with and use what you learned in Focus on Speaking (page 46) to reflect on the procedure for learning it. Your topic could be a sport, a hobby, a game, a skill like cooking, or something else. Check with your teacher for approval of your topic and ideas.

B. Survey five students to discover what they would find challenging when learning the procedure you have chosen. Create a bar chart to shade in their positive (yes) answers. A sample question might be, "What do you think you would find challenging about learning to sail?" You may add details to the sub-questions, such as *remembering* the parts of the boat, *understanding* warning signs, *applying* navigation lessons, *analyzing* wind directions, *evaluating* speed, and *creating* a route.

SKILLS	RESPONSES				
	STUDENT 1	STUDENT 2	STUDENT 3	STUDENT 4	STUDENT 5
remembering					
understanding					
applying					
analyzing					
evaluating					
creating					

C. Once you have your data, structure your presentation. Include about seven steps using the imperative and linking words you learned in Focus on Speaking (page 46). Use what you learned in Focus on Accuracy (page 35) to add things that students *can, could, might,* and *should* do as they learn.

> Today, I'm going to discuss seven steps to help you learn how to ...,
> then I will share information on what other students think would be most
> challenging. First, ...

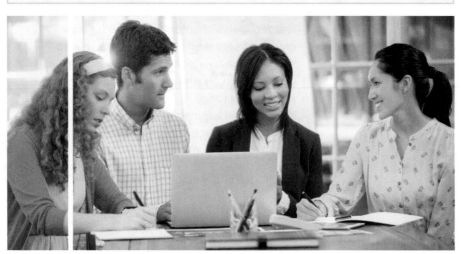

D. After you have outlined your steps, use what you learned in the Warm-Up Assignment (page 42) to discuss the data in your chart.

> Most of the data shows .... The data shows few instances of .... Only one student thought .... Overall, this bar chart suggests ....

E. After all students have finished their presentations and asked for questions, ask for feedback so you can improve your presentation skills.

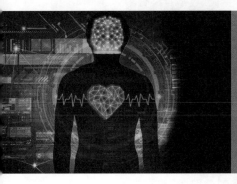

Critical Connections

Much of this chapter has been about things that you do to *help* your brain. Now, consider how you can *damage* your brain, and share your ideas in a group.

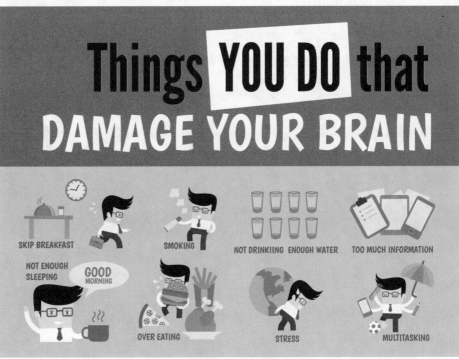

A. Look at the chart *Things You Do That Damage Your Brain*. Work in a small group to discuss the problems. Together, use what you learned in Focus on Critical Thinking (page 31) to create a mind map about the main ideas, supporting details, and examples. Each student should choose one of the problems.

B. Use what you learned in Focus on Speaking (page 46) to talk about procedures you should follow to avoid damaging your brain, and use what you learned in Focus on Accuracy (page 35) to tell students what they should or should not do, using modals (e.g., *Helmets should fit tightly.*).

C. Practise, then present your procedure to another group. Discuss to make sure your steps are easy to follow.

CHAPTER 3

Selling Dreams

The future belongs to the young and curious but with social media, some individuals and companies have become extremely skilled at promoting dishonest ideas and using propaganda to extend their influence. You are probably influenced by what you see and do online, but you also help shape the online world. When you post a positive comment, make an ethical purchase, or recommend a worthy website, you and millions of others define what is valuable on the Internet. How much are you using the online world and how much is it using you?

In this chapter,
you will

- learn vocabulary related to marketing and propaganda;

- listen for how speakers organize ideas;

- learn strategies to propose solutions to problems;

- explore ways to talk about the past;

- use stress and intonation to enhance meaning;

- practise answering questions;

- discuss ideas about how to create a marketing campaign with a partner and present the campaign to a group.

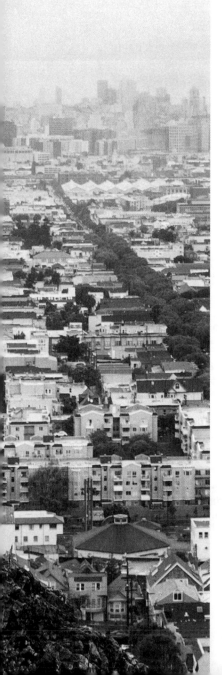

GEARING UP

A. Look at the marketing infographic about ten ways you encounter advertisements and answer the questions.

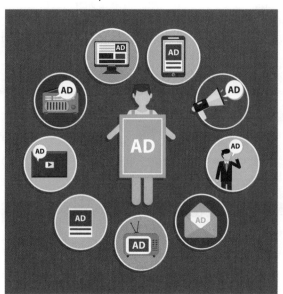

1. Which of the marketing methods have you encountered this week?

   _____

2. Which of the methods are *most* effective in shaping your opinions?

   _____

3. Which of the methods are *least* effective in shaping your opinions?

   _____

4. Choose two of the methods and think of a product that it's best to advertise using one method rather than the other.

   _____

B. Discuss your answers with a partner.

Below are the key words you will practise in this chapter. Check the words you understand, then underline the words you use. Highlight the words you need to learn.

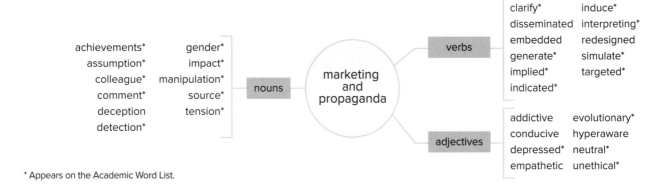

nouns — marketing and propaganda

achievements* gender*
assumption* impact*
colleague* manipulation*
comment* source*
deception tension*
detection*

verbs

clarify* induce*
disseminated interpreting*
embedded redesigned
generate* simulate*
implied* targeted*
indicated*

adjectives

addictive evolutionary*
conducive hyperaware
depressed* neutral*
empathetic unethical*

* Appears on the Academic Word List.

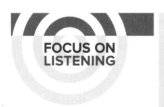

**FOCUS ON
LISTENING**

Listening for How Speakers Organize Ideas

Sometimes when you listen, it takes a moment to understand what is being discussed, particularly when the topic is technical. You start by picking up key words to identify the topic, and then get a sense of the speaker's point of view. But to really understand, it helps to recognize the *structure*—or organization type—of the talk.

A. Look at the chart and match the organization types to the typical signal words you are likely to hear.

ORGANIZATION TYPES		SIGNAL WORDS
❶ **CAUSE AND EFFECT:** explaining how one thing leads to another	*d*	a) after, at last, at that time, before, during, since, until, while
❷ **CHRONOLOGICAL:** discussing ideas with reference to time		b) means, can be defined as, the same as, like
❸ **COMPARISON:** showing similarities among two or more ideas or things		c) in brief, in conclusion, in short, as a whole, to sum up, to summarize
❹ **CONTRAST:** explaining how ideas or things are different		d) accordingly, as a result, because, consequently, due to, therefore
❺ **DEFINITION:** explaining the meaning of a word or idea		e) next, then, first, second, third, finally
❻ **PROCESS:** explaining an order of events		f) also, likewise, similarly, similar to, compared to
❼ **SUMMARY:** making brief points about a larger discussion		g) although, differ, however, but, yet, on the other hand, at the same time

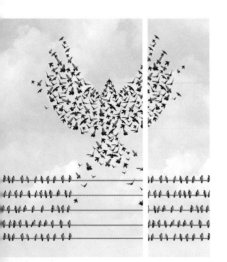

B. Listen to three short paragraphs and decide what organization type is used in each one.

❶ _____

❷ _____

❸ _____

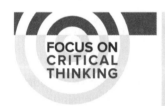

Speakers often use a mixture of organization types in a single talk.

C. Write three sentences, each using different types of signal words from task A. Practise saying your sentences with a partner. Ask your partner to guess what organization type you are using for each one.

❶ _____

❷ _____

❸ _____

FOCUS ON CRITICAL THINKING

Using Strategies to Propose Solutions

You are often given problems to solve in university. Solving these problems develops your critical thinking so you can solve real-world problems for the rest of your life. When you propose solutions, you need to be systematic, starting with understanding the problem. Then you can try multiple strategies to arrive at the best solution. But you also need to make sure a new solution doesn't cause more problems.

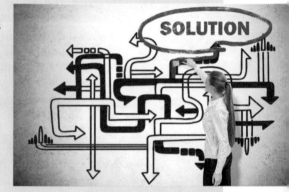

A. Listening 2 (page 59) considers the idea of how people become addicted to and distracted by their phones, such as when driving. Match the strategies to the solutions.

STRATEGIES		SOLUTIONS
❶ change by adding or taking away something	_d_	a) have more advertisements about the dangers of distracted driving
❷ change a process	_____	b) make it illegal to use phones while driving on roads
❸ change attitudes	_____	c) make phones unreachable by others when they are inside cars
❹ find a compromise	_____	d) build in a car sensor that turns off the driver's phone when the car is in motion
❺ introduce rules/laws	_____	e) let people use their phones while driving but only for directions

B. A problem referred to in Listening 1 is the promotion of cigarettes even though scientific studies have long shown that they increase the risk of heart disease and cancer. Today, there are similar health concerns about the overuse of sugar, particularly in fast foods and soft drinks. With a partner, choose one of the five strategies from task A and identify an existing or new solution that might be used to discourage people from using too much sugar.

STRATEGY: _____

_____

SOLUTION: _____

_____

_____

Sometimes solutions have both positive and negative consequences. For example, in 1935, Australian scientists tried to solve the problem of beetles eating sugar cane plants by introducing Hawaiian cane toads. But a negative consequence was that cane toads caused the deaths of many native animals. There are now 200 million cane toads in Australia.

C. Consider the problem of Internet advertising that irritates you. A simple solution would be to ban it. But that would bring consequences. Look at the mind map and, with a partner, identify three positive or negative consequences.

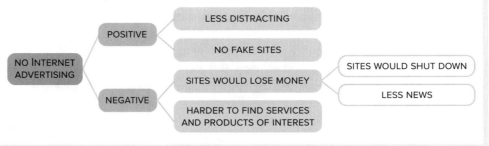

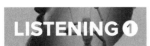 **LISTENING ①** **Understanding Propaganda**

Are you a victim of propaganda? Propaganda uses persuasion in a negative way because the individuals or motives behind propaganda are sometimes hidden, and the means of changing people's minds are usually dishonest. Have you ever been convinced to think or do something, but later realized that it was because you received dishonest information?

VOCABULARY
BUILD

In the following exercises, explore key words from Listening 1.

A. Use the key words in the box to complete the sentences adapted from Listening 1.

achievements	deception	gender	implied	manipulation

❶ *Black propaganda* is based on _____, perhaps making it seem that a competitor is promoting something bad.

2 The public will often follow a famous person's _____ endorsement.

3 Listing false _____ is part of the *cult of leadership,* used to increase a leader's power and prestige.

4 A group affected by propaganda could be a segment of the population, like old people or young people, or a particular _____.

5 Using _____, propaganda frequently ignores the truth, or at least the *whole* truth.

B. Using the words in the box, identify the correct synonym for each set of words.

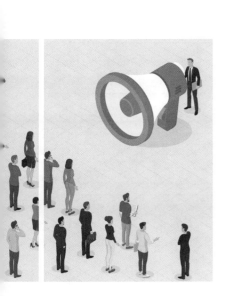

Propaganda includes a lot of professional jargon. When you study a new area of knowledge, explore its jargon.

disseminated	simulate	source	targeted	unethical

1 fake, pretend, imitate _____

2 corrupt, illegal, wrong _____

3 aimed, directed, pointed _____

4 foundation, basis, cause _____

5 spread, circulated, distributed _____

Before You Listen

A. Propaganda is all about shaping a message that will convince people to believe in certain things or to act in certain ways. Before you listen to a lecture on propaganda techniques, think about what the word *propaganda* means to you. Write two examples of occasions when you thought propaganda was used in an attempt to shape your or others' thinking.

1 _____

_____

2 _____

_____

B. Here is the first segment of the lecture you will listen to in Listening 1. Read it carefully and highlight the key words that indicate what you are likely to learn more about. Read it again and identify the type of organization it uses.

> Today, in this lecture, we will be talking about marketing. Marketing is an important way for us to connect producers with consumers. Most marketing is transparent, informative, and quite often entertaining. Good marketing not only helps us choose the products and services we need, it also makes us feel confident about our choices. But today we're examining another side of marketing: propaganda. Propaganda is used to shape and influence public opinion, most often through emotional appeals. In this way, it's not any different from simple persuasion. But propaganda goes further by manipulation and by frequently ignoring the truth, or at least the *whole* truth.

TYPE OF ORGANIZATION: _____

C. *Persuasion* is the name for a number of techniques you use to get people to adopt new ideas. Persuasion involves giving reasons, and perhaps adding emotions. Persuasive speech might be found in everything from conversations about what to have for lunch to advertisements trying to get someone to vote for a particular candidate. How would you persuade someone to try a dangerous sport? Pick a sport with a partner and brainstorm different ideas you might use.

_____

_____

While You Listen

D. This lecture deals with several new ideas. While you listen, write definitions of each of the propaganda techniques and terms.

PROPAGANDA TECHNIQUES	DEFINITIONS
❶ demonization	*portrays an individual or a group as being bad or evil*
❷ appeals to prejudice	
❸ cult of leadership	
❹ ad nauseam statements	
❺ appeals to fear	
❻ bandwagon	
❼ selective omission	
❽ glittering generalities	
❾ white propaganda	
❿ black propaganda	
⓫ grey propaganda	

After You Listen

E. Check your answers to task A. Was one or more of the techniques from Listening 1 used to shape your thinking? Discuss your answers with a partner and explain the technique(s) that was (were) used.

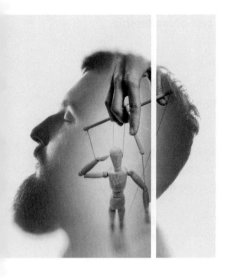

F. Read the following sentences from Listening 1 and identify the best examples of the words in **bold**.

① **Bandwagon** as a propaganda technique is an appeal to follow the crowd: to join a group or activity because others have.

   a) You and your best friend each join different political parties.

   b) You join a political party because everyone else seems to be joining.

   c) You avoid joining political parties because you think too many others are joining.

② It's common to think of **propaganda in terms of *white*,** *black* and *grey*.

   a) An example of white propaganda is oil producers saying spilled oil is natural.

   b) An example of white propaganda is oil producers pretending not to drill for oil.

   c) An example of white propaganda is oil producers publishing lies about competitors.

③ But propaganda goes further by manipulation and by frequently ignoring the truth, or **at least the *whole* truth**.

   a) They said he was arrested and the newspapers confirmed it.

   b) They said he was arrested, but it was an innocent mistake.

   c) They said he was arrested, but didn't explain he was found innocent.

④ Moreover, the **ways consumers are being manipulated** may not be easy to understand.

   a) Larger sizes are placed on the right side of shelves to encourage right-handed people to choose them.

   b) People are told to buy larger sizes because it can save them more money.

   c) People are given coupons that offer them a discount on larger sizes.

⑤ When people became aware of the dangers of smoking, one tobacco company response was to create **so-called *natural* brands**.

   a) It's dangerous to say that tobacco companies cause people to smoke.

   b) The new brands might have been natural, but they were not danger-free.

   c) It's good to respond and anything that is natural must be good for you.

⑥ Understanding marketers' propaganda techniques and **channels** is the first step to avoid being unfairly influenced.

   a) Channels refer to how often you watch one or more TV programs.

   b) Channels include things like toys with company labels on them.

   c) Channels are the paths that unwanted ideas tend to take.

⑦ Good marketing not only helps us choose the products and services we need, it also **makes us feel confident** about our choices.

   a) I'm not sure this is the right one but the clerk told me I should buy it.

   b) I don't really think it's useful to do any research before shopping.

   c) After reading all about the product, I'm sure I made the right purchase.

8 Piling up these false achievements was part of the **cult of leadership**, used to increase a leader's power and prestige.

a) I think my boss is the worst person in the world and deserves less praise.

b) My boss is part of a cult and wants me to join it, but I've refused.

c) Every small thing my boss accomplishes is mentioned in our company newsletter.

G. Philosopher Eric Hoffer (1898–1983) wrote, "Propaganda does not deceive people; it merely helps them deceive themselves." Think about people who do unhealthy things like smoke. Why do they choose to believe advertising propaganda that tells them it's fashionable to smoke?

_____

_____

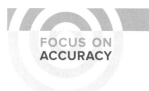

MyBookshelf > My eLab > Exercises > Chapter 3 > Understanding Propaganda

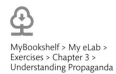

FOCUS ON ACCURACY

Talking about the Past

One of the most common questions you hear is, "What happened?" Answering this question involves using past tenses. These include forms such as *I ran, I was running, I have run, I have been running,* and *I had run.* Understanding the differences between these past forms can help you phrase ideas properly in the Warm-Up and Final Assignments.

Past tenses describe what happened before the present moment.

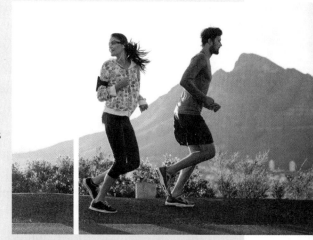

TENSES	FORMS	USAGE	EXAMPLES
1 simple past	Add –*ed* to the base form of most regular verbs. Irregular verbs: *was, had, did, said* ...	Events that began and ended in the past Key words: yesterday, last week, ago, in 2016 ...	They texted on how to survive.
2 past progressive	Past tense of *be* + –*ing* form of the verb	Events that were continuing to happen over a period of time in the past Key words: *when* and *while* to show the passage of time	They were texting on how to survive.
3 present perfect	Present tense of *have* + past participle form of the verb	Shows that the action has happened but may continue Key words: *since* and *for* to show the passage of time	They have texted on how to survive.

A. Fill in the blanks with the simple past or the past progressive tense of the verbs in parentheses.

1 I (sit) _____ in my friend's car and we

(listen) _____ to the radio when we

(hear) _____ a political announcement.

2. One political party (criticize) _____ another and at one point the speaker (say) _____ that his opponent was an animal.

3. "Ah!" I (say) _____. "That's demonization!"

4. But when I looked over at my friend, she (shake) _____ her head.

5. "What's the matter," I (ask) _____. I thought she didn't know what I (refer) _____ to.

6. Pointing to the man who (speak) _____, she said, "He is my father."

B. Use the simple past or the present perfect tense of the verbs in parentheses.

1. I (find) _____ that other people's moods affect me.

2. My friend (send) _____ me a message last week by email after I (wish) _____ her a happy birthday.

3. I (know) _____ this friend for ten years.

4. But the message (confuse) _____ me because it (seem) _____ so short; was she upset?

5. I should (guess) _____ that there was another reason.

C. Answer these questions with sentences that are true for you.

1. What is one of the most important things you have done?

_____

_____

2. What were you doing when you learned you were accepted at your school?

_____

_____

3. What is something that happened when you turned sixteen?

_____

_____

MyBookshelf > My eLab > Exercises > Chapter 3 > Focus on Accuracy

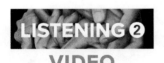

Brain Hacking

VIDEO

How much time do you spend picking up your phone or other digital devices to check for messages or play games? If you're like most people, the answer is, "A lot of time." You might be surprised to find that you're not the only one interested in those messages. Many companies rely on your addiction to your phone to make money from you.

In the following exercises, explore key words from Listening 2.

A. Collocations are words that commonly go better with certain words than with others. Choose the word from the box that forms a natural collocation with each set of three words.

addictive	colleague	comment	generate	impact

❶ big, minimal, serious _____

❷ close, trusted, professional _____

❸ automatically, quickly, randomly _____

❹ brief, fair, critical _____

❺ extremely, highly, very _____

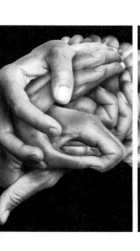
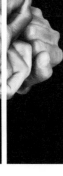

B. Use the following words to complete the sentences in the paragraph.

embedded	evolutionary	hyperaware	indicated	redesigned

Internet addiction has led to people becoming _____ of the

negative impacts of constantly using one's phone, particularly for checking and

sending messages. It seems to be an _____ trait that we

check our messages to avoid being left out of a group. Of course, there's often

critical information _____ among the hundreds of messages

most people receive each day, but recent studies have _____

that we use our phones to calm our anxieties in a cycle that creates more

anxiety. While many software companies are delighted with the attention,

others have _____ phone applications to allow users

to avoid receiving too much information.

C. Use the pairs of words in parentheses to write new sentences.

❶ (embedded / generate)

_____

_____

❷ (comment / redesigned)

_____

_____

❸ (indicated / impact)

_____

_____

Before You Listen

A. *Nomophobia* is a term coined by Iowa State University researchers to describe people who are afraid of not having access to their smartphones. Part of their research included a survey with the following five questions. Complete the survey, then compare your answers with a partner to see if you think the same way or differently.

STATEMENTS	YES	NO
❶ I would feel uncomfortable without constant access to information through my smartphone.		
❷ Running out of battery power in my smartphone would scare me.		
❸ If I were to run out of credits or hit my monthly data limit, I would panic.		
❹ If I could not use my smartphone, I would be afraid of getting stranded somewhere.		
❺ If I did not have my smartphone with me, I would feel weird because I would not know what to do.		

Reference: Yildirim, C. & Correia, A-P. (2015). Exploring the dimensions of nomophobia: Development and validation of a self-reported questionnaire. *Computers in Human Behavior, (49)*, 130-137

B. Read the introduction from Listening 2. Decide on the type, or types, of organization of the paragraph.

> Have you ever wondered if all those people you see staring intently at their smartphones—nearly everyone, everywhere, and at all times—are addicted to them? According to a former Google product manager you are about to hear from, Silicon Valley is engineering your phone, apps, and social media to get you hooked. He is one of the few tech insiders to publicly acknowledge that the companies responsible for programming your phones are working hard to get you and your family to feel the need to check in constantly. Some programmers call it "brain hacking" and the tech world would probably prefer you didn't hear about it.

While You Listen

C. As you listen, add details to each of the problems identified by the speakers. Listen again to identify additional details.

PROBLEMS	DETAILS
❶ Checking your phone is like playing a slot machine.	*It becomes addictive; you keep looking for interesting news.*
❷ Snapchat includes a feature called streaks.	
❸ Harris was bombarded with email and calendar invitations amid the overload of working at Google.	
❹ The constant distractions of emails and apps weaken relationships and focus.	

PROBLEMS	DETAILS
⑤ We don't feel good about how we are using computer apps.	
⑥ Parents don't understand their children's anxieties, fears, and loneliness in using phones.	
⑦ Tech companies remain secretive about what they do to keep users engaged with their screens.	
⑧ Meaningless rewards are timed to make you want more.	
⑨ The more you use your screens, the more information marketing companies collect about you.	
⑩ Continuous scroll convinces people to keep reading longer.	
⑪ The cortisol hormone (hydrocortisone) makes people more anxious about checking their phones.	
⑫ Corporations and creators of content have, since the beginning, wanted to make their content as engaging as possible.	
⑬ Companies like Apple will not accept phone apps that discourage use of other apps.	

After You Listen

D. Use what you learned in Focus on Critical Thinking (page 53) to propose solutions to these three problems from task C. With a partner, discuss positive and negative consequences of any solution.

① Children become addicted to streaks.

SOLUTION: _____

POSITIVE CONSEQUENCES: _____

NEGATIVE CONSEQUENCES: _____

② Apps make us feel less in control.

SOLUTION: _____

POSITIVE CONSEQUENCES: _____

NEGATIVE CONSEQUENCES: _____

③ Information about your search history is shared with companies.

SOLUTION: _____

POSITIVE CONSEQUENCES: _____

NEGATIVE CONSEQUENCES: _____

E. Choose the best phrase to complete each sentence.

1. The metaphor of *a slot machine* is meant to point out _____.
   a) how it can be a gamble to buy a phone
   b) how many people like to gamble
   c) the power of occasional rewards

2. The phrase *playbook of techniques* refers to _____.
   a) different strategies app designers can use
   b) a professional sport's set of strategies
   c) ways you can overcome phone addiction

3. The question, *Who does the new app help?*, relates to _____.
   a) the specific part of the population it's meant for
   b) the public benefit or the company's benefit
   c) how often people who hate it still use it

4. The reference to *brain stem* refers to people's _____.
   a) nervous system
   b) primitive emotions
   c) state of mind

5. The difference between gossiping on a phone and using social media _____.
   a) has to do with the people working to keep you engaged
   b) relates to how harmful gossip can be regardless of the device
   c) ignores the fact that everyone uses some kind of social media

6. Brown's study of neuroscience means _____.
   a) he failed to graduate as a doctor to practise medicine
   b) everyone today is trying to become an app designer
   c) his perspective on apps is biological and psychological

7. The fact that you don't pay Facebook to use their services means _____.
   a) you are getting an excellent deal
   b) others are happy to pay for you
   c) you are not a customer of Facebook

8. The purpose of Cooper being attached to a computer is _____.
   a) to allow him to play games directly without his hands
   b) to monitor changes in his heart rate and perspiration
   c) to reduce the number of times he checks his phone

9. Scanning teenagers' brains is being used _____.
   a) to understand changes over a twenty-year period
   b) to design apps that improve their cortisol (hydrocortisone) levels
   c) to reduce their levels of anxiety

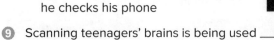

⑩ The purpose of apps like *Onward* is _____.

    a) to reduce people's use of their phones

    b) to increase people's use of their phones

    c) to let people use other computer devices more

F. Could the same principles behind the problems identified in task D be used for good purposes; for example, making programs that would make language learning more addictive? How might that work? Discuss your ideas in a group.

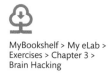

MyBookshelf > My eLab >
Exercises > Chapter 3 >
Brain Hacking

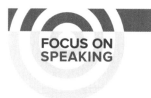

FOCUS ON SPEAKING

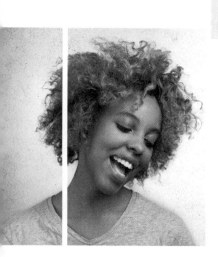

Using Stress and Intonation

A piece of common wisdom is *It's not what you say, but how you say it.* In terms of stress and intonation, this can refer to how you can shape your message by adding emphasis to parts of words (stress) or raising and lowering the tone of selected words in sentences (intonation). Stress is also important for showing the difference between some words that are spelled the same but have different meanings based on what syllable is stressed.

A. In sentence intonation, content words are usually stressed and function words are not stressed.

CONTENT WORDS	EXAMPLES	FUNCTION WORDS	EXAMPLES
MOST NOUNS	colleague, impact, source	AUXILIARY VERBS	am, can, weren't
MOST VERBS	achieve, imply, simulate	CONJUNCTIONS	and, but, while
ADJECTIVES	addictive, targeted, unethical	DETERMINERS	a, some, the
ADVERBS	deceptively, quickly, unethically	PREPOSITIONS	after, around, in
		PRONOUNS	he, me, you

B. Read these sentences and highlight the content words. Then try saying each sentence, stressing the highlighted words by saying them louder or at a higher or lower pitch. Practise with a partner and ask your partner which of your sentences sound more natural.

❶ As I said, when we sampled people throughout the nation, this is the response that we get.

❷ So we're going to start with a very simple first study.

❸ Whatever the other person said, they just agreed with them.

❹ None of them had ever done that before, but we just simply asked them how they did it afterwards.

C. Read the sentences aloud, adding intonation to the word in bold in each one. How does this change the meaning of each sentence? Match each sentence to its explanation.

SENTENCES		EXPLANATIONS
❶ **I** don't like sending texts.	_____	a) I might just like writing them.
❷ I **don't** like sending texts.	_____	b) I might love it or hate it ... who knows?

© ERPI • Reproduction prohibited

SENTENCES		EXPLANATIONS
❸ I don't **like** sending texts.	_____	c) Other people might like doing it, but I don't.
❹ I don't like **sending** texts.	_____	d) I might prefer sending things like emails.
❺ I don't like sending **texts**.	_____	e) I'm not interested in doing it.

MyBookshelf > My eLab >
Exercises > Chapter 3 >
Focus on Speaking

WARM-UP ASSIGNMENT
Discuss a Marketing Campaign

Now it's time to research ideas with a partner using what you have learned
so far in this chapter. You will discuss ideas about how to create a viral marketing
campaign to raise awareness of one propaganda technique.

A. With a partner, choose one
of the propaganda techniques
you explored in Listening 1:
demonization, cult of leadership,
ad nauseam statements, appeals
to fear, appeals to prejudice,
bandwagon, selective omission,
or glittering generalities.

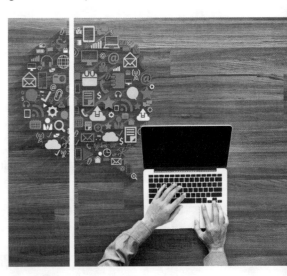

B. Use what you learned in Focus
on Critical Thinking (page 53)
to consider the problem of a new
app. Imagine that this app uses
the propaganda technique you
chose for dishonest purposes. For
example, it might be used to attack
a particular group, to promote a particular leader, or to encourage people
to use or consume unhealthy products or activities.

C. Brainstorm ideas about what you could say to counter the purpose of the app.
Use this framework:

TALKING POINTS	YOUR IDEAS
Describe the app (what does it do?) (E.G., A game that is prejudiced against a group).	
Describe the target audience. (Who would use it?)	
What technique does the app use to get its message across?	
Why is the technique wrong?	

D. After you and your partner are finished brainstorming ideas, think about
positive and negative consequences to choose the best solution or solutions.
Save your notes for the Final Assignment.

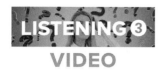

LISTENING ③
VIDEO

Contagion, Affirmation, and Lies: The Psychology of Social Media

A *contagion* usually refers to a dangerous disease that easily spreads from person to person. But dangerous ideas can also spread in the same way. Social media makes this simple because it's easier to insult someone and express strong emotions when you are not physically present. Have you ever written something online that you wouldn't say to someone's face?

VOCABULARY BUILD

In the following exercises, explore key words from Listening 3.

A. Read the sentences adapted from Listening 3 and insert an arrow ↓ where the key word (in parentheses) goes.

❶ (assumption) This that emotion is communicated primarily non-verbally is a very powerful idea .

❷ (depressed) The study showed that people tend to communicate much less than people who are happy .

❸ (detection) We're now doing a task ; we're going to see if we can watch emotion spread from one person to another .

❹ (empathetic) We knew he was because of the way he helped those who were having more problems .

❺ (conducive) It turns out that a group is much more to the spread of a contagion than just a dyad (pair) .

B. Match each of the key words to its synonym (word with the same meaning). Then work with a partner and use each key word in a sentence.

KEY WORDS		SYNONYMS
❶ interpreting	_____	a) unbiased
❷ induce	_____	b) explain
❸ clarify	_____	c) understanding
❹ tension	_____	d) pressure
❺ neutral	_____	e) persuade

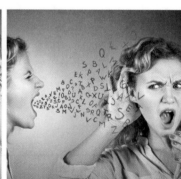

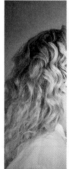
MyBookshelf > My eLab > Exercises > Chapter 3 > Vocabulary Review

Before You Listen

A. In 2016, Brandon Cardinal was about to start his shift at work when he got a text that said, "You're fired." The story made the news because it seemed a bad and impersonal way to share such important information. With a partner, think of three reasons people prefer to communicate by text rather than speaking in person.

_____

_____

_____

B. Read the introduction to Listening 3 and answer the questions. After, check your answers with a partner to see if you both agree.

> Well, one of the biggest questions around emotion and text is that text removes all of that. So, text is this really non-verbally poor channel. And when we have something to say like this or like that, the fact that there's a screen between us gets rid of all of that. And this assumption that emotion is communicated primarily non-verbally is a very powerful, very old assumption. And the modern legacy probably comes from Paul Ekman, a very famous, a huge-impact social psychologist. He was interested in emotion and facial expression. And so, we have been studying and thinking about how the face, the body, and the non-verbal cues express emotion.

1 Who is Paul Ekman?

_____

2 What assumption is made about emotion?

_____

3 Why are texts a poor channel?

_____

4 How is emotion expressed?

_____

_____

While You Listen

C. Listening 3 discusses human psychology as well as an experiment that tries to explore two questions. The first question is "Do texts sent by mobile and other devices show the sender's emotional state, even when the sender is not talking about emotions?" The second question is "Are those emotions contagious?" That is, when people are working on tasks and feeling happy or sad, do they influence other people reading their texts, even if they are not talking about emotions? As you listen, try to answer these questions. Listen a second time to check your answers and add details.

1 What is the speaker's perception of emotion in texts?

_____

_____

2 What examples does the speaker give for his ideas about emotion in texts?

_____

_____

3 How does the experiment try to make some of the subjects sad?

_____

_____

④ How does the experiment try to make some of the subjects have neutral emotions?

_____

_____

⑤ What is the result of the study?

_____

_____

D. Listen again to the last part of the presentation, in which students ask questions. As you listen, make notes on Hancock's answers. Listen again and add details.

STUDENTS' QUESTIONS	HANCOCK'S ANSWERS
Student #1: Can you just **clarify** real quick? You said they talk and that they text. Was there verbal talking, or texting?	
Student #1: So there were no physical cues at all?	
Student #2: So how was **tension** different from negative affect?	
Student #3: When they followed up to do their texting, were they talking about neutral topics? Was there something they were supposed to talk about or were they getting indignant ...?	
Student #4: Do you find the negative feelings are more contagious than happy feelings or are they kind of similar?	
Student #5: Did the neutral groups and the partners get to talk at all?	
Student #6: What were they texting on?	
Student #6: No, no, I mean the device.	

After You Listen

E. Reconsider your answer to task A. Did the "You're fired" text message show emotion?

_____

F. Read the following statements and indicate whether you think each one is true or false. For each false statement, write the true statement.

STATEMENTS	TRUE	FALSE
1 Most people have always known that texts are good for communicating. _____ _____		
2 One way we indicate emotions in texts is through the degree of punctuation. _____ _____		
3 Depressed people are more likely to agree in text messages. _____ _____		
4 Arguments are more likely to occur in person than in emails because you can get other cues to emotions. _____ _____		
5 The reason for having the tissues in the room was because some people were likely to cry. _____ _____		
6 The experiment was only text-based, with no verbal communication among the subjects. _____ _____		
7 Emoticons are perfectly named because they accurately display a sender's emotions. _____ _____		
8 The subjects were not aware of what they were being evaluated on. _____ _____		

G. Now that you know that your texts can convey information about your emotions, what kinds of texts should you send or not send? Check the types of messages you think are OK to send, then compare your choices in a group to see if others agree. If they disagree, ask why.

_____ announcements   _____ complaints

_____ apologies   _____ compliments

_____ big secrets   _____ congratulations

_____ birthday wishes   _____ party invitations

Answering Questions

Answering questions is something you do all the time. But answering questions in a presentation is different. You have to be aware of the key types of questions and decide when and how to answer them, or whether to answer them at all. Understanding this can also help you ask better questions in the lectures and presentations you attend.

There are many types of questions and they have different purposes.

QUESTION TYPES AND PURPOSES	EXAMPLES	HOW TO DEAL WITH THEM
❶ **ADMINISTRATIVE QUESTIONS**: Usually to deal with a technical format or understand the format.	Could you turn up the volume, please? Will you be taking questions during the presentation?	Quickly deal with the problem or explain why you cannot (e.g., "Sorry, this is the best we can do.")
❷ **CHALLENGE QUESTIONS**: Often disruptive, questions from speakers who want to talk about their own ideas rather than listen to yours.	I think I know a lot more about this topic than you, so do you mind letting me share my ideas with the audience?	Suggest that the speaker save questions and comments until later and perhaps speak to you privately.
❸ **CLARIFICATION QUESTIONS**: Questions that aim to better understand a point that the speaker may not have fully explained.	Could you please explain the difference between the first one and the second one?	If you think it's a good question, pause and explain. If not, and the rest of the audience understands, say you'll come back to it later during the question period.
❹ **FURTHER INFORMATION QUESTIONS**: Questions that build on what you've said. You may or may not have time to answer them.	This is all very interesting but I'm wondering if you could tell us what you think it will be like a hundred years from now?	Answer according to how much time you have. During a presentation, you can suggest saving it for the question period.
❺ **OFF-TOPIC QUESTIONS**: Questions that are not related to the topic.	You speak very well but I wonder if you get nervous when you talk and if you have any tips for me?	Explain that the question is interesting, but not the focus of what you're talking about now. Suggest speaking together later.
❻ **RHETORICAL QUESTIONS**: Questions for which an answer is not expected. These are simply to make a point or to challenge the speaker.	We all agree that telephones will disappear in fifty years, don't we?	Suggest that it's an idea that you might discuss with the person later.

A. Imagine you are giving a presentation based on Listening 3 about emotions in text messages. Match the questions with the best responses.

QUESTIONS		RESPONSES
❶ I'm sorry, I can't see the image on the screen; could you move over?	_____	a) That's an interesting question, but not for today's lecture.
❷ I completely disagree with everything you're saying. Could I start by making three points.	_____	b) Good question. I meant this year.
❸ When you said "Now," were you talking about today or did you mean this year?	_____	c) I know you're trying to make a point, but let's move on.
❹ You mentioned texts; would your study also apply to emails?	_____	d) Certainly. Is that better now?

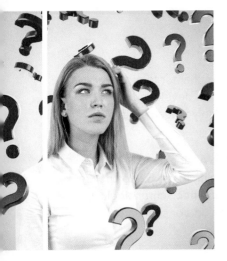

QUESTIONS		RESPONSES
5 Do you believe aliens are trying to communicate with us through secret messages on our phones?	_____	e) Yes, the two are quite similar in many ways.
6 You'd agree that no one was texting a hundred years ago, wouldn't you?	_____	f) Perhaps you could save your comments for the end of/after the presentation.

Three important rules when answering questions are to be *brief*, to be *clear*, and to be *polite*. Be brief by leaving out unnecessary information. Be clear by rephrasing part of the question and using signal words that you learned in Focus on Listening (page 52) to help your audience understand. Be polite by treating every question like it is worthy of respect—even if it is odd, off topic, or asked in an impolite way.

B. Rewrite the following answers to make them brief, clear, and polite. After, practise the questions and your answers with a partner to see if they could be briefer, clearer, and more polite.

1 QUESTION: I'm sorry, I know you've explained your three points once, but could you try to explain them again?

BAD ANSWER: Yes, I was talking about three inventions. The three inventions were wonderful. They included the invention of the electric computer, the transistor, and the memory storage system. They were all firsts. They were developed in 1939, 1947, and 1949. They led to the development of modern computers.

BETTER ANSWER: _____

_____

_____

2 QUESTION: Would you say that the invention of texting was a natural outcome of the invention of email?

BAD ANSWER: Well, let me think about that. I suppose, on reflection, I'd have to use my background in computing and long-term use of phones to answer in the negative in response to that question of yours.

BETTER ANSWER: _____

_____

_____

3 QUESTION: This all sounds like complete garbage and you're a complete fool to believe it, aren't you?

BAD ANSWER: Maybe you're the fool and just can't understand good ideas when you hear them.

BETTER ANSWER: _____

_____

_____

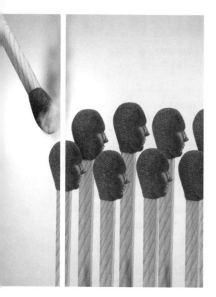

FINAL ASSIGNMENT
Present a Marketing Campaign

Now it's your turn. Use everything you have learned in this chapter to present a marketing campaign with your partner, using the ideas you developed in the Warm-Up Assignment (page 65) and the question expertise you learned in Academic Survival Skill (page 70).

A. With your partner, review your ideas from the Warm-Up Assignment. Based on your ideas, use what you learned in Focus on Listening (page 52) to choose the best way or ways to organize your ideas: cause and effect, chronological, classification, comparison, contrast, definition, process, and/or summary.

_____

_____

B. Use what you learned in Focus on Critical Thinking (page 53) to describe a marketing campaign that will address the problem you identified.

Your marketing campaign needs to

- define the propaganda technique you identified in the Warm-Up Assignment and explain why it's a problem. Use what you used in Focus on Accuracy (page 58) to talk about the past;

- explain how you are going to raise awareness of the problem through a marketing campaign. For example, you may suggest a letter campaign, a website, an online infomercial, a video, or something else. (You just have to *explain* one of these, not create it.)

C. Divide the responsibilities to explain the app and the problem propaganda technique. Explain the viral campaign you would use to confront the problem. Use what you learned in Academic Survival Skill to understand and answer questions. As you talk, use what you learned in Focus on Speaking (page 64) to use stress and intonation to make your meaning clear.

D. As you listen to other presentations, ask questions during the presentations and after. Listen to others' questions and vary the question types so that the presenters have the opportunity to answer at least one of each of the six types of questions identified in Academic Survival Skill: administrative, challenge, clarification, further information, off-topic, and rhetorical questions. Use what you learned in Focus on Critical Thinking to identify the positive and negative consequences of the presenters' solutions.

> It's hard to answer questions during a presentation, but it's a valuable skill to develop!

E. After, comment on each presenter's delivery, messages, and skill in answering questions. Consider what others have done well so you can improve.

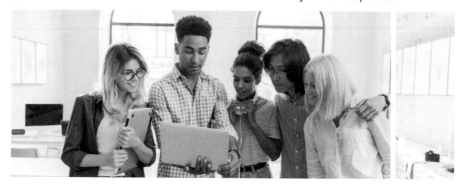

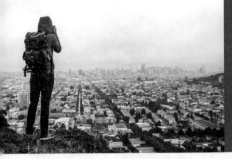

Critical Connections

In 1791, theatre owner Richard Daly (1758-1813) bet he could make a nonsense word popular. He had several people write the nonsense word *quiz* on walls around the city and, within two days, countless people were discussing it. The word *quiz* soon took on one of its modern meanings: "to ask questions." This story may not be true, but it's an example of how viral marketing works. Something interesting captures people's attention and spreads as they discuss it.

A. Use what you learned in Focus on Critical Thinking (page 53) to consider the problem of how you could promote a new word.

① Work with a partner and think of seven nonsense words. Then decide what each might be used for. For example, each one might be the name of a new start-up company, a new product, or a new service.

OUR NONSENSE WORDS	PURPOSES
❶	
❷	
❸	
❹	
❺	
❻	
❼	

② Choose the best of the nonsense words and explain whether it is the name of a company or the name of a product or a service. Write an explanation.

_____

_____

_____

③ Think of ideas to make the nonsense word go viral. What would be the best idea for promoting it? Would you create a song; put a video on YouTube; create an event that the media would report on? Try to think of a few other creative options and choose the best one.

Your best idea: _____

_____

B. Meet with another pair of students and share your ideas. Ask questions about how the viral marketing strategy would work. As you discuss, use what you learned in Focus on Speaking (page 64) to vary your stress and intonation. Use what you learned about question types in Academic Survival Skill (page 70) to ask and answer questions. After, share your best ideas in a group.

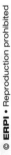

CHAPTER 4
Changing Business

Would you like to be a business innovator? How about creating a business brand? Innovative businesses carefully create brands by shaping how the public thinks about them, their products, and their services. In an increasingly competitive world, businesses struggle to stand out and offer new ideas. People are no different, and it may be time for you to think of yourself as a brand. The qualities, skills, and interests that shape who you are set out the differences of your personal brand. Once you have a better idea of who you are, you can begin changing the world.

In this chapter,
you will

- learn vocabulary about business and innovation;

- listen to identify bias;
- learn to summarize key information;
- practise using the passive voice;

- learn when to use formal and informal language;
- develop interview skills;
- profile a business innovator and conduct an interview.

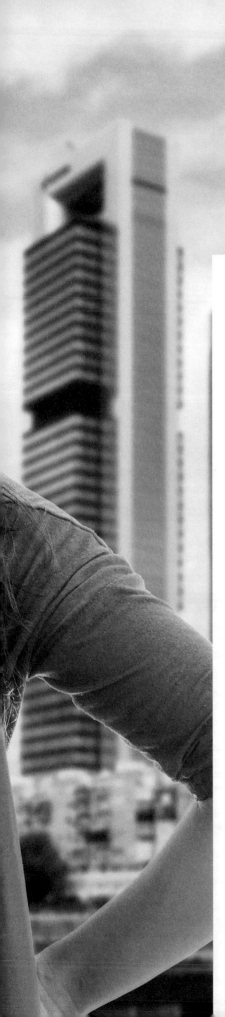

GEARING UP

A. Look at the steps in the infographic that show the process of moving from an idea to selling a finished product in stores. Then, answer the questions.

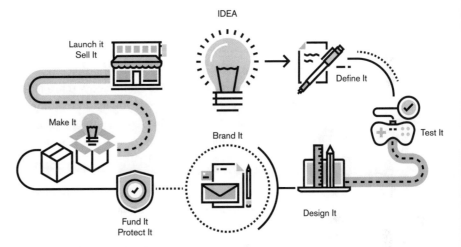

❶ Why is it necessary to *define* an idea after thinking of it?

_____

❷ Testing and designing a product often involve showing prototypes (samples) to others. Why do businesses do this?

_____

_____

❸ Besides using your own money to fund a new product, what other ways could you pay your costs?

_____

_____

❹ In a larger company, which step in the process would you most like to be involved in? Why?

_____

B. Work in groups. Compare your answers with those of other students to see if they have other ideas.

Below are the key words you will practise in this chapter. Check the words you understand, then underline the words you use. Highlight the words you need to learn.

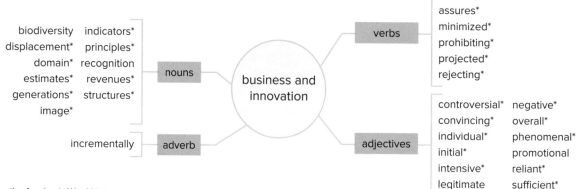

biodiversity   indicators*
displacement*   principles*
domain*   recognition
estimates*   revenues*
generations*   structures*
image*

incrementally → **adverb**

nouns → business and innovation

verbs →
abandoned*
assures*
minimized*
prohibiting*
projected*
rejecting*

adjectives →
controversial* negative*
convincing*   overall*
individual*   phenomenal*
initial*   promotional
intensive*   reliant*
legitimate   sufficient*

* Appears on the Academic Word List.

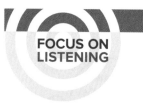

Listening for Bias

Are you biased? You don't have to think about it; the answer is *yes*. You're biased because you tend to have unconscious thoughts about the world based on what you've learned. For example, you are likely biased in favour of the foods you grew up eating. But when you listen to someone speak, it's important to be able to understand what biases they might bring to a lecture or a conversation and why they might have them. Sometimes, strong biases can stop them—and you—from understanding the truth.

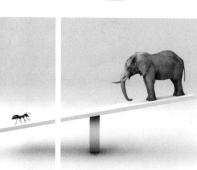

A. Consciously or unconsciously, biased speakers often use strategies to try to change how you think. Look at the biased strategies and connect each one to an example.

BIASED STRATEGIES		EXAMPLES
❶ ignores or dismisses important facts	_____	a) Using oil is wrong because everyone hates the oil industry and thinks it makes people sick.
❷ uses overly positive or negative words	_____	b) I'm sure you have other opinions, but there's only enough time for me to share my ideas.
❸ only offers opinions and emotional perspectives	_____	c) This is absolutely the greatest invention ever, and people will love using it for the rest of their lives. You should buy two!
❹ oversimplifies or overgeneralizes information	_____	d) I know that most environmentalists argue that we consume too much, but as a businessperson, I disagree.
❺ limits discussion of a topic	_____	e) Unethical businesses are OK; think of the world as an apple with a couple of bad spots that don't change its taste.

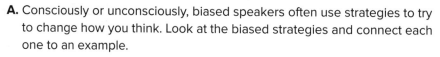

A hidden bias is often referred to as a hidden agenda.

When you listen for bias, you need to consider the speaker's purpose. Sometimes this is obvious, such as a teacher teaching or a salesperson selling. Sometimes the bias is hidden.

B. Listen to three speakers and work with a partner to identify the bias and purpose of each speaker, as well as the biased words each one uses.

① SPEAKER'S BIAS: _____

_____

SPEAKER'S PURPOSE: _____

BIASED WORDS: _____

② SPEAKER'S BIAS: _____

_____

SPEAKER'S PURPOSE: _____

BIASED WORDS: _____

③ SPEAKER'S BIAS: _____

_____

SPEAKER'S PURPOSE: _____

BIASED WORDS: _____

C. In a group, share a few sentences, talking about something that you strongly like or dislike. Your group members then identify any biases you have, including the points in task A.

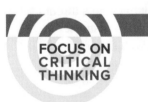

FOCUS ON CRITICAL THINKING

Summarizing Key Information

Because you cannot remember every detail of everything you read or hear, summarizing is an important academic skill. Summarizing key information is useful to improve your abilities to understand, to express yourself, and to take notes. A summary should be shorter than the original passage and written in your own words. Use these steps during, or after, listening to someone speak:

- Identify the main ideas.
- Focus on answering *who, what, when, where, why,* and *how* questions.
- Include your opinions, but keep them separate.

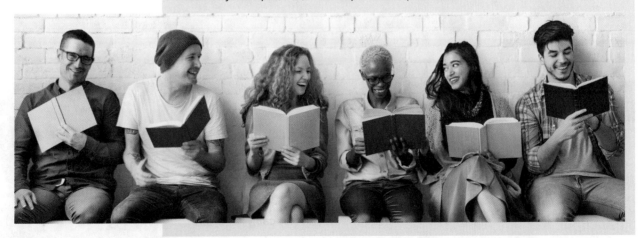

A. Besides main ideas and *wh-* questions, what parts of a talk should you note and which should you ignore? Work with a partner to complete the table.

PARTS OF A TALK	NOTE	IGNORE
1 conclusions		
2 examples		
3 ideas that are repeated		
4 information on a chart		
5 numbers		
6 long lists		
7 people's titles, like *Ms., Dr., Prof.*		
8 topic sentences		

> Topic sentences often contain the main ideas.

B. Read the following paragraph adapted from Listening 2 (page 84). Highlight the main ideas and points that answer *who, what, when, where, why,* and *how* questions.

> The earliest use of coffee was around mosques, to keep those who are calling worshippers for prayer awake. And then people started gathering around mosques to consume coffee. And that changed the social order, in that instead of the leaders being the ones who would disseminate information on how society functions, people would gather around coffee houses and they would start sharing information. So, it became a threat to the way society was organized. And it was actually quite dramatic when coffee got to the Ottoman Empire. In the early days, if you were found drinking coffee, you were first caned and then, if you were caught drinking coffee for the second time, you were basically sewn in a bag and thrown into a river.

> Summaries of longer passages follow the same principles. You may write a few shorter summaries and then put them together for study notes.

C. Use what you identified in task A to write a one- or two-sentence summary of the paragraph. Remember to use your own words and cut unnecessary information. After you finish, practise saying your sentences with a partner.

_____

_____

LISTENING ❶ **Creating Your *Me* Brand**

You may not realize it, but you already have a brand. Your identity is a reflection of the clothes you wear, your hairstyle, the things you own and use—even the friends you make. But does this really represent you? How do your personal experiences shape you and play a part in creating what you can call your brand?

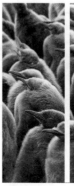
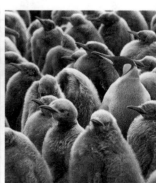

In the following exercises, explore key words from Listening 1.

A. Consider the context of these sentences adapted from Listening 1 and fill in the blanks with words from the box.

indicators	individual	overall	projected	recognition

1 Brand _____ is tied up in many details beyond a logo, a slogan, or a jingle.

2 An _____ who is different from his or her competitors is in a better position to compete in the workplace.

3 Starbucks' brand image is _____ by its colours.

4 People get a general idea about your age and even your income level from your clothing and _____ appearance.

5 Billionaires often dress in casual clothes, so possessions or personal style are not always strong _____ of someone's wealth.

B. Match each word from the box with its three synonyms.

abandoned	image	initial	minimized	principles

1 beliefs, codes, values _____

2 discarded, uncontrolled, wild _____

3 early, first, original _____

4 diminished, lessened, reduced _____

5 appearance, look, representation _____

C. Write sentences using the pairs of words in parentheses.

1 (abandoned / principles)

_____

2 (individual / image)

_____

3 (initial / recognition)

_____

Before You Listen

A. Famous people are their own brands. Their names and faces are like their logos, promoting who they are and what they represent. When you consider the following professions, who are the individuals you think of, and what does each person represent?

PROFESSIONS	INDIVIDUALS	WHAT THEY REPRESENT
1 actor		
2 athlete		

PROFESSIONS	INDIVIDUALS	WHAT THEY REPRESENT
❸ businessperson		
❹ musician		
❺ politician		

B. Read the beginning of Listening 1, answer the questions, then discuss your answers with a partner.

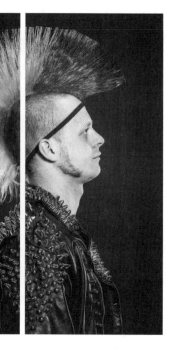

> Today, in this lecture about business, we will be discussing marketing, but starting from an unusual point of view. That point of view is *you*. At some point in our life, each of us asks, "Who am I?" Even as I say the words, you probably have a series of images appearing in your mind about who you are. We define ourselves in many ways: by nationality, by profession, by the things we like to do, be it riding motorcycles, playing hockey or studying dance. What I would like to do during this lecture is explore these and other qualities in terms of a business model. Essentially, I want to explore principles of business that have to do with branding and will ask you to consider yourselves in terms of a *me* brand.

❶ Based on what you learned in Focus on Listening (page 76), what is the speaker's bias?

_____

_____

❷ If you were a brand, what product or service would you represent?

_____

_____

❸ What is something you might like to do to stand out from the crowd; that is, be different than everyone around you?

_____

_____

While You Listen

C. Read the topic sentences and use what you learned in Focus on Critical Thinking (page 77) to summarize each section in one or two sentences. Listen again to check your summaries and to add details.

TOPIC SENTENCES	SUMMARIES
❶ Today, in this lecture about business, we will be discussing marketing, but starting from an unusual point of view.	*You are your own brand, as defined by your activities and experiences.*
❷ Before we go into the personal qualities that shape each of us and that play a part in creating what we can call our brands, let's discuss what a brand is.	
❸ I'm sure you can quickly think of a number of different companies or organizations and how they are branded.	

TOPIC SENTENCES	SUMMARIES
4 Brand recognition is tied up in many details beyond a logo, a slogan or a jingle. Jingles—short snippets of song to promote a product—were popular when most people got their news and advertisements from radio, but they are less popular today.	
5 So far we've been talking about brands and branding as they relate to companies and organizations.	
6 It's an interesting idea and one that a lot of people have embraced over the past few years, particularly as social media have allowed people to "sell" themselves, so to speak, through online services like Facebook and LinkedIn, where you can create a profile of yourself through a formal or informal curriculum vitae, or resumé.	*Creating a profile on social media is a form of personal branding.*
7 First, let's address *you* at your most basic level.	
8 But few of these things are really important in branding yourself—unless they work to your advantage in some particular way.	
9 I'm going to continue to frame these ideas in business contexts, so in this case, we can say that the personal impression that you give is like a packaging design on a box, or the cover of a book.	
10 Regardless of what you look like and how others perceive you, aspects of your personal appearance can shape you, as does your personal history.	
11 In a business context, for purposes of your personal brand, past relationships will have a lot to do with how you work with others.	*You need to question your relationships with others.*
12 What are your beliefs and values?	
13 Education and work experience can also shape your concept of your identity, that is, your personal brand.	*Educational and business experiences add to your personal brand.*
14 At the same time, many people who have *not* graduated from university have gone on to create their own companies and have done well.	*Bill Gates is defined by his business successes.*
15 We started off discussing the idea of the *me* brand.	

After You Listen

D. Review your notes and think of two ways that a personal brand differs from a business brand.

1 _____

2 _____

E. Check your comprehension by referring to your summaries from task C to choose the best phrases to complete these statements.

1. One of the main purposes of a business brand is _____.
   a) to connect consumers to products and/or services
   b) to show how successful a company has become
   c) to show that a company is different than an individual

2. When a company chooses a slogan, it _____.
   a) never rethinks it
   b) rarely improves it
   c) often changes it

3. Jingles are less popular now because _____.
   a) radio is a less common advertising medium
   b) most of the good tunes have already been taken
   c) people get tired of listening to the same songs

4. The example of Starbucks is meant to show _____.
   a) how easy it is to find a nearby coffee shop
   b) how a logo is used in multiple applications
   c) why few people go to other coffee shops

5. Tom Peters' points on creating a *me brand* are mostly about _____.
   a) understanding yourself
   b) differentiating yourself
   c) competing with yourself

6. Others are likely to make a quick judgment about you _____.
   a) based on your accent
   b) from what they've heard
   c) within three seconds

7. The example of billionaires dressing in casual clothes suggests they _____.
   a) are more worried about their personal brands
   b) don't understand their personal brands
   c) are less worried about their personal brands

8. An example of your personal beliefs is _____.
   a) worrying about what to wear each morning
   b) thinking the world is inherently fair or unfair
   c) wondering if others like the way you speak

9. The speaker suggests that going to an important university is _____.
   a) more important than doing well there
   b) less important than being a top student elsewhere
   c) the only reason certain people get the best jobs

10. The speaker mentions *hobbies* and *interests* as things that _____.
    a) take away from your personal brand
    b) should not be mixed with business
    c) can shape your personal brand

F. You've probably heard popular slogans such as "I'm lovin' it!" and "Just do it!" and can identify the companies they represent. Write a slogan that captures your personal brand. Discuss your slogans in a group and choose the best ones.

MyBookshelf > My eLab >
Exercises > Chapter 4 >
Creating Your Me Brand

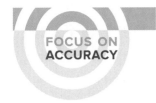

FOCUS ON
ACCURACY

Using the Passive Voice

"Your computer was broken this morning." When you hear a sentence like this, your first question is likely to be, "Who broke it?" This points out what is often a problem with the passive voice. It doesn't specify the *actor*—the person or thing that has done the action. When you listen or speak about actions, it's important to know when and when not to use the passive voice.

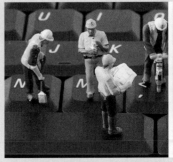
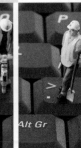

A. In some cases, there are good reasons for using the passive. Connect the reasons with the examples.

REASONS FOR USING THE PASSIVE VOICE		EXAMPLES
❶ to explain something when the actor is unknown	_____	a) Electric power lines were installed first in New York.
❷ to explain something when the actor is unimportant	_____	b) The electric chair was promoted by Edison.
❸ to avoid responsibility	_____	c) Electricity is used by everyone.
❹ to share a general truth	_____	d) Hundreds of years ago, electricity was little understood.
❺ to emphasize the thing or person that's receiving the action	_____	e) In Denmark, electricity is commonly produced through the motion of wind turbines.
❻ to speak about scientific processes	_____	f) Mistakes were made.

The passive voice presents problems for speakers and listeners when the reasons for using it are not clear. If a speaker is using the passive voice and you cannot understand why, ask the speaker to explain and identify the actor.

B. Read these sentences and write questions about unclear or missing information. After, take turns with a partner saying the statements and asking the questions.

❶ Studies were done to show that most people prefer certain company brands.

_____

❷ You have been identified as one of our ideal customers!

_____

© **ERPI** • Reproduction prohibited

③ Because of an error, your tickets were cancelled.

_____

④ Slogans were invented to make products and services memorable.

_____

⑤ Pictures were used in place of slogans when many people could not read.

_____

C. Sometimes the passive voice is vague. Read the sentences and write questions about the unclear information.

❶ A letter is supposed to be sent to the company lawyer.

_____

❷ Lunch may be eaten in the office cafeteria.

_____

❸ The job might be gone if you don't apply today.

_____

❹ She has to be seen by someone in human resources.

_____

❺ An answer had better be left with the receptionist.

_____

MyBookshelf > My eLab >
Exercises > Chapter 4 >
Focus on Accuracy

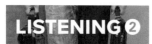 **LISTENING ❷**   **Innovation and Its Enemies**

While you may embrace change, new ideas always have their enemies—those who try to stop a disruptive product or service. Often, opposition is for selfish reasons, such as to crush competition. Coffee, household electrical systems, and ways of working are examples of innovations that have faced strong opposition.

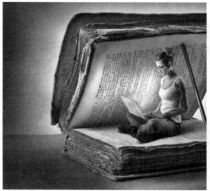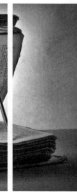

VOCABULARY BUILD

In the following exercises, explore key words from Listening 2.

A. Match the key words to the set of words that form collocations, then practise using the collocations in sentences.

KEY WORDS		WORDS THAT FORM COLLOCATIONS
❶ controversial	_____	a) of people, of water
❷ displacement	_____	b) strongly, immediately

KEY WORDS		WORDS THAT FORM COLLOCATIONS
❸ generations	_____	c) changing, increasing
❹ incrementally	_____	d) current, older
❺ rejecting	_____	e) decisions, politically

B. Complete the sentences adapted from Listening 2 using the words in the box.

biodiversity	domain	intensive	structures	sufficient

❶ Even though it was a good idea, it wasn't getting _____ political support.

❷ Coffee also undermined some economic _____ in society, because it was a threat to the consumption of milk, beer, and wine.

❸ This was an academic paper that was free for everyone to read because it was in the public _____.

❹ Unlike tea, which could easily dry at home, coffee roasting is actually quite technologically _____.

❺ He went on to head the development of the United Nations Convention on _____, studying how to address genetically modified organisms.

Before You Listen

A. Read an opening excerpt from Listening 2. Highlight the main ideas and the points you would include in a summary. Then, write a one- or two-sentence summary.

> This season on *The Current*, our project The Disruptors has been looking at the often-unforeseen forces that change the way we live. Of course, it's often a technological breakthrough that changes our day-to-day life in ways that we cannot have imagined. Even when that change is for good, there's a pattern in history that when technology disrupts, it's greeted by opposition. Society's inborn fear of innovation has some deep roots, from pratical issues such as the fear of technology replacing jobs to fears about the loss of identity and fears of social upheaval. New technologies—from tractors to GMOs, recorded music to margarine—have all been met with resistance.

SUMMARY: _____

_____

B. Based on your summary, answer these questions.

❶ Besides the three fears mentioned above, what is one other reason people oppose innovations?

_____

_____

❷ Besides tractors, genetically modified organisms (GMOs), recorded music, and margarine, what are three other modern innovations?

_____

_____

③ Choose one of the innovations you identified in question 2 and explain the reasons some people may oppose it. Discuss your answers in a group.

_____

_____

_____

While You Listen

C. Listen to Calestous Juma's responses to Anna Maria Tremonti's interview questions and take notes to summarize his answers. After, listen again to check your notes.

ANNA MARIA TREMONTI	CALESTOUS JUMA
❶ Why was margarine, of all things, such a controversial thing both politically and technologically?	• *opposed by the dairy industry* • *preferred by the poor because it was cheaper*
❷ And even in Canada, Canada banned margarine until 1948. But then there were laws about the colour of margarine. Note: Sometimes a speaker makes a point and the listener understands that it is a request to explain.	
❸ In fact, people did ... They had a little colour bead that they would put in the margarine and mix it all up. How strong was the scientific case against margarine in terms of health and safety at the time?	
❹ Even now, nearly 150 years after it was created and invented, there is still a debate about the relative merits of margarine versus butter. Why can battles over the acceptance of something new like that drag on for so long?	
❺ What are people afraid of when it comes to new technology?	
❻ When people argue against adopting a new technology, what else comes into play beyond facts?	
❼ Interesting, interesting. When personally did you see this kind of resistance to new ideas?	• *local rejection of cassava despite a desperate need for a new source of food*
❽ You went on to head the development of the UN Convention on Biodiversity in its early days in the nineties, and with it the discussion about how to address genetically modified organisms. What did you learn from being in the middle of the GMO controversy?	• *vested interests protect incumbent (existing) industries*
❾ You got caught up in a controversy yourself two years ago, over failing to disclose discussions with Monsanto about a paper that you wrote about the risks of rejecting biotechnology. What happened there?	• *this was a paper that was in the public domain*

ANNA MARIA TREMONTI	CALESTOUS JUMA
⑩ Before we move on from food, why do you call coffee a disruptive innovation?	
⑪ And why is that disruptive? Or why was that disruptive?	
⑫ Well, Germany called it unpatriotic. Because it was a threat to beer?	
⑬ I want to ask you about electricity as well.	
⑭ It's extraordinary to think that an industrial fight, I was going to say sparked, and I don't mean a pun …	
⑮ OK. We're listening to Charlie Parker with the tune "Donna Lee." Between 1942 and 1944, Charlie Parker and essentially all other musicians in the US were not making records. Why was that?	
⑯ It's interesting, because it is a good example of an industry where people did lose jobs because of the technology. But as the technology became better, it created whole new areas of work.	

After You Listen

D. There were biases against the following five innovations. Explain who was opposed to each one and why. Include the false reasons for opposing the innovation and the true reasons for opposition. After, discuss your answers with a partner.

① MARGARINE

OPPOSED BY: _____

FALSE REASON: _____

TRUE REASON: _____

② CASSAVA

OPPOSED BY: _____

FALSE REASON: *none given* _____

TRUE REASON: _____

③ GENETICALLY MODIFIED ORGANISMS (GMOs)

OPPOSED BY: _____

FALSE REASON: _____

TRUE REASON: _____

cassava

4 **COFFEE**

OPPOSED BY: _Ottoman Empire; German king_ _____

FALSE REASON: _soldiers ..._ _____

TRUE REASON: _____

5 **ALTERNATING CURRENT**

OPPOSED BY: _____

FALSE REASON: _____

TRUE REASON: _____

6 **RECORDED MUSIC**

OPPOSED BY: _____

FALSE REASON: _none given_ _____

TRUE REASON: _____

E. In Listening 2, an example of a disruptive technology is alternating current (AC), the electricity system used by most home appliances worldwide. Inventor Thomas Edison (1847–1931) favoured his own version of electricity called direct current (DC), now mostly used in batteries. He fought AC's introduction, saying that it "will kill a customer within six months after he installs a system of any size." Can someone be an innovator and still oppose innovations by others? Why or why not? Discuss with a partner.

F. An audio clip (transcript below) in the interview features Eleanor Roosevelt (wife of an American president) talking about the butter substitute, margarine. Use what you learned in Focus on Listening (page 76) to identify Roosevelt's bias on the topic, including biased words she uses. Then, choose a food you like or dislike and talk about it in a group so your group members can identify your bias.

> Years ago, most people never dreamed of eating margarine. But times have changed. Nowadays, you can get a margarine like the new Good Luck, which really tastes delicious. That's what I've spread on my toast. I thoroughly enjoy it.

_____

_____

_____

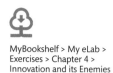

MyBookshelf > My eLab >
Exercises > Chapter 4 >
Innovation and its Enemies

**FOCUS ON
SPEAKING**

Using Formal and Informal Language

"How do you do?" "How you doing?" Both phrases are common greetings but they differ in terms of their level of formality. When deciding whether to use formal or informal language, it's important to adapt your vocabulary and grammar to the context of a conversation, the person with whom you are speaking, and the topic of the conversation.

Formal words tend to be longer than informal words. Informal language features more phrasal verbs. Informal language also features many slang expressions, while formal language does not.

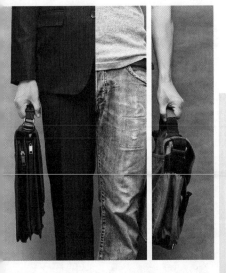

A. Match the formal words to the informal words and expressions.

FORMAL WORDS		INFORMAL WORDS AND EXPRESSIONS
1 ascertain	_____	a) get in touch with
2 fabricate	_____	b) put up with
3 oppose	_____	c) make up
4 contact	_____	d) start
5 commence	_____	e) find out
6 tolerate	_____	f) go against

In terms of grammar, here are three differences between formal and informal language:

1. Formal language tends to feature complete sentences; informal language often includes incomplete sentences.

2. Formal language emphasizes correct grammar; informal language is less concerned with correct grammar.

3. Formal language uses the passive voice more often; informal language doesn't and tends to use more contractions and drops some words if they are commonly understood.

Knowing *when* to use formal or informal language is also important.

• Use formal language when there is a need to be exact, even in informal situations. Informal language is more common in situations that are not critical.

• Use formal language to show respect when speaking to people in authority and to show your own professionalism. This includes when you speak to your teachers and when you speak about the field you are studying.

• Use formal language with friends when the topic is serious, or understanding is critical.

B. Rewrite the following sentences adapted from Listening 2, making the formal ones informal and the informal ones formal. Practise the sentences with a partner, comparing your formal and informal language.

1 That got me really kind of mixed up a little bit, as a kid, that math was something over my head.

As a child, I was confused and thought mathematics was difficult. _____

_____

2 It is often technological breakthroughs that change our day-to-day lives in ways that we cannot have imagined.

_____

_____

3 Well, Germany squealed about it being unpatriotic because it was bad for beer.

_____

_____

C. The *context* refers to the situation or place where a conversation takes place, and the person you are speaking with or listening to determines the use of formal or informal language. Think of three contexts and three people who would call for the use of formal language.

CONTEXTS: _____

PEOPLE: _____

MyBookshelf > My eLab >
Exercises > Chapter 4 >
Focus on Speaking

WARM-UP ASSIGNMENT
Profile a Business Innovator

Now it's your turn to research and discuss a business innovator using the formal language rules you learned in Focus on Speaking. This Warm-Up Assignment will prepare you to take part in an interview in your Final Assignment.

A. Work in pairs and choose a business innovator. For example,

- Jeff Bezos, founder of Amazon
- Richard Branson, founder of Virgin Group
- Jessica Alba, actress and co-founder of The Honest Company
- Deepa Mehta, director, screenwriter
- Joseph-Armand Bombardier, inventor
- Oprah Winfrey, media founder

Ask your teacher if you can use another local or international business innovator you know.

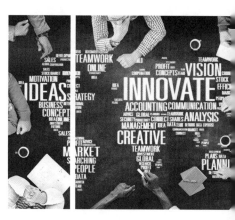

B. Discuss what you already know about the business innovator you selected. Do additional research online to find out about the innovator's background and accomplishments, using what you learned in Focus on Listening (page 76) to determine if your research sources are biased or not. Create a mind map to describe your business innovator. For example, here is one for Martine Rothblatt:

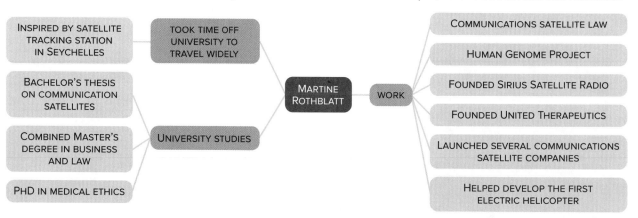

C. Take turns explaining your business innovator. Use what you learned in Focus on Critical Thinking (page 77) to summarize the innovator's achievements and what you learned in Focus on Accuracy (page 83) to use the passive voice when needed to express your ideas.

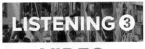

LISTENING ③ VIDEO

Fake Online Reviews

How often do you read fake reviews of restaurants or hotels? The answer is probably more often than you think! Fake reviews online are a way for businesses to attract more customers. People often trust reviews because they seem to come from the public and are assumed to be unbiased. But how do you know you can trust a review?

VOCABULARY BUILD

In the following exercises, explore key words from Listening 3.

A. Look at each list of words and choose the word that does not belong.

1. estimates, decides, projections, assessments

2. prohibiting, forbidding, exception, excluding

3. promotional, publicity, ignorance, persuasive

4. reliant, unsupportive, dependent, trusting

5. revenues, earnings, payments, income

B. Create common collocations by filling in the blanks with words from the box. After, practise the phrases in sentences with a partner.

assures	convincing	legitimate	negative	phenomenal

1. _____ excuse

2. _____ results

3. _____ view

4. _____ argument

5. _____ success

MyBookshelf > My eLab > Exercises > Chapter 4 > Vocabulary Review

Before You Listen

A. Read the following excerpt from Listening 3, and answer the questions.

> The better the reviews, the more we trust the business. For companies, that means a better bottom line. One extra star in a restaurant review and revenues can go up by as much as 9 percent. With so much money on the line, no wonder companies might be tempted to fudge their reputations. But how easy is it to fake it? We're using our Cheezed Off food truck to find out. Like every new business, Cheezed Off needs a website with lots of convincing photos, and that means a trip to our graphics department for a logo and a look.

1. Based on the context, what does "bottom line" mean?

_____

2. The phrase "on the line" can mean "connected by telephone". Based on the context, what does it mean here?

_____

Cheesed off is slang for angry.

③ Based on the context, what does *fudge* mean?

_____

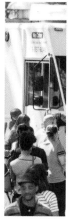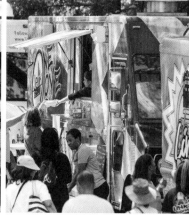

B. Imagine you are looking at reviews for a restaurant or a hotel you might want to visit. What might make you think that a review is fake? Discuss with a partner to see if you have different ideas.

A review is likely fake if _____

_____

While You Listen

C. Use what you learned in Focus on Critical Thinking (page 77) to write important points that can be made into a summary. Remember to pay particular attention to topic sentences, numbers, and repeated ideas.

COMMENTS AND INTERVIEWS	SUMMARY POINTS
① We're in the back alleys of North Toronto getting ready to assume a whole new identity.	*building a fake food truck to test fake advertising*
② Do you ever read online reviews?	*interviewee points:*
③ Online review sites work hard to gain your trust. Just check out this Hotels.com ad.	*guest interviews*
④ The better the reviews, the more we trust the business.	*more stars = more business*
⑤ CBC graphic designer	*discussion about*
⑥ CBC web designer: So, we've set up the website with a whole bunch of ...	*fake website as bait to*
⑦ What's our Twitter handle?	*fake Twitter and Facebook sites*
⑧ Next step in our creation of a fake business? We make a promotional video.	
⑨ Our ultimate goal is to see how easy it is to get some fake reviews and fake buzz for our fake truck.	*40* *500views.com:* *companies such as Universal and Sony*
⑩ fiverr.com	
⑪ True and fake reviews for a Chicago hotel	*only 1*

COMMENTS AND INTERVIEWS	SUMMARY POINTS
⑫ Jeff Hancock studies online behaviour, especially online fakery.	*54%*
⑬ Computer program Review Sceptic	*90%* *fake =*
⑭ Fake written and video reviews	*the examples are convincing*
⑮ Our hidden cameras take you inside an industry promising to help us fake it until we make it.	*companies will* *New York:*
⑯ Emizr worker explains ...	
⑰ ... fake reviews undermine our trust in the kindness of strangers and they could lead to some real trouble.	*dentist, lawyer, doctor reviews*
⑱ Most reviews are done out of revenge.	*most reviews are negative; positive ones …*
⑲ Yelp, Urban Spoon, Google	*Yelp catches* *Urban Spoon:* *Google:*
⑳ tigerdirect.ca	*changed*
㉑ Meantime, it's the end of the road for Cheezed Off.	*Conclusion:*

After You Listen

D. Look at your answer in task B. After making notes about Listening 3, would you change your answer in any way?

_____

_____

E. Based on the notes you made in task C, write answers to the questions. After, compare your answers with a partner to see if you both agree.

① Why do the interviewees on the street use online reviews?

_____

_____

② What is a reason one of the interviewees gives for trusting online reviews?

_____

_____

③ Why do businesses want more stars?

_____

_____

④ What's the goal of creating the Cheezed Off food truck?

_____

_____

⑤ How do Yelp, Urban Spoon, and Google differ in terms of dealing with fake reviews?

_____

_____

⑥ What does the article lead you to believe about fake online reviews?

_____

_____

F. The conclusion offers advice. Write three points for people concerned about fake reviews.

① _____

② _____

③ _____

G. Write a short summary of the main points of the video. Share your summary with a partner.

SUMMARY: _____

MyBookshelf > My eLab >
Exercises > Chapter 4 >
Fake Online Reviews

_____

Academic
Survival Skill

Developing Interview Skills

Interviews are all about getting information, finding out a story, or giving someone a chance to respond to questions. You may have had an interview to get into university or when applying for a job. You may also interview someone for class assignments, news, or opinions, either in person, over the phone, or on camera. It's important to learn the language of interviews.

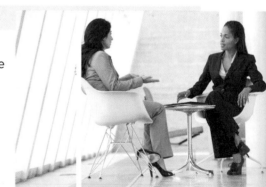

A. In Listening 2 (page 84), interviewer Anna Maria Tremonti uses a range of different question types. Read the questions and the explanations, and write questions you would ask a business innovator using the same format.

INTERVIEW QUESTIONS	EXPLANATIONS	YOUR QUESTIONS
❶ What are people afraid of when it comes to new technology?	An open-ended question invites a longer answer.	

INTERVIEW QUESTIONS	EXPLANATIONS	YOUR QUESTIONS
❷ And you weren't paid for that either, were you?	A closed-ended question invites a shorter answer.	
❸ You got caught up in a controversy yourself two years ago, over failing to disclose discussions with Monsanto about a paper that you wrote about the risks of rejecting biotechnology. What happened there?	A long statement is followed by a short question asking for an explanation.	
❹ But then there were laws about the colour of margarine.	Interviewers sometimes make statements and expect interviewees to talk about them.	
❺ So, in other words, the controversy around you is emblematic of what you're talking about.	A paraphrase of what the speaker said can be followed by, "Is that right?" but the question is usually understood.	
❻ Before we move on from food, why do you call coffee a disruptive innovation?	Transition phrases like "before we move on" help ready the speaker for the next question.	

B. For each of the following points, choose the best example of what you'd say or do during a formal interview.

❶ Be polite and formal, especially during introductions and closings.

   a) Thanks for taking the time to hang out and chat! / OK, that's all.

   b) Thank you for the opportunity to interview you. / Thank you for speaking with me.

❷ Use body language that is respectful and shows your interest.

   a) Relax and put your feet up on the table, like me.

   b) Please, have a seat and make yourself comfortable.

❸ Use some closed-ended questions.

   a) Are you writing a book about your business successes?

   b) What are your thoughts about a book on your business successes?

❹ Use some open-ended questions.

   a) What is the future of social media in business?

   b) Does social media have a future in terms of business?

❺ Ask follow-up questions.

   a) Let me start by asking whether you like every part of your job.

   b) You mentioned you love your job; could you tell me more about that?

❻ Use transitions to move to a new topic.

   a) If I can switch topics for a moment, what do you wish you'd done differently?

   b) What is the best business strategy? What do you think of IBM as a company?

Just like taking notes during lectures, it's also important to revise your notes soon after an interview.

C. Think of a time you have been interviewed (such as in a phone survey) or have interviewed someone else, and answer these questions. Compare your answers in a group.

1 What was the purpose of the interview?

_____

2 What is an example of a closed-ended question from the interview?

_____

3 What is an example of an open-ended question from the interview?

_____

FINAL ASSIGNMENT
Interview a Business Innovator

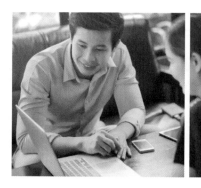

Now it's your turn. Use everything you have learned in this chapter to take part in an interview in which you play the role of the business innovator you researched in the Warm-Up Assignment (page 90). You will also take on the role of interviewer, finding out about other students' business innovators.

A. Choose a student other than the partner from the Warm-Up Assignment. Find out who (the business innovator) you will be interviewing. Once you do, take a few minutes to write interview questions based on what you learned in Academic Survival Skill (page 94). You should have a mix of the following:

• formal and informal language _____

_____

• closed-ended questions _____

_____

• open-ended questions _____

_____

• follow-up questions _____

_____

> Check to see whether the interview questions and answers show bias.

Remember to introduce yourself and welcome the interviewee and speak politely and formally, based on what you learned in Academic Survival Skill and Focus on Speaking (page 88).

B. For follow-up questions, you can use a mix of secondary questions based on your closed- and open-ended questions as well as additional questions based on the answers you hear.

C. At the end of the interview, briefly summarize what your interviewee has said, using what you learned in Focus on Critical Thinking (page 77). Thank your interviewee and switch roles.

D. After the interviews are complete, ask for feedback on three things you might improve.

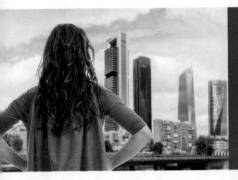

Critical Connections

Listening 2 (page 84) talked about many innovations that have faced opposition by different groups. Many of these groups have used false stories and misleading evidence to support their claims. Working with a partner, imagine that an innovative new device called HeadCom will replace computers and smartphones with a computer chip directly implanted into your brain.

1. Use what you learned in Focus in Critical Thinking (page 77) to summarize the benefits of the innovation. Use what you learned in Focus on Speaking (page 88) to discuss it in formal language with a partner, using examples of the passive voice that you learned in Focus on Accuracy (page 83).

2. List three groups who might oppose the new innovation and give a reason why each one might object.

GROUPS	NAMES	REASONS	REASONABLE	UNREASONABLE
GROUP 1:				
GROUP 2:				
GROUP 3:				

3. Decide if each group's bias against HeadCom is reasonable or not. Choose one reason and think of an argument against it, in favour of HeadCom. Discuss your ideas with a partner and choose the best ones.

CHAPTER 5

Applying Science

The scientific method evolved as a way of better understanding the world through careful observation, measurement, and experimentation. These processes help develop theories. The scientific method is also vital to inventing new devices and processes and improving old inventions. Scientific thinking begins with curiosity and, if all goes well, ends with understanding facts, such as the knowledge that the Earth goes around the sun, not the opposite. You use scientific thinking to solve problems and to make decisions. But some people ignore science and cling to ignorance and superstition.

How do you use science to help you make decisions about what you do and what you believe?

In this chapter, you will

- learn vocabulary about the scientific method;
- listen for cause and effect;
- use linking words to talk about cause and effect;
- learn how to evaluate a presentation;
- learn to develop an argument;
- cite sources in a discussion;
- explore a scientific issue and discuss cause and effect in a group

GEARING UP

A. A fishbone diagram outlines causes and effects. Imagine that the problem (effect) in the diagram is pollution. Answer the questions with a partner.

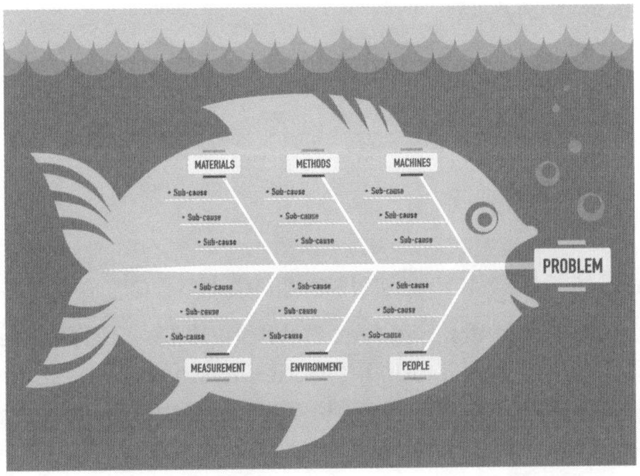

1. In the production of electricity, some materials, like *coal*, and some methods, like *burning* cause pollution. Does the use of wind-turbine towers produce any pollution?

   _____

   _____

2. It is easy to recognize how *machines* and *people* cause pollution, but how can *measurement* of pollution be a problem?

   _____

   _____

3. How can the *environment* add to pollution problems? Hint: Consider people who live in very hot or very cold countries.

   _____

   _____

4. The fishbone diagram was developed to examine industrial problems, such as the challenges of building a new car. In a group, briefly discuss what materials, methods, machines, measurement, people, and the environment might do to cause problems in building an electric car rather than a gasoline-powered one.

Below are the key words you will practise in this chapter. Check the words you understand, then underline the words you use. Highlight the words you need to learn.

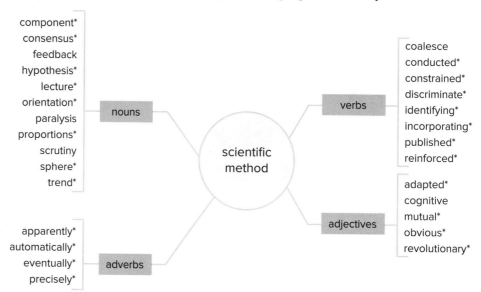

nouns

component*
consensus*
feedback
hypothesis*
lecture*
orientation*
paralysis
proportions*
scrutiny
sphere*
trend*

verbs

coalesce
conducted*
constrained*
discriminate*
identifying*
incorporating*
published*
reinforced*

scientific
method

adjectives

adapted*
cognitive
mutual*
obvious*
revolutionary*

adverbs

apparently*
automatically*
eventually*
precisely*

* Appears on the Academic Word List.

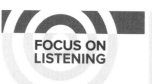

Listening for Cause and Effect

In 1666, scientist Sir Isaac Newton (1643–1727) witnessed an apple falling and wondered why it didn't fall sideways or up. These thoughts helped him develop the first theory of gravity. In this case, there was a *cause*—an apple falling. The *effect* was Newton developing his theory.

When people talk about *cause* and *effect*, they tend to use connecting words and phrases such as:

- as
- because
- due to
- owing to

A. Look at these examples of cause-and-effect sentences from Listening 1 and Listening 2 and highlight the cause-and-effect words and phrases.

1 As the word suggests, you are making your findings *public*.

2 If the prayers and sacrifices had no effect, the man might have decided his house was cursed.

3 We're not encouraged from the time that we're children to smell things. The result is that we don't really use our noses.

4 The lack of light was caused by a burnt-out light bulb.

5 We kind of deprive dogs of smells in our homes because we clean everything.

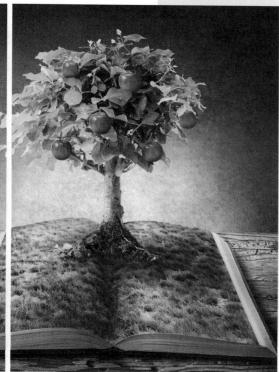

B. Make sure that there is a reasonable connection between the cause and the effect. Sometimes it is just a case of *correlation*, when two things happen to occur at the same time, but are not related. Read the sentences below and decide whether each one shows correlation or cause and effect.

SENTENCES	CORRELATION	CAUSE AND EFFECT
1 I was at work when the storm started.	✓	
2 I went home and saw the damage that had occurred.		
3 Due to the high winds, the roof of the house blew away.		
4 However, since it was the middle of the day, no one was home.		
5 Thanks to friends, I was able to find a place to stay for a few weeks.		
6 I tried to get a quick insurance payment, but it took a surprisingly long time.		
7 But because of fundraising in the community, I was able to rebuild within weeks.		
8 Everything is back to normal now and I've made a lot of friends.		

C. Listen to a paragraph about the ice ages—times when large parts of the Earth were covered by ice. Then write down the causes and the effects. Discuss your answers with a partner to see if you agree.

CAUSES: _____

EFFECTS: _____

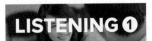

LISTENING ❶   **The Scientific Method**

What do you know about the scientific method? From its roots with the Greek scientist Aristotle (384–322 BCE), the scientific method evolved over the course of centuries as people explored new ways to measure and understand the natural world.

VOCABULARY BUILD

> ❗ Feedback is an example of a compound word. Compound words can be confusing because their meanings are not always obvious from the words that make them up.

A. Collocations are words that are commonly found in combination. Match each key word with words that form collocations.

KEY WORDS		WORDS THAT FORM COLLOCATIONS
1 scrutiny	_e_	a) speculative, testable, working
2 feedback	_____	b) broad, emerging, unspoken
3 hypothesis	_____	c) constructive, negative, valuable
4 lecture	_____	d) appear, look, seem
5 obvious	_____	e) careful, close, rigorous
6 consensus	_____	f) formal, impromptu, guest

B. Complete each sentence by using an arrow ↓ to indicate where the word in parentheses should go.

1 (consensus) Second , he looked for general , or agreement .

2 (conducted) The fourth step was when you an experiment .

3 (incorporating) Aristotle challenged this notion by measurement into his method .

4 (published) Finally , as a sixth step , you your findings .

5 (obvious) On the surface , it made sense .

C. Write sentences using the pairs of words in parentheses.

1 (revolutionary / published)

_____

_____

2 (scrutiny / consensus)

_____

_____

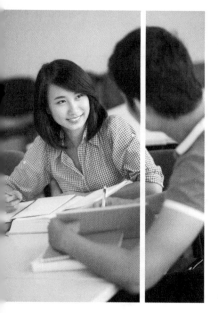

Before You Listen

A. Before listening to a lecture on the scientific method, read a paragraph from the beginning of the lecture, describing a common problem. The words and phrases in bold indicate the different steps in the scientific method to solve it. With a partner, review the steps and discuss another problem that you would solve following the same steps, such as how you would go about finding a lost phone.

"You enter your home—let's say your front hallway—and it's dark. You try to turn on a light switch but no light comes on. Not having any light in the hallway is a problem, so you **consider** a few things that might be **causing** it. You **do a little research** and see if other lights in your home work. They do. You then **decide that the problem might be** that the hallway light bulb has burned out. You find a new light bulb and change it. OK! It works. You've **solved** the problem. Later, you run into a friend and casually **mention** that the light wasn't working but that you identified and solved the problem."

While You Listen

B. Because this lecture describes a method, you can expect to learn about steps. While you listen, identify the steps and then write notes to explain each one. Listen again to add details.

STEPS IN THE SCIENTIFIC METHOD	NOTES/EXPLANATIONS
STEP 1: IDENTIFY A PROBLEM	

STEPS IN THE SCIENTIFIC METHOD	NOTES/EXPLANATIONS
STEP 2: LOOK FOR A CAUSE	
STEP 3: DO RESEARCH	
STEP 4: HYPOTHESIZE WHAT THE PROBLEM MIGHT BE	
STEP 5: APPLY THE SOLUTION AND SEE IF IT WORKS	

After You Listen

C. Review your notes. Based on what you've learned, do scientists usually start with causes or effects? Discuss your answer with a partner to see if you agree.

D. Choose the phrase that best completes each sentence, according to Listening 1.

1 Inductive reasoning refers to starting with _____.

   a) small details and developing a theory

   b) no details and relying on a theory

   c) large details and questioning a theory

2 Deductive reasoning refers to starting with _____.

   a) asking many people what they might think

   b) a question that has not ever been answered

   c) a general theory and then looking for evidence

3 Studying existing writings about a subject is called _____.

   a) doing a literature review

   b) making a bibliography

   c) creating an appendix

4 Aristotle held sway over scientific thinking _____.

   a) until he died

   b) for a long time

   c) for less than ten years

5 Arab scientist Ibn al-Haytham (965–1040) wrote a revolutionary book on _____.

   a) paper

   b) optics

   c) leather

6 Ibn al Haytham suggested the need to avoid, as much as possible, human observation as a _____.

   a) replacement for clocks

   b) form of measurement

   c) way of seeing things

7 Ali al-Rahwi (854–931) introduced the first peer review, in which results were _____.

   a) available for anyone in the public to look at

   b) kept secret for a period of one year

   c) first sent to other scientists for their comments

8 Galileo explained the need to question _____.

   a) nothing

   b) everything

   c) other scientists

9 Galileo refused to believe that the moon had anything to do with _____.

   a) the Earth

   b) the stars

   c) the tides

10 The scientist Copernicus offered scientific proof that _____.

   a) the Earth went around the sun

   b) the Earth and the sun went around each other

   c) the sun went around the Earth

MyBookshelf > My eLab > Exercises > Chapter 5 > The Scientific Method

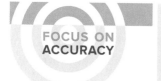

FOCUS ON ACCURACY

Linking Cause and Effect

When you talk about causes and effects, you use linking words to connect ideas. The most common of these linking words is *because*, e.g., "We stopped going to the moon **because** we wanted to build an international space station." Here are some things to know about using linking words.

- **Because** can be used with any combination of tenses.

- **Now that** is used for present causes of present or future situations.

- **Since** expresses a known cause. Note: *Since* is also used to indicate time.

- **Therefore** shows a result.

- **Consequently** has the same meaning as *therefore*, but it also gives a sense of occurring after a time.

- **So** often shows a result, but usually links clauses.

- **Such** and **so** show that something is to a high degree and may be used with **that**.

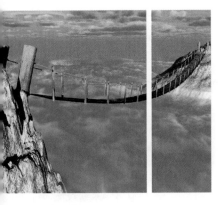

A. Based on the above explanations, read the sentences and use linking words to create new sentences. As a theme for your sentences, use the topic "bridges" or another topic approved by your teacher. After, practise the sentences with a partner to check that you have used the linking words correctly.

1 **Because** dogs have a good sense of smell, they're used to detect bombs.

Because bridges cross deep spaces, they have to be built high up.

2 Dogs are used to detect bombs **because** they have a good sense of smell.

_____

3 **Now that** we understand dogs' sense of smell, we can use it for medicine.

_____

4 **Since** dogs cost less than machines, it makes sense to use them.

_____

5 The dog was lost. **Consequently**, we found him.

_____

6 The dog was lost, **so** we looked for him.

_____

7 He was **such** a good dog **that** we gave him a treat.

_____

8 He was **so** pleased **that** he ran around the room.

_____

B. Use an arrow (↓) to indicate where in the sentence the linking word(s) in parentheses should occur.

1 (because) Many people believe in fairies of old stories about them .

2 (since) Fairies probably don't exist , there is no scientific evidence for them .

3 (so) However , there are mysterious small lights that are sometimes seen over marshes or swamps people believe they're fairy lights .

4 (so ... that) They are common people can often walk close to see them before they disappear .

5 (consequently) Early superstitions said they were lights carried by fairies who first wanted to attract people and drown them .

6 (now that) scientific experiments have been done , we understand the lights are caused by the decay of vegetation .

7 (therefore) , although some people will continue to believe in fairies , they shouldn't believe that they carry lights over marshes and swamps .

C. Rewrite the following pairs of sentences, using the linking words in parentheses to connect them. Add or delete words and punctuation as necessary. After, practise saying the sentences with a partner to check that you are using the rules correctly.

1 (because) The scientific method became popular. It better explained everyday mysteries.

_____

2 (such ... that) It was a different way of looking at things. It inspired people to conduct countless experiments.

_____

_____

3 (so) Galileo didn't believe the moon affected the tides. He never bothered to investigate them.

_____

_____

4 (since) Some people would rather be famous than right. They fake their experiments.

_____

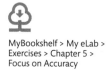

MyBookshelf > My eLab > Exercises > Chapter 5 > Focus on Accuracy

5 (now that) We have scientific experts on TV. More people are learning about science.

_____

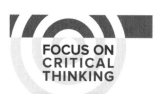

FOCUS ON CRITICAL THINKING

Evaluating a Presentation

Whom do you trust? When you listen to a speaker on a new topic, you are likely to evaluate the truth and value of the information. In academic situations, you need to make your evaluations based on whether speakers are authorities on the topic, whether their ideas are up to date, and what purposes the speakers have in sharing their ideas.

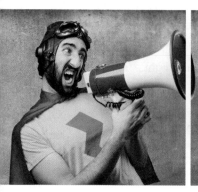

Authority

- Find out whether the speaker has professional qualifications related to the topic.
- If the speaker is not a professional, decide whether the ideas are supported by facts or research.
- Check to see if the speaker has written or spoken about the topic elsewhere.
- Decide if the information is original (primary research) or simply reports on research done by others (secondary research).

Up to date

- Find out whether the speaker's information is recent or not. If it's recent, is it from a reliable source?

Purpose

- Find out the speaker's purpose for sharing ideas. For example, a professor explaining scientific principles is probably more trustworthy than a stranger sharing an opinion. This is because the professor is likely impartial and has little to gain whether you agree with the ideas or not. On the other hand, the stranger might have hidden reasons for wanting to convince you of something. A professor might suggest electric cars are good for the environment based on research to educate you. The stranger might say the same thing, but only in order to sell you an electric car.

A. Read the following paragraph from Listening 2 introducing Alexandra Horowitz. With a partner, decide how you would evaluate what she says based on the points about *authority*, being *up to date*, and *purpose*.

> To some, the world is divided into two groups: dog people and non-dog people. And, as you can hear, Alexandra Horowitz is definitely a dog person. When she was writing her *New York Times* best-seller, *Inside of a Dog*, she became enraptured with how dogs take in the world, which, she says, they do through scent. And that got her thinking. Sure, dogs have fifty times more olfactory receptors in their noses than we do, and yes, they can detect a teaspoon of sugar in two Olympic-pools worth of water. But you wonder, could she develop her own sense of smell to become more like a dog? Dr. Horowitz runs the dog-cognition lab at Barnard College in New York City and she's written a new book called *Being a Dog: Following a Dog into the World of Smell*.

_____

_____

_____

_____

_____

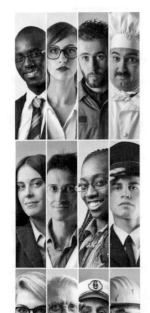

B. With a partner, briefly think about another authority you both know. It could be a friend, a relative, an acquaintance, or a celebrity. It could be someone in a particular profession. Rate the person's authority on the topic, being up to date, and having a clear purpose for sharing expertise. Evaluate each point on a scale from 1 to 10. After, discuss your rating.

TOPIC: _____

____ **AUTHORITY** (e.g., professional? research-based? talked or written about it before?)

____ **UP TO DATE?** (e.g., how recent?)

____ **PURPOSE:** _____ (e.g., to inform, to persuade, to sell, to discourage)

LISTENING ②   Being a Dog

The philosopher Ludwig Wittgenstein (1889–1951) once observed, "If a lion could talk, we would not understand it." The idea is that a lion's way of seeing the world is so different from our own that we would have nothing to communicate and few common interests. But what about other animals? Most pet owners feel close to their animals and consider that they understand each other and perhaps see the world the same way. Do you have a pet? Do you think you can communicate with it?

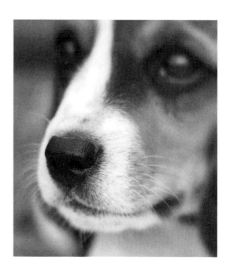

VOCABULARY BUILD

A. Choose the correct words from the box to complete the sentences.

component	constrained	discriminate	identifying	precisely

An important _____ of any doctor's tool kit is his or her senses.

A doctor's senses are used to _____ fine differences in

colour, texture, and smell. Of course, a young doctor's senses might be

_____ by a lack of training, but they are useful for getting a general

idea. For diagnoses that must be done more _____, a doctor

turns to _____ patient problems with a wide range of clinical tests.

B. Each of these key words has a core form called a *root word*. Write the root word and a short definition or synonym for each one. Look up those you do not know in a dictionary.

KEY WORD	ROOT WORD	DEFINITION OR SYNONYM
❶ apparently		
❷ constrained		
❸ identifying		
❹ precisely		
❺ automatically		

Before You Listen

A. Before you listen to an interview about a dog's sense of smell and what that means to the dog, discuss these questions with a partner and write short answers.

  ❶ How does a dog's sense of smell compare to a human's sense of smell?

_____

2 How effective are electronic noses compared to dogs' noses?

_____

3 Besides other dogs, what other animals can dogs locate using their sense of smell?

_____

B. Read the following paragraph from Listening 2 and identify an example of a cause and examples of different effects.

> About twenty years ago, there were a couple of examples of dogs that were bothering their owners by sniffing a part of their body repeatedly. And a couple of these people went to have that part of their body checked out at a doctor and found malignant melanomas. And it looked like the dogs had smelled the cancerous cells on their skin. Since that time, there have been a lot of research programs seeing if dogs can be trained on the breath, blood, or urine samples of cancer patients.

CAUSE: _____

_____

EFFECTS: _____

_____

While You Listen

C. The first time you listen, try to get the main ideas. Listen a second time to write details about Dr. Horowitz's answers to the points in your own words. Listen a third time to check your notes.

POINTS	MAIN IDEAS AND DETAILS
1 Before you began this journey, what part of your dog's experience were you hoping to tap into?	• _especially dogs because of their olfactory (smell) sense_
2 What is it about the dog's nose that makes it so good at smelling?	• _more olfactory receptor cells and more kinds of receptors_
3 You also talk about when they actually take a sniff, that they do it differently than we do.	
4 So, they're not blowing away what they're actually trying to smell.	• _side slit exhales create a puff of air = new odour molecules into their nostrils_
5 It really is a remarkable smelling machine, the dog's nose.	

POINTS	MAIN IDEAS AND DETAILS
6 Right. I think it's a high barrier.	
7 You also pointed out in your book that we kind of deprive dogs of smells in our homes ...	
8 Well, you talk about that in your book. About looking at these local landmarks. Tell me about the study on the pee posts in the park and what you found.	• *wolves mark territory, domestic dogs don't*
9 Well if it's not territorial, what are they doing?	
10 So, leaving calling cards.	• *Precisely.*
11 What was the most impressive dog-smelling feat you encountered?	• *Dr. Sam Wasser / Conservation Canines / a dog, Tucker, whom he uses to identify the location of orcas through their scat*
12 That's astounding. So he can track animals by their poop.	
13 Amazing. Well, you also talk about dogs that are being used to smell disease and even cancer.	• *a doctor found malignant melanomas (cancer)*
14 How good are they?	• *better than instruments and earlier detection*
15 You describe a hilarious scene in your book ...	• *wanted to understand what it's like to be an olfactory creature*
16 But did you actually smell what the dog was smelling in the park?	• *practice might make you more sensitive*
17 So you're saying that it's mostly just practice. We just don't do it.	• *dogs don't have a language like people so they have a different experience*
18 So you're saying not only stop and smell the roses, but smell everything else you can at the same time.	• *maybe you can smell the hand of the person who last touched that rose*

After You Listen

D. Work with a partner to list and discuss seven things you have learned about dogs and their sense of smell.

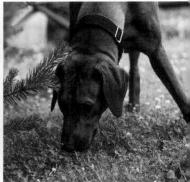

_____

_____

_____

_____

_____

_____

E. Use your notes from task C to match phrases and identify the main ideas from the interview.

PHRASES		
1 Dogs have a better sense of smell because ...	_____	a) so she tried smelling the same things as her dog.
2 One measure of the success of dogs' sense of smell is ...	_____	b) dogs spend more time smelling.
3 Unlike wolves that constantly mark their territory,	_____	c) of anatomical and behavioural differences from humans / more receptors.
4 Horowitz wanted to experience smells like a dog ...	_____	d) if they tried harder to notice smells.
5 People could likely improve their sense of smell ...	_____	e) electronic machines are not as good for things like smelling bombs.

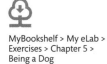

MyBookshelf > My eLab > Exercises > Chapter 5 > Being a Dog

F. In a group, reflect on the interview. Do the interviewer, Bob McDonald, and Dr. Horowitz both show authority, up-to-date information, and clear purpose?

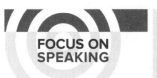

FOCUS ON SPEAKING

Developing an Argument

In academic speaking and listening, an argument is more than just disagreeing with others. Instead, an argument is about presenting evidence in a way that changes other people's minds and makes them believe or do something different. There are techniques you can use to develop an effective argument. In preparation for the Warm-Up Assignment, learn these techniques to help you evaluate and influence others' opinions, facts, emotions, and actions.

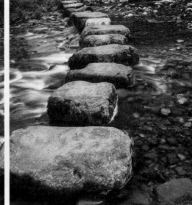

A. Developing an argument often follows five steps. Read the steps and number them in the correct order.

_____ Choose your point of view.

_____ Identify a topic that has more than one point of view.

_____ Summarize your argument and, if necessary, ask your listener(s) to take an action or make a decision.

_____ Think of how you can explain your facts and give examples.

_____ Research evidence to support your point of view with three or more facts.

B. The following statements are based on the five steps in task A. Number them to develop an argument, then practise the argument with a partner.

_____ Although there are challenges to living on Mars, we can do it and the first step is trying to understand that we can use science to help us.

_____ Many people wonder whether it's possible to send someone to Mars.

_____ Research suggests going to Mars is possible but we need to take action now to achieve that dream, by sending robots to Mars to build homes and farms.

_____ Research shows that Mars has water at its frozen poles, minerals that could be used for manufacturing, and carbon in the air that could be used to make plastics and fuel.

_____ I believe that it's both possible and something we need to do.

C. _Confirmation bias_ is the tendency for people to embrace points that support what they believe and reject facts that don't. What is a current fact that some people reject? Why might they reject it?

_____

_____

_____

_____

MyBookshelf > My eLab >
Exercises > Chapter 5 >
Focus on Speaking

WARM-UP ASSIGNMENT
Explore a Scientific Issue

Now it's your turn to explore a scientific issue and use cause-and-effect points to support a point of view.

A. With a partner, choose a topic on a scientific issue and identify a cause and three or more effects. You may use one of the topics below or check with your teacher if you can choose another one. For the statement you select, choose your point of view for or against the statement.

- The study of animals has many practical benefits.
  CAUSE: studying animals   EFFECTS: medical knowledge
- Climate change will make life on Earth impossible for humans.
  CAUSE: increasing pollution   EFFECTS: increasing storms
- Increased Internet use will make people less smart.
  CAUSE: dependence on   EFFECTS: less conversation
  the Internet for information
- Medicine will help people live to the age of two hundred.
  CAUSE: medical advances   EFFECTS: working longer
- Land-based fish farms will lead to cheaper foods.
  CAUSE: creation of new fish habitats   EFFECTS: efficient harvesting

B. Draw a fishbone diagram like the one in Gearing Up (page 99) to list the *cause* and three or more effects.

C. Use what you learned in Focus on Speaking (page 111) to talk about the effects and develop them into an argument by adding a recommendation for something people should or shouldn't do, such as supporting more animal research.

D. Evaluate your argument based on what you learned in Focus on Critical Thinking (page 106). Consider whether your information shows authority and is up to date. What purpose might you have in sharing such information?

Academic Survival Skill

> There are many citation and reference formats. Find the one most common in your area of study.

Citing Sources in a Discussion

Speeches, lectures, and discussions often develop their arguments by featuring evidence from a book, video, article, or other media. When you refer to such content in a talk, it's important to give credit to the author or authors. Referring to where the information came from is called *citing* a source. In your talk, it's called a *citation*. The term *citation* is related to a *reference*. A reference is a written description of where a listener can find more information on the topic you mentioned.

A formal reference using the American Psychological Association (APA) format, which you would use in an essay, is:

- Horowitz, A. (2016) *Being a dog: Following a dog into the world of smell*. New York: Scribner.

Compare that to a spoken citation from Listening 2 (page 107):

- Dr. Horowitz has written a new book called *Being a Dog: Following a Dog into the World of Smell*.

The following are other ways to cite this same source. It's not always necessary to use the writer's first name or to list the city in which it was published or the publisher.

- In 2016, writing in *Being a Dog: Following a Dog into the World of Smell*, Alexandra Horowitz says …
- Alexandra Horowitz, author of a 2000 book, *Investigations*, writes about the "adjacent possible," saying …
- *Being a Dog: Following a Dog into the World of Smell*, a book by Horowitz published in 2016, suggests that dogs …
- Having read Horowitz's 2016 book, *Being a Dog: Following a Dog into the World of Smell*, I know that her idea of dogs' sense of smell is …

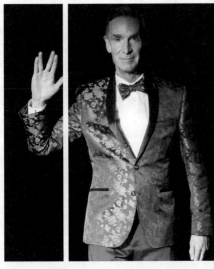

Bill Nye, The Science Guy

A. Read the following details about three references, and write an informative citation sentence that you would say for each. Include the quote and cite the relevant details.

DETAILS	REFERENCE SENTENCE CITING DETAILS
❶ "There are obviously still things we can learn from the moon." Mansbridge, P. (2016, May 1) One on one: Bob McDonald, host of CBC's *Quirks and Quarks. CBC.* Retrieved from http://www.cbc.ca newsmansbridge-one-on-one-bob-mcdonald-host-of-cbc-s-quirks-and-quarks-2016-part-1-1.3560896	
❷ "Gadget fixation is part of the problem, not part of the solution." Chatfield, T. (2016, Summer). The Classroom of the future. *New Philosopher.* 35–37.	
❸ "Algebra is the single most reliable indicator of whether or not you will pursue a career in math and science. It's not clear that it's cause and effect, but algebra not only enables you to think abstractly about numbers, it enables you to think abstractly about all sorts of things." Burdette, K. (2017), "Science Guy" Bill Nye's new mission. *Fortune.* Retrieved from: http://fortune.com/2017/03/30/bill-nye-science-guy-netflix-originals/	

B. Work with a partner and practise your sentences to see what you could improve.

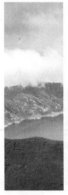
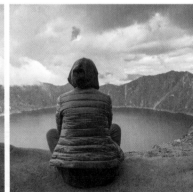

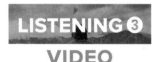

LISTENING ❸

VIDEO

One on One: Bob McDonald

If you could ask a scientist any question you wanted, what would you ask? Bob McDonald is a Canadian scientist and journalist who regularly answers the public's questions about scientific issues that concern them. He explains his ideas in easy-to-understand language, using engaging metaphors.

VOCABULARY BUILD

A. Reading words in context can help give an idea as to their meaning. Read sentences adapted from Listening 3 and fill in the blanks with words from the box.

adapted	eventually	mutual	paralysis	proportions

❶ Objects in space, when they do come together, are grabbed by gravity, their _____ gravity, and they'll spin around when they hang on.

2 So their shoulder joints are different from ours. They're _____ for the arms to be up.

3 But all rivers lead to the sea. Then the water _____ becomes salty.

4 There's a condition that we have in our brain called sleep _____. It's like a switch that switches off your motor cortex, which controls all your body movements.

5 They have long arms and short legs. So the _____ of the bones are different.

B. Read the key words and their synonyms (in parentheses). Use each key word in a sentence that illustrates its meaning.

1 coalesce (join)

_____

2 orientation (direction)

_____

3 reinforced (strengthened)

_____

4 sphere (ball)

_____

5 trend (tendency)

_____

MyBookshelf > My eLab > Exercises > Chapter 5 > Vocabulary Review

Before You Listen

When answering the question about the total amount of water on Earth, Bob McDonald gives a lot of detail. To simplify, you can summarize it in terms of the main idea, the cause, and the effects:

MAIN IDEA: water on Earth remains stable
CAUSE: water came from the original cloud that formed our solar system and the Earth
EFFECTS: volcanoes released water vapour

A. Read the paragraph and highlight the parts that show the main idea, the cause, and the effects.

> This is a fascinating question because the water we have today, which is dihydrogen monoxide by the way, that's its chemical formula, two hydrogen, one oxygen, is the same water we've always had. So the water came from the original cloud that formed our whole solar system and the Earth. So it was embodied within the Earth when the Earth coalesced out of that. So it spouted out of volcanoes.

While You Listen

B. Watch Peter Mansbridge interview Bob McDonald. After each question, take notes on the main ideas, the causes, and the effects. Watch again to add details.

QUESTIONS	MAIN IDEAS, CAUSES, AND EFFECTS
1 But how has it been, how is it returning?	**MAIN IDEA:** *freshwater changes to salt water and back again* **CAUSE:** *evaporation* **EFFECTS:** *it recycles through clouds, streams, rivers, lakes, and oceans; it changes form*
2 How delicate is the balance?	**MAIN IDEA:** **CAUSE:** **EFFECTS:**
3 I don't know whether you saw Suzuki the last couple of weeks.	**MAIN IDEA:** **CAUSE:** *environmentalists like David Suzuki* **EFFECTS:**
4 I've noticed that each time a volcano erupts, it always seems to be followed by an earthquake soon after. In your opinion, is there any correlation?	**MAIN IDEA:** **CAUSE:** *cracks in the surface of the Earth* **EFFECTS:**
5 In a word, are we getting any closer to predicting earthquakes?	**MAIN IDEA:** *predicting earthquakes has to be precise* **CAUSE:** **EFFECTS:**
6 Randy Chappel: My question is, why don't they fly to the moon anymore?	**MAIN IDEA:** **CAUSE:** *change in priorities* **EFFECTS:**
7 But in terms of the moon, there are obviously still things we can learn from the moon.	**MAIN IDEA:** **CAUSE:** *ideas for using the moon for new purposes* **EFFECTS:**
8 Dogs will seem to be dreaming of being out for a good run when they have constant movement of extremities at times while sleeping. What is going on in dogs' brains?	**MAIN IDEA:** **CAUSE:** *differences in dogs' brains* **EFFECTS:**
9 We know the speed of sound and light, but what is the speed of sight? I can open my eyes at night and see stars millions of miles away. How fast does that image travel?	**MAIN IDEA:** *the speed of sight* **CAUSE:** **EFFECTS:** *looking is slower because …*
10 The depictions I see of our solar system have all the planets more or less on exactly the same plane. Why is this?	**MAIN IDEA:** *planets are on the same plane (level)* **CAUSE:** **EFFECTS:**

QUESTIONS	MAIN IDEAS, CAUSES, AND EFFECTS
⑪ Is there anything in the universe that does not spin?	**MAIN IDEA:** **CAUSE:** *gravity* **EFFECTS:**
⑫ What shape are the bone cells of primates and apes?	**MAIN IDEA:** *differences in human and animal bones* **CAUSE:** **EFFECTS:**

After You Listen

C. Read the following statements and indicate whether you think each one is true or false. For each false statement, write the true statement.

STATEMENTS	TRUE	FALSE
❶ Ice ages occur approximately every 10 thousand years. _____		
❷ Volcanoes are the cause of big earthquakes. _____		
❸ The trouble with predicting earthquakes is that a wrong prediction could cause chaos. _____		
❹ The moon may eventually be used as a base to travel to Mars. _____		
❺ There is no form of water to be found on the moon. _____		
❻ Sleep paralysis happens to avoid you acting out your dreams. _____		
❼ The difference between the speed of light and the speed of sight has to do with your nerves. _____		
❽ The universe is like a pancake, with everything on the same plane. _____		
❾ Very few things in the universe actually spin. _____		
❿ Animal and human bones are similar because we all do the same things. _____		

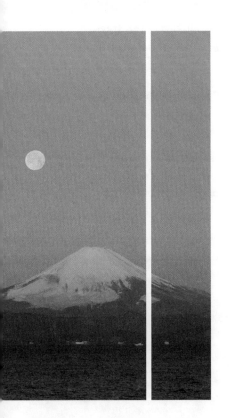

D. Beyond basic understanding, comprehension involves being able to explain what you learn. Take one of the main points from task C and explain the cause and effects to a partner. Use what you learned in Academic Survival Skill (page 113) to practise citing the source of your information. For example, "According to a video interview with Bob McDonald …"

E. Many of the answers to the questions in that interview are now available on the Internet. Does having access to more knowledge and answers make people smarter? Why or why not? Discuss in a group.

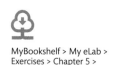

MyBookshelf > My eLab >
Exercises > Chapter 5 >
One on One: Bob McDonald

FINAL ASSIGNMENT
Discuss Cause and Effect in a Group

Now it's your turn. Use everything you have learned in this chapter to develop your Warm-Up Assignment (page 112) argument about a scientific issue to present your ideas in a group.

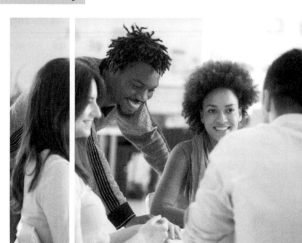

A. Review the argument you and your partner developed in the Warm-Up Assignment.

B. Research additional evidence to support your point of view with three more facts. Find support in the form of an online article or video that you can cite in your discussion according to the formats you learned in Academic Survival Skill (page 113). Use the linking words you learned in Focus on Accuracy (page 104) to structure your argument.

C. With your partner, choose responsibilities for each part of the presentation. Summarize your argument and, if necessary, ask your listeners to take an action or make a decision.

D. Present your argument in a group, and listen to other students' presentations. Then discuss the presentations, using what you learned in Focus on Critical Thinking (page 106) to question whether the other groups' examples show authority, are up to date, and have a clear purpose, such as encouraging you to take an action.

E. After, ask for feedback from other students in your group about your presentation and discussion points to see what you can improve.

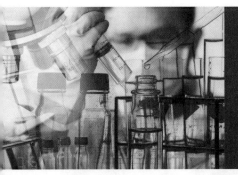

Critical Connections

Now you have a chance to connect skills you've learned in this chapter to think critically about a new problem. Read the information below and then answer the questions.

A. Beck (2015) suggests there is a mismatch between what scientists and the public believe about scientific facts. Read the points below and highlight *scientists* or *public* to show whom you agree with more. Then, with a partner, discuss reasons why the public and scientists differ on their support for each point.

- **Genetically modified foods**: 88 percent of scientists say they're "generally safe" to eat; 37 percent of the public agrees.

- **Vaccines**: 86 percent of scientists believe they should be required in childhood, compared to 68 percent of the public.

- **Climate change**: 94 percent of scientists say it's a "very serious" or "somewhat serious" problem; 65 percent of the public agrees. And 87 percent of scientists blame humans; 50 percent of the public does too.

- **Evolution:** 98 percent of scientists say they believe humans evolved over time, compared to 65 percent of the public.

Reference: Beck, J. (2015, July 9). Americans believe in science, just not its findings. *Atlantic*. Retrieved from https://www.theatlantic.com/health/archive/2015/01americans-believe-in-science-just-not-its-findings/384937/

B. Choose one of the points in task A and find a short video about it online. Use what you learned in Focus on Critical Thinking (page 106) to decide if the information in the video is from an authority and is up to date. Also, decide the speaker's purpose in sharing the information. Make notes, including a citation for the video.

C. In Focus on Speaking (page 111), you learned about how to develop an argument. Cite your video and share what you learned about its evidence, facts, and examples. Based on what you learned, suggest an action your listeners should take. Practise, then present your argument in a group and discuss.

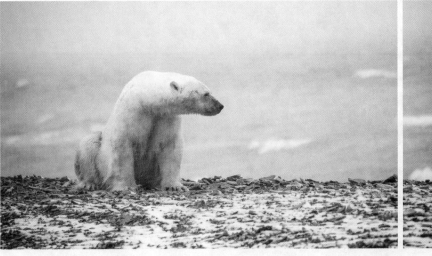

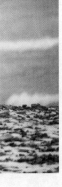

CHAPTER 6

From Numbers to Ideas

In the children's story, *Nigel's Numberless World*, a boy frustrated with math gets his wish for all numbers to disappear. The consequences, affecting the measure of time, baking temperatures, and sports scores, are serious. Nigel soon regrets his wish.

Mathematics is an important part of everyday life but many people fear that our lives are being reduced to numbers alone. Big data, collected from countless statistics about us, is used to make computer-based decisions in areas from policing, to medical care, to the evaluation of job performance. Similarly, companies use big data to market products and services. How do numbers and data shape your world?

In this chapter, you will

- learn vocabulary about math and data;
- listen to recognize certainty;
- identify logical fallacies;
- learn to create cohesion for communicating;
- discuss pros and cons;
- learn informal debating strategies;
- prepare for and take part in an informal debate.

GEARING UP

A. Data analytics is about using statistics to understand and make decisions. Look at the infographic and answer the questions.

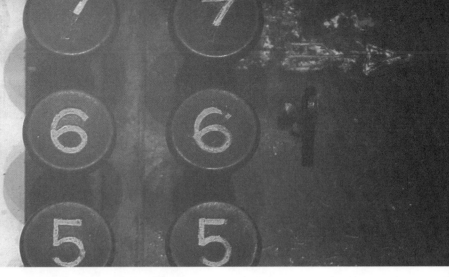

1 Big data analysis uses information about you to discover patterns and trends. What is an example of information that is collected about you?

_____

_____

2 Data mining helps companies find specific information from large volumes of data, like government censuses. Why might a company want to know the incomes and languages spoken by people in a certain area?

_____

_____

3 Data storage is digital, which means it can be kept forever. What is the danger of digital data versus data printed in books?

_____

_____

B. Discuss the questions and your answers with a partner.

Below are the key words you will practise in this chapter. Check the words you understand, then underline the words you use. Highlight the words you need to learn.

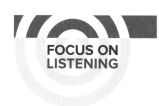

affirmation   exclusion*
assumption*   incidence*
bias*   regulation*
clarity*   reluctance*
consequences* substitutions*

nouns → **math and data**

→ **verbs**

accumulate*   extract*
converse*   implement*
eliminate*   instituted*
exposed*   transcended

→ **adjectives**

condescending prime*
inconsistent* rigorous
inevitable*   stationary
integral*   underlying*
marginal*   unfocused*
predictive*   widespread*

* Appears on the Academic Word List.

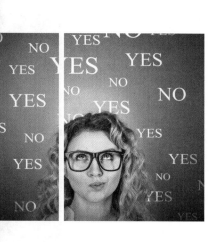

FOCUS ON LISTENING

Identifying Certainty

Do speakers really understand their topics? One way to tell is to listen for key words and expressions that show the degree of doubt or confidence they have in their own words. Knowing this information helps you evaluate a speaker's ideas and decide whether you should challenge them. It's not just about what people say, it's how they say it.

Speakers use many phrases to signal doubt and confidence. These range from mild questions like *Really?* to strong statements like *Absolutely!*

A. Here are eight common expressions that people use to express doubt or confidence. Rate them from 1 (most doubtful) to 8 (most confident). After, compare your answers with a partner to see if you agree.

_____ I'm not sure, but …

_____ I know it's true.

_____ I think …

_____ I'm fairly confident.

_____ Most people believe …

___1___ I don't know.

_____ I'm pretty sure that …

___8___ I'm absolutely certain.

B. Read the following sentences adapted from Listening 1 and highlight the words that express doubt or confidence. Then rewrite each sentence to express more confidence.

❶ Cryptography can be considered an art.

Cryptography is an art.

❷ I guess that didn't fool anyone for long.

_____

③ I'm not sure that would be easy in my house.

_____

④ It sounds like something only a computer could do.

_____

⑤ I'm not certain I understand.

_____

⑥ Perhaps you won that debate.

_____

❼ I know this comes back to secret codes.

_____

❽ I'm fairly certain secret codes are better today.

_____

C. One of the most common ways to express doubt or confidence is through facial expressions and body language. In a group, practise different facial expressions and body language, and decide which ones show the most doubt and which show the most confidence.

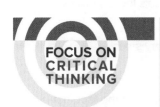

FOCUS ON CRITICAL THINKING

Identifying Logical Fallacies

When you debate, the most common challenge is knowing how to respond when you disagree with other speakers. But a more important challenge is recognizing argument techniques that are *logical fallacies*—arguments that don't make sense. When you can recognize logical fallacies, and put labels on them, it helps you dismiss a speaker's weak argument and focus on more important ideas.

A. Work with a partner to match the logical fallacies to the definitions.

LOGICAL FALLACIES		DEFINITIONS
❶ *ad hominem* attack	_____ d _____	a) explaining why something happened using the wrong reasons
❷ circular arguments	_____	b) pretending to be shocked about something
❸ false cause	_____	c) numbers that might be correct but that don't tell the whole truth
❹ misleading statistics	_____	d) criticizing the person making the argument, rather than the argument itself
❺ personal incredulity	_____	e) statement that can't be believed because it's too broad
❻ sweeping generalization	_____	f) arguments that use their own reasoning

B. Read the sentences from Listening 1 and number them according to the six logical fallacies in task A.

___1___ Ah, you're just saying that because you're a mathematician!

_____ There simply isn't any security anymore.

_____ It makes me afraid to use credit cards or shop online.

_____ Computers can figure out anything to do with numbers. And if a computer can do that, then it can figure out the numbers of a secret code, primes or no primes.

_____ I recently read that last year, ransomware attacks increased by 100 percent! (Actually, there was only one ransomware attack last year and two this year.)

_____ Obviously, people's computers get hacked more and more because hackers are so sophisticated. (Actually, it's because people have weak passwords.)

C. Imagine you are having a debate about the best smartphone. Read the examples of each logical fallacy in task B and then take turns saying them to a partner. Your partner should identify each sentence's logical fallacy and then explain why each is wrong.

1 If you don't use a smartphone, you must not be very smart.

_____

2 Smartphones are good because everyone has one. And the fact that everyone has one shows how popular smartphones are.

_____

3 Smartphones have black screens because black is the colour people like best.

_____

_____

4 More United Arab Emirates citizens own smartphones than any other country's population, which means people there must like to talk a lot.

_____

_____

5 I can't believe anyone wouldn't have a smartphone!

_____

6 Smartphones are like any other toy; people will get bored with them.

_____

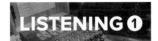

Prime Secrets

What do the nine photos of numbers have in common? They are all prime numbers that can only be divided by the number one and themselves. Prime numbers have an important role in modern secret codes used to keep online financial transactions secure from hacking (illegal access to others' data). But there is a race among code makers to keep ahead of codebreakers.

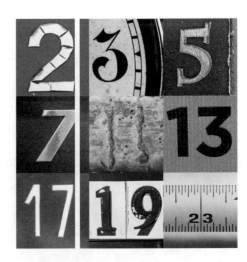

VOCABULARY BUILD

In the following exercises, explore key words from Listening 1.

A. Choose the key word in the box that forms collocations with each set of words below.

accumulate	exposed	extract	inevitable	reluctance

1. become, dangerously, heavily: _____
2. steadily, rapidly, tend to: _____
3. information, quickly, try to: _____
4. initial, considerable, apparent: _____
5. absolutely, appears to be, virtually: _____

B. Use the words in the box to complete the sentences.

converse	incidence	integral	prime	substitutions

1. A _____ example of a secret code is the password on your phone.
2. Secret codes are _____ to the banking industry.
3. If you take time to _____ with coding experts, you can learn a lot.
4. Using _____ of numbers for letters is an easy way to create a code.
5. The _____ of computer hacking is increasing year after year.

Before You Listen

A. Part of Listening 1 is an informal debate. A debate begins with a *proposition*, a statement that debaters must be for or against. Read the following proposition from Listening 1 and discuss it with a partner, each taking a position *for* or *against* it.

> It's inevitable that any secret code created by humans will be hacked by humans.

ARGUMENT FOR: People will always find ways to break new codes.

ARGUMENT AGAINST: Some codes will remain unbreakable.

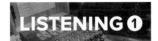

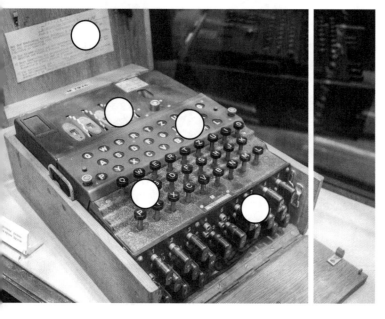

B. Read about the Enigma coding machine and try to understand how it made codes difficult to break. Write the numbers of the three parts of the machine described in the text on the photo.

It's a bit complicated, but try to imagine a typewriter keyboard[1] along with a series of spinning wheels, or rotors[2]. Each rotor has the twenty-six letters of the alphabet, numbers, and other symbols. Every time you type a letter, the rotor turns once so typing the same letter again would end up coding another letter. This other letter appears on a display[3] above the keyboard on the Enigma machine. The person receiving the message would need to know the order of the rotors. It was an incredibly complex way to code.

While You Listen

C. Listening 1 is divided into an explanation and a debate. Listen to the explanation and note the key points.

EXPLANATIONS	KEY POINTS
❶ Yes, it certainly is an art but, over time, the science parts of secret codes have become an integral part of daily life.	*secret codes: integral to daily life*
❷ When I was younger, I heard a friend converse with her mother in their first language.	
❸ Prime numbers are numbers that can only be divided by one and themselves.	
❹ Absolutely. Some very old substitution ciphers used random numbers in place of letters.	
❺ I guess that didn't fool anyone for long? No, and nor did other ciphers with letter or symbol substitutions.	
❻ Ah, you're just saying that because you're a mathematician!	*an* ad hominem *attack*
❼ No, history is quite clear on this.	
❽ I'm fairly certain secret codes are better today, aren't they? Yes, certainly. There are lots of clever ones, like book codes.	
❾ Sometimes people used common books, like dictionaries or Shakespeare plays.	
❿ Cipher machines were developed over the years, but the most effective ones of the twentieth century were developed in Germany.	
⓫ How did the machine work? It's a bit complicated, but try to imagine a typewriter keyboard …	
⓬ Yes. Polish mathematicians were the first to make progress on understanding it.	
⓭ It sounds like something only a computer could do.	

D. Now, listen to the debate portion of Listening 1 and decide if each point is for, against, or neutral to the proposition. Listen again to add details.

DEBATE	FOR, AGAINST, OR NEUTRAL TO THE PROPOSITION		
❶ Let me start by saying that the news is full of stories about people getting their computers hacked. DETAILS:	☐ FOR	☐ AGAINST	☐ NEUTRAL
❷ That's a sweeping generalization, Craig, and there are a few other problems with your argument. DETAILS:	☐ FOR	☐ AGAINST	☐ NEUTRAL
❸ What about other hacking? DETAILS:	☐ FOR	☐ AGAINST	☐ NEUTRAL
❹ People have a reluctance to use passwords that are more complicated than, for example, the word *password*. DETAILS:	☐ FOR	☐ AGAINST	☐ NEUTRAL
❺ But it's getting worse! DETAILS:	☐ FOR	☐ AGAINST	☐ NEUTRAL
❻ You need facts. In this case, it comes back to the magic of prime numbers—incredibly large prime numbers. DETAILS:	☐ FOR	☐ AGAINST	☐ NEUTRAL
❼ But computers can figure out anything to do with numbers. DETAILS:	☐ FOR	☐ AGAINST	☐ NEUTRAL
❽ ... an advanced computer might be able to extract the answer. DETAILS:	☐ FOR	☐ AGAINST	☐ NEUTRAL

After You Listen

E. Review your discussion with your partner about the proposition in task A. Have you changed your mind about some of the points you made after listening and taking notes during tasks C and D? Why or why not?

F. Indicate whether these statements are true or false, according to Listening 1. For the statements that are false, write the true statements.

STATEMENTS	TRUE	FALSE
❶ The purpose of the debate is to create a better secret code. _____ _____		
❷ Ruth Cole became interested in codes because she spoke two languages when she was young. _____ _____		

STATEMENTS		TRUE	FALSE
❸	Cryptography is the study of codes and ciphers.		
❹	Mary, Queen of Scots' cipher was used to capture others in the murder plot.		
❺	There are only 168 prime numbers.		
❻	In English, "e" is the most common letter and "q" is the least common.		
❼	For a book code, the two books would have to be exactly the same—not different editions.		
❽	The Enigma machine was one of the first computers built by Alan Turing.		
❾	The largest prime numbers are millions of numbers long.		
❿	It can take a year for a modern computer to break a code using two of the largest prime numbers.		

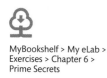

MyBookshelf > My eLab >
Exercises > Chapter 6 >
Prime Secrets

G. Based on what you understand from Listening 1, are you more comfortable or more concerned with the security of your banking and other data? Explain your reasons in a group.

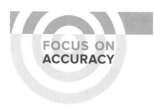

FOCUS ON
ACCURACY

Creating Cohesion

The term *cohesion* refers to the ways ideas stick together. Cohesion is particularly important for listeners to understand the connections from one idea to another and the flow of an argument, such as in an informal debate. Key parts of cohesion are the use of pronouns and dependent and independent clauses connected by conjunctions. Using and listening for cohesive elements improves your communication skills.

Pronouns

Pronouns take the place of nouns and help you avoid repeating the same noun. The most common ones are personal pronouns and possessive adjectives including *I*, *you*, *he/she*, and *my, your, his/her*.

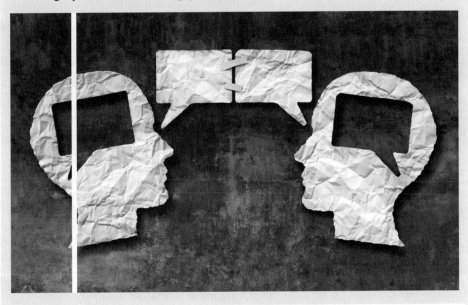

See My eLab Documents for a list of pronouns and possessive adjectives.

A. Read this paragraph from Listening 2 and highlight all the pronouns and possessive adjectives. After, discuss with a partner what each pronoun stands for. Consider how awkward the paragraph would sound if each pronoun were replaced with the word or phrase it stands for.

> Well, you have to understand that I came from mathematics. I was a mathematician, which is to say, I was essentially an artist. Mathematicians live on their own islands of beauty of axioms and logical arguments, inference. And it's this weird place where, you know, if someone points out an error that you're making, you're thinking, you thank them. And it's not true for most of the world. And I had this extremely naive concept when I left academics for finance in 2007 that I could somehow, you know, continue in this way of sort of imparting clarity. But when I got there, I mean, almost immediately the crisis started.

Clauses

Clauses are either *independent*, standing as sentences on their own, or *dependent*, missing one or more parts of speech that would let them form a sentence. Combinations of clauses form simple, compound, and complex sentences, and are connected with conjunctions.

SIMPLE (ONE INDEPENDENT CLAUSE): I don't consider ramen noodles to be food.

COMPOUND (TWO OR MORE INDEPENDENT CLAUSES): I don't consider ramen noodles to be food but my kids consider them delicious.

COMPLEX (ONE OR MORE INDEPENDENT CLAUSES AND ONE OR MORE DEPENDENT CLAUSES): I don't consider ramen noodles which my teenagers love, to be food.

B. Use the conjunction in parentheses to connect the two clauses in each sentence. Replace repeated words with pronouns where necessary. After, highlight the dependent clause in each of your sentences.

1 (when) Cathy realized how mathematics could hurt people. Cathy spent some time working in finance.

Cathy realized how mathematics could hurt people when she spent some time working in finance.

2 (before) She spent time working in finance. The 2008 financial crisis.

_____

3 (or) We talk about privacy online. Even in conversations we have with people.

_____

4 (because) Thanks for asking me. I wrote this book almost in direct response to that.

_____

5 (and) Cathy became a data scientist. Cathy was among those people who were in the start-up community.

_____

_____

C. Combine what you know about pronouns and clauses to write three sentences about mathematics.

1 SIMPLE SENTENCE: _____

2 COMPOUND SENTENCE: _____

3 COMPLEX SENTENCE: _____

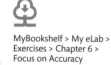

MyBookshelf > My eLab >
Exercises > Chapter 6 >
Focus on Accuracy

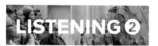

LISTENING ②   Weapons of Math Destruction

Big data is used to predict human behaviour, such as the likelihood of crimes. But if data predicts that a neighbourhood is more likely to have crimes, more officers will be sent there. Then, would the police officers be more likely to harass people about less important problems like littering? Would you want more police in your neighbourhood?

VOCABULARY BUILD

In the following exercises, you will explore key words from Listening 2.

A. Read the sentences and choose the best word to fill in the blank based on the context.

implement	instituted	predictive	underlying	unfocused

1 A _____ factor for becoming a scientist is having an interest

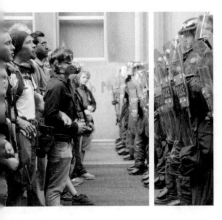

in mathematics.

2 People who are _____ cannot handle the details necessary for math.

3 After the school _____ chess classes, math scores improved.

4 If you want to _____ a new routine, consider creating a schedule.

5 An _____ cause of failure in math is not knowing the times table.

B. Choose the best word from the box to complete each set of synonyms.

clarity	consequences	eliminate	inconsistent	widespread

1 uneven, unpredictable, unreliable _____

2 exclude, remove, reject _____

3 clearness, simplicity, precision _____

4 extensive, general, common _____

5 costs, concerns, penalties _____

C. Write sentences using the pairs of words in parentheses and practise saying them with a partner to check your pronunciation and usage.

1 (eliminate / underlying) _____

_____

2 (consequences / implement) _____

_____

3 (instituted / widespread) _____

_____

Before You Listen

A. In Listening 2, mathematician Cathy O'Neil says the *weapons of math destruction* are characterized by three properties: they are widespread, they are secret, and they are destructive. An example is the collection of images and video from government and private cameras on streets. In what ways might they be widespread, secret, and destructive?

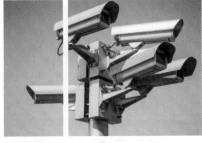

1 WIDESPREAD: _____

_____

2 SECRET: _____

_____

3 DESTRUCTIVE: _____

_____

The phrase "weapons of math destruction" is a pun on "weapons of mass destruction."

B. O'Neil talks about moving from teaching university to finance just before the 2008 financial crisis. Read the paragraph and answer the following questions.

> The essential story is that they traded money for lies of a mathematical variety. It was the very opposite of what I thought mathematics was supposed to be used for. So, it really shamed me and disillusioned me. The thing is, the financial crisis didn't seem to give us pause.

1 What might she mean by "they traded money for lies of a mathematical variety"?

_____

2 What does she think mathematics should be used for?

_____

3 The phrase *give us pause* means "make us think." What does she mean by her last sentence?

_____

C. Computers use algorithms—sets of rules for problem solving. These rules may ignore human values, especially in the banking industry. Think of another example of where algorithms might be used elsewhere in society. With a partner, discuss whether algorithms are dangerous or not.

_____

_____

While You Listen

D. Listen once and note Cathy O'Neil's answers to the interviewer's questions. Listen again to add details and to consider how confident Cathy is in her replies.

INTERVIEWER'S QUESTIONS	O'NEIL'S ANSWERS
1 I asked Cathy why the lessons of 2008 didn't make us rethink the power we give algorithms in our society.	*we invest in algorithms that are problems and no one takes responsibility*
2 Could you give me an example of how algorithms are used in ways that might have a real impact on someone; for example, as a consumer?	
3 Can you expand on that, because one of the things that you talk about is how algorithms tend to affect people in poverty more than the wealthy?	
4 But how is it that opinions and values end up getting embedded in the models themselves?	

INTERVIEWER'S QUESTIONS	O'NEIL'S ANSWERS
5 So, are there things coming from your perspective specifically as a mathematician that you find particularly concerning about algorithms?	
6 Right. And then isn't part of the problem, as well, that once we start using these weapons of math destruction in more and more areas, they kind of have knock-on effects or spiral effects?	
7 I understand that you have been asked, from time to time, to teach ethics to data scientists. So, what do you tell them?	
8 How do we change this trajectory that we're on?	

After You Listen

E. Check your answers to tasks A, B, and C. Would you change any of your answers? How? Discuss any changes and reasons with a partner.

F. Choose the phrase that best completes each sentence.

1 When O'Neil talks about thanking others for pointing out her errors, she _____.

  a) notes how finance encourages it

  b) contrasts it with the real world

  c) means it's what she likes to do

2 In using the phrase *drinking the Kool-Aid* (everyone foolishly believing in something dangerous), O'Neil means _____.

  a) no one wanted to be healthy anymore

  b) everyone was thirsty for new ideas

  c) others didn't care about consequences

3 O'Neil notes that almost all algorithms are scoring systems that influence _____.

  a) things like how much you pay for insurance

  b) the way people are starting to think in real life

  c) the training of future finance professionals

4 The problem with assessing teachers on their students' test scores is _____.

  a) some less-abled students might get their teachers fired

  b) that teachers are not always allowed to write the tests

  c) that it is the teachers who should be assessed instead

5 The arrest records of different groups of people show how statistics _____.

  a) are always fair   b) can be biased   c) mean nothing

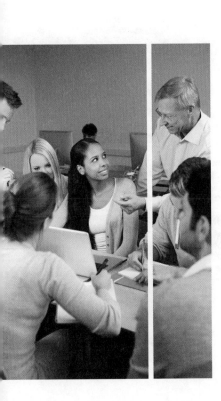

6 Because people are unaware of policing algorithms, _____.

   a) they don't need to worry about them

   b) everyone is treated exactly the same

   c) they are unable to protest unfairness

7 The Nutella (chocolate/nut spread) example is meant to show _____.

   a) how biases can affect algorithms

   b) why children aren't mathematical

   c) how algorithms can affect biases

8 The idea of Twitter being used to estimate popularity is an example of _____.

   a) a fair bias

   b) a stupid proxy

   c) an unusual algorithm

9 One of the problems with data scientists is their _____.

   a) failure to apply ethics to their work

   b) inability to learn mathematics

   c) lack of understanding of computer science

10 The example of sending application letters with different names is _____.

   a) to reach more people   b) to find the best applicant   c) to understand racism

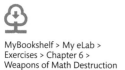

MyBookshelf > My eLab >
Exercises > Chapter 6 >
Weapons of Math Destruction

G. O'Neil mentions she uses algorithms—decision processes—to plan meals. Think of an example of something you plan, and consider how you make your decisions. Do you have an algorithm? What are your biases? Discuss your answers in a group.

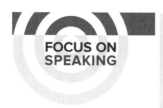

FOCUS ON SPEAKING

Discussing Pros and Cons

When you listen to a speaker share a new idea, it's natural to consider the pros (advantages) and cons (disadvantages). But deciding whether an idea has more advantages or disadvantages is only the first step. You also need to be able to talk about them, particularly if a speaker's decision affects you.

When considering an argument over two points of view, such as in a debate, you can begin by asking, "What are all the pros and cons?" You can then brainstorm as many ideas as possible without considering which ideas are best, or useful.

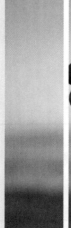
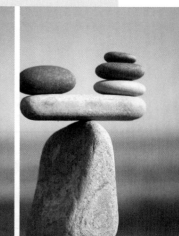

Each time you think of a pro point, try to think of a parallel con point with the opposite point of view.

A. Listening 2 mentions issues with police using big data. Review the table and add one *pro* and one *con* point.

POLICE USE OF BIG DATA			
PROS	**1** predicting crimes based on arrest records	**2** using police resources wisely	**3**
CONS	**1** over-policing of some neighbourhoods	**2** ignoring crimes by other groups in other areas	**3**

In a discussion or informal debate, you can use your pro and con points to help build your side of the argument and to ask for clarification or to challenge the other speaker.

B. Read the following questions and decide which are asking for clarification, and which are challenging the points. Then, write one more clarification question and one more challenge question on the points you added to task A.

QUESTIONS	CLARIFY	CHALLENGE
1 When you say, "Use police resources wisely," what do you mean by "wisely"?		
2 Isn't predicting crime based on arrest records just bullying people who may have once made mistakes?		
3 How would you define *over-policing*?		
4 With the phrase, "crime by other groups," aren't you just avoiding naming specific groups?		
5 No one really believes big data is dangerous, right?		
6 Prime numbers, which are ...?		
7		
8		

C. Choose the pros or cons from task A and let your partner take the opposite points. Discuss the ideas using clarification and challenge questions from task B, as well as the following expressions to present new points:

• Although what you say might be true, another way of looking at it is ...

• An argument for/against this idea is ...

• Another point of view is ...

• A different side to the issue is ...

• Everyone knows that ...

• Many people agree that ..., but others say ...

• On one hand, ... but on the other hand ...

• There's little doubt that ...

MyBookshelf > My eLab >
Exercises > Chapter 6 >
Focus on Speaking

WARM-UP ASSIGNMENT

Prepare for a Debate

Now it's your turn to brainstorm the pros
and cons of one of the issues from this chapter.

A. With a partner, choose a topic for debate
from Listening 1 and Listening 2:

- ethics in finance
- algorithms for making predictions
- computer hackers
- secret codes
- test scores for evaluating teacher performance
- emotional biases in decision-making

B. Develop the topic into a proposition on which you and your partner can have
different points of view. For example, for ethics in finance, you may choose
to discuss the proposition, "Everyone who works in finance should have to take
an ethics course."

PROPOSITION: _____

C. Use what you learned in Focus on Speaking (page 134) to develop a list
of seven pros and seven cons.

PROPOSITION:	
PROS	**CONS**
❶	❶
❷	❷
❸	❸
❹	❹
❺	❺
❻	❻
❼	❼

D. Discuss the pros and cons with your partner and use clarification and challenge
questions to improve your points. As you discuss the points, use what you
learned in Focus on Listening (page 122) to make your statements and questions
sound more confident and less doubtful. Save your notes and ideas to use
in the Final Assignment.

Too Much Math, Too Little History

Economics is concerned with the production, consumption, and transfer of wealth. In simpler terms, it asks questions about how you and others earn, save, and spend your money. Economists tend to use two ways to build models that help them understand the world of wealth: history and math. But which is more important and why? That is the debate in Listening 3.

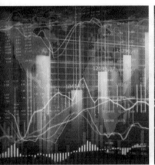

VOCABULARY BUILD

In the following exercises, explore key words from Listening 3.

A. What do the words in bold mean to you? Complete the sentences with information that is true for you.

1 A **marginal** concern that I don't care about is _____

_____ .

2 A common **regulation** at school that I don't like to follow is _____

_____ .

3 One activity that I do that gives me **affirmation** is _____

_____ .

4 Something that I have practised in a **rigorous** way is _____

_____ .

5 The **exclusion** of this one thing that would make my life more difficult is

_____ .

B. Read the sentences and use an arrow (↓) to indicate where each word in parentheses belongs. Then, discuss each sentence with a partner to explain the meaning of the key words. Use a dictionary to look up words you don't know.

1 (assumption) He has made the   that people behave in economic ways ; that is , always thinking about money in terms of their own best interests .

2 (bias) Because she is older , she has a   toward the belief that the prices people pay , on average , are fair because they are set by the marketplace .

3 (condescending) His worst character flaw was that he was   , always looking down on people .

4 (stationary) Many economic principles change , but some are   and stay the same .

5 (transcended) The economic decline of the Great Depression (1929–1939) was only   by government spending and investment .

C. Often, speakers use words in more than one way. An example in Listening 3 is the key word *exclusion*. When the speaker uses the following three words, what does each mean? If you are not sure, look up the words in a dictionary.

1 exclude: _____

MyBookshelf > My eLab > Exercises > Chapter 6 > Vocabulary Review

2 exclusion: _____

3 exclusionism: _____

Before You Listen

A. Read the beginning of Listening 3, introducing the debate, and write a short summary.

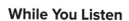
In British English, mathematics is shortened to maths. Elsewhere, it is math.

> Ladies and gentlemen, it's my job to try and persuade you, together with my colleague, Dr. Ha-Joon Chang, of the truth of this proposition, that there is too much maths and too little history in economics as it's currently taught and conceived. And let us start off with an obvious question: why do people study economics? Basically, to understand how economies work. And there are two different ways of understanding that. I mean, there's maths and there's history. And they stand at opposite poles in terms of epistemology (the theory of knowledge).

SUMMARY: _____

_____

B. Listening 3 mentions several concepts that may be unfamiliar if you're not studying economics or business. However, understanding the full details of each one is not necessary to get a general idea of what the speaker is saying. Read the concepts and their definitions and check the ones you are already familiar with.

☐ PLATONIC: a way of thinking of everything as numbers. Note: The more common meaning is "an affectionate relationship that isn't intimate."

☐ PAUL KRUGMAN / CRASH OF 2008–2009: a banking crisis based on bad loans

☐ BOB LUCAS / NORMATIVE THRUST OF MATHEMATICAL ECONOMICS: focusing on the math of economics, ignoring other factors

☐ REALITY VERSUS CONVENIENCE: models that are based on the real world versus ones based on what is easy to measure

☐ HUBRIS: excessive self-confidence

☐ HORSES FOR COURSES: different ideas or people are suited to different things

While You Listen

C. Listen to Lord Robert Skidelsky present his side of the debate on math versus history in economics. As you listen, check the boxes to indicate whether the points that Skidelsky mentions are pro or con history in economics, or pro or con math. Listen again to write the main point of each section.

SKIDELSKY'S POINTS	HISTORY OR MATH: PRO OR CON
❶ Let's take maths first. Two things that maths tries to do, claims to do.	HISTORY: ☐ PRO ☐ CON MATH: ☐ PRO ☐ CON MAIN POINT: *math is logical and can be used to prove some ideas in economics*
❷ But because the social system to which they apply maths is so complex, too complex to obtain reliable proof, they're tempted by the first or what I would call the platonic view of the subject.	HISTORY: ☐ PRO ☐ CON MATH: ☐ PRO ☐ CON MAIN POINT:

SKIDELSKY'S POINTS	HISTORY OR MATH: PRO OR CON
3 Economists fell in love with the old idealized vision of an economy in which rational individuals interact in perfect markets.	HISTORY: ☐ PRO ☐ CON MATH: ☐ PRO ☐ CON **MAIN POINT:**
4 Now, an economic model is not like that of, like, a model of an airplane that is, in reality, in a miniaturized form.	HISTORY: ☐ PRO ☐ CON MATH: ☐ PRO ☐ CON **MAIN POINT:**
5 As soon as you get into an assumption-based mathematical modelling, you are actually inserting the problems you think are important and also inserting your view on how they ought to be discussed and excluding other views on how they ought to be discussed.	HISTORY: ☐ PRO ☐ CON MATH: ☐ PRO ☐ CON **MAIN POINT:**
6 What then is the role of history in economics? I would argue that the role of history is that of a reality check.	HISTORY: ☐ PRO ☐ CON MATH: ☐ PRO ☐ CON **MAIN POINT:**
7 The general reason for the exclusion of history is quite insidious. It arises from the belief that everything to be learnt from history has already been incorporated into the latest textbooks.	HISTORY: ☐ PRO ☐ CON MATH: ☐ PRO ☐ CON **MAIN POINT:**
8 So much for the history of economic thought.	HISTORY: ☐ PRO ☐ CON MATH: ☐ PRO ☐ CON **MAIN POINT:**
9 Now, but the point of studying the history of economic thought is precisely to realize that the important debates in economics have never been resolved and continue to vex us today.	HISTORY: ☐ PRO ☐ CON MATH: ☐ PRO ☐ CON **MAIN POINT:**
10 Knowledge of the history of economic thought can help us avoid hubris or absolute confidence in our own favoured school of thought.	HISTORY: ☐ PRO ☐ CON MATH: ☐ PRO ☐ CON **MAIN POINT:**
11 To take a less obvious example, and this I think is controversial, the marginalist revolution of the 1870s ...	HISTORY: ☑ PRO ☐ CON MATH: ☐ PRO ☐ CON **MAIN POINT:** *economic activity is embedded in a web of social institutions, customs, beliefs, and attitudes*
12 Concrete outcomes are undoubtedly affected by these background factors.	HISTORY: ☐ PRO ☐ CON MATH: ☐ PRO ☐ CON **MAIN POINT:**

SKIDELSKY'S POINTS	HISTORY OR MATH: PRO OR CON
⓭ Finally, history shows us how economic ideas reflect power structures.	HISTORY: ☐ PRO ☐ CON MATH: ☐ PRO ☐ CON MAIN POINT:
⓮ I would like to champion the view of horses for courses, for choosing those bits of economics appropriate to different problems and situations.	HISTORY: ☐ PRO ☐ CON MATH: ☐ PRO ☐ CON MAIN POINT:
⓯ On the [one] hand, if you want to forecast the conditions of supply and demand for a particular product or a particular sector of the economy, …	HISTORY: ☐ PRO ☐ CON MATH: ☐ PRO ☐ CON MAIN POINT:
⓰ But, having said that, the banishing of history from standard economics curricula is a symptom of a loss of pluralism and imagination in the discipline.	HISTORY: ☐ PRO ☐ CON MATH: ☐ PRO ☐ CON MAIN POINT:

After You Listen

D. When you present an argument in a debate, it needs to make sense to your listeners. Read Skidelsky's key debate points, then number them in the correct order.

_____ Although mathematics can show logic and proof, these are too simple to model the real world.

___8___ Based on this thinking, universities need to teach students both history and mathematics.

_____ History provides examples of what economic policies have and haven't worked.

___1___ Math and history are two ways of looking at economics.

_____ But economic activity is embedded in a web of social institutions, customs, beliefs, and attitudes.

_____ Math provides logical proof.

_____ Models used in economics tend to be based on assumptions.

_____ These assumptions simplify problems so they are easier to deal with.

E. Based on what you learned in Focus on Speaking (page 134) and your answers to tasks C and D, decide if the following statements are pros or cons for the proposition that history is more important than mathematics in economics.

STATEMENTS	PROS	CONS
❶ New businesses, like start-ups, don't have a historical background.		
❷ People's economic behaviour is not always in keeping with mathematical rules.		
❸ When you look at averages among a group of people, you ignore what is individual about each of them.		

STATEMENTS		PROS	CONS
❹	Stock market crashes will occur again if we don't learn from the mistakes that led to previous ones.		
❺	Mathematics is the best tool for predicting the future.		
❻	How people behaved economically a hundred years ago is different compared to how they act today.		

MyBookshelf > My eLab >
Exercises > Chapter 6 >
 Too Much Math, Too Little History

Academic
Survival Skill

F. Skidelsky's final comment is "Awareness of the past should make our discipline less arrogant and more useful." In a group, discuss whether an understanding of history is important to the fields you each wish to study. Explain why or why not.

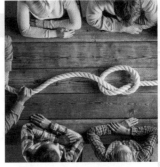
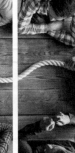

Informal Debating

You think of pros and cons every day. It's a normal way of arriving at sensible decisions. In an informal debate, you use facts to support these kinds of pros and cons, developing them into your point of view. In informal debates, you also use techniques like offering analogies that compare parts of your arguments to things that are easier to understand.

A. There are many different structures for debates, but most feature a proposition that one side supports and the other tries to refute/rebut/argue against. Rewrite this question from Listening 2 as a proposition, making it a statement and cutting out unnecessary words.

> Could you give me an example of how algorithms are used in ways that might have a negative impact on someone; for example, as a consumer?

_____

A formal debate has strict rules and timing for each team.

B. Consider your proposition and the structure for informally debating it below. Complete the notes.

DEBATE STRUCTURE		NOTES
❶	Share the proposition and explain your point of view—for or against.	*We agree with (the proposition) that algorithms are …*
❷	Argue with three or more points. Strengthen your arguments with analogies.	**POINT 1:** *Algorithms that raise the prices of insurance based on predictions are like betting games at a casino where the odds are against the players.* _____ _____ **POINT 2:** _____ _____ **POINT 3:** _____ _____

DEBATE STRUCTURE	NOTES
❸ Anticipate the other side's arguments and think of counter-arguments.	POINT 1: Now, you might argue that ... _____ _____ POINT 2: Although you might say ... _____ _____ POINT 3: I'd have to disagree with your point about ... _____ _____
❹ Offer a conclusion that summarizes your points.	We feel that our ideas show ... _____ _____

❗ Remember what you learned in Focus on Critical Thinking (page 123) to spot logical fallacies.

C. It's tempting to go through the arguments point by point, but it's better to summarize them and take a thematic (overall idea) approach. Look at the following arguments and fill in the missing information with your own ideas.

ARGUMENT	THEME	REBUTTAL
❶ Algorithms are natural and we use them in our daily lives, such as planning meals.	*Algorithms are natural.*	*Although you try to confuse meal planning with financial algorithms ...*
❷ Algorithms are necessary for finance, policing, and employment, which is why we need them.	*Lumping details together doesn't make the argument stronger.*	
❸ Algorithms are here to stay and nothing you can say will make them disappear.		

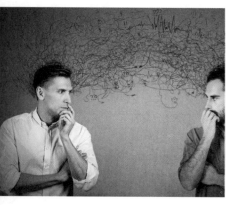

FINAL ASSIGNMENT
Participate in an Informal Debate

Now it's your turn. In small groups use everything you have learned in this chapter to prepare for, and participate in, informal debates on the topics you prepared in the Warm-Up Assignment (page 136).

A. Working with your partner and another pair of students, form a group to debate the topics you developed in the Warm-Up Assignment. Take some time to prepare points for the other pair's proposition.

B. Begin by sharing your point of view on your proposition and offering three points of evidence, using the format in Academic Survival Skill (page 141). Use what you learned in Focus on Accuracy (page 128) to make your opening points cohesive and clear.

C. Let the other pair rebut your points and present three points of their own.

D. Rebut the other team's points, considering the pros and cons you learned about in Focus on Speaking (page 134) and the logical fallacies you learned in Focus on Critical Thinking (page 123). Remember to use what you learned in Focus on Listening (page 122) to evaluate the other speakers' degrees of doubt and confidence in what they are saying. Offer a conclusion that summarizes your points.

E. After the other team offers their conclusion, discuss the points and reflect on what you could improve, including your debating skills.

> In a debate, it's easy to forget to listen because you're thinking of what you will say next. Listen to the other side so you're ready to argue against their points.

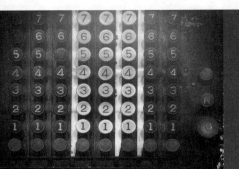

Critical Connections

This chapter talked about how mathematics and data are used and abused in areas as diverse as police work and economics. Every student studies some math but many stop before they get to university. Should mathematics be taught throughout every student's education?

A. Consider this proposition and use everything you learned in this chapter to discuss the pros and cons with a partner.

> Everyone should study mathematics throughout school and university.

B. Complete the chart, listing the pros and cons of the proposition.

PROS	CONS

C. Work with a partner, each of you taking one side, and informally debate the proposition.

D. After you have finished, brainstorm new ideas that build on your informal debate. For example, perhaps different kinds of math should be taught, such as more financial awareness, or math for computer programming.

CHAPTER 7

Thinking Machines

Will a machine ever be as smart as you? Inventor Ray Kurzweil suggests that machines will develop like humans and adds that, "self-aware, self-improving machines will evolve beyond humans' ability to control or even understand them." Although this seems like a wild idea, many computer scientists agree, and predict surprising abilities for artificial intelligence, or AI, over the next hundred years. In the meantime, semi-intelligent AI-enabled programs will continue to take on and automate a wide range of jobs from cleaning homes, to building things in factories, to evaluating medical data. But truly human-like intelligence in machines is likely to remain as science fiction.

In this chapter, you will

- learn vocabulary about artificial intelligence;

- listen to recognize paraphrases;

- play the devil's advocate;

- learn new brainstorming techniques;

- make and understand comparisons;

- learn to apply turn-taking to your conversations;

- brainstorm and discuss AI topics.

GEARING UP

A. Look at the infographic about the many professions that robots with AI might someday have, then answer the questions.

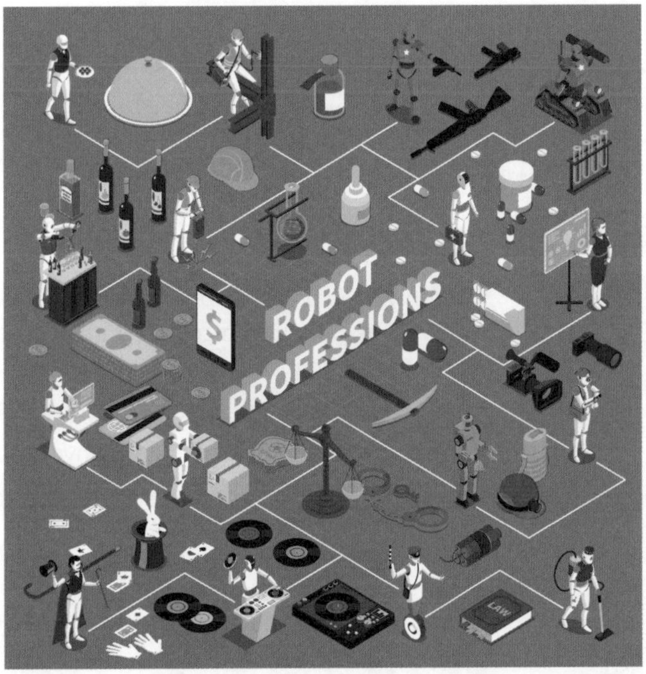

① Intelligent robots are likely to take on many dangerous jobs, like mining and construction. What jobs for robots might cause danger to people?

_____

_____

② Intelligent robots might serve as entertainers. Would you find robot magicians and DJs more interesting than human ones? Why or why not?

_____

③ What would be the advantages and disadvantages of a robot teacher?

_____

_____

④ Which of the jobs in the infographic would put the most people out of work if intelligent robots took over their work?

_____

B. Compare your answers in a group to see where you agree and disagree.

Below are the key words you will practise in this chapter. Check the words you understand, then underline the words you use. Highlight the words you need to learn.

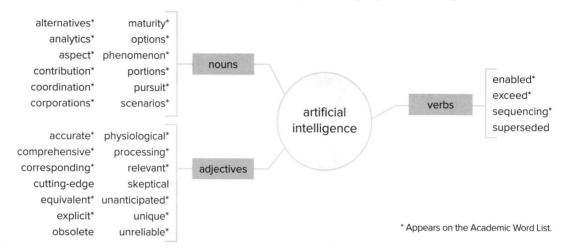

nouns
alternatives*
analytics*
aspect*
contribution*
coordination*
corporations*
maturity*
options*
phenomenon*
portions*
pursuit*
scenarios*

artificial intelligence

verbs
enabled*
exceed*
sequencing*
superseded

adjectives
accurate*
comprehensive*
corresponding*
cutting-edge
equivalent*
explicit*
obsolete
physiological*
processing*
relevant*
skeptical
unanticipated*
unique*
unreliable*

* Appears on the Academic Word List.

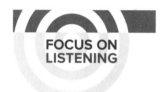

FOCUS ON LISTENING

Recognizing Paraphrases

When you listen, it's important to recognize when a speaker paraphrases a word or an idea. Speakers also paraphrase sentences, paragraphs, or even entire speeches in the form of a summary. Recognizing paraphrases helps you take notes on the key points of a talk.

The simplest paraphrase is a synonym of a single word. For example, in the phrase "virtuous, or good," *good* is the paraphrase, or simpler word, for *virtuous*. Paraphrases are often signalled by a drop in tone, especially in the middle of a sentence. Sometimes just a signal word, like *or*, is dropped, especially when hyphens and parentheses surround the paraphrase.

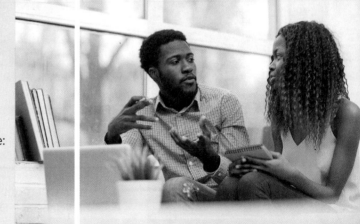

Signal words to listen for include:

- also known as
- in other words
- means/meaning
- that is to say

A. Highlight the paraphrase and practise saying these sentences with a partner, dropping your tone for the transition word and paraphrase.

① AI, that is to say, artificial intelligence, may impact our future.

② Science fiction—predictions of the future—often fears innovation.

③ The next stage (step) in human evolution may be higher-level thinking machines.

▶

B. Listen and indicate whether a word, phrase, or sentence is being paraphrased.

	WORD	PHRASE	SENTENCE
1			
2			
3			
4			
5			
6			

One important way to paraphrase is to summarize a talk, usually signalled by phrases such as:

• All this is to say

• To summarize this

• What this all means is

C. Listen to a paragraph and paraphrase it, writing a one-sentence summary.

_____

_____

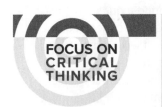

FOCUS ON CRITICAL THINKING

Playing the Devil's Advocate

Imagine this situation: Someone has a great idea and everyone else agrees. But there's a problem with the idea. Should you speak up? If you decide *not* to speak up, you are part of *groupthink*, the tendency for people to follow an idea because they assume everyone else supports it. But if you do speak up, you're taking on the role of *devil's advocate*—someone who challenges others' ideas.

Devil's advocate is an important role in business and industry where someone is often appointed to try to tear apart popular ideas in hopes that they can be improved. You will use what you learn about playing devil's advocate in Listening 1, Listening 3, and the Warm-Up and Final Assignments.

Acting as a devil's advocate involves different strategies to challenge what others are thinking. You do not always need to have alternative answers, but you can encourage others to look for them.

A. Look at these five strategies and consider how you would challenge someone who was suggesting that the work of police officers could be automated and/or replaced by robots. Choose the best point for each one.

1 QUESTION ASSUMPTIONS: What is the basis of the argument?
   a) Is the reason for this to save money spent on police officer salaries?
   b) Do people naturally prefer high-technology types of machines?

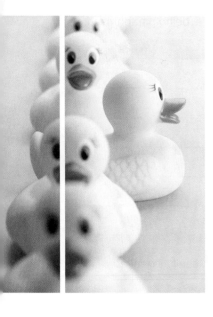

2 CONSIDER OTHER PERSPECTIVES: Is there another way of looking at the problem or proposal?

    a) Instead of replacing police officers, could we have longer prison sentences?

    b) Instead of replacing police officers, could we automate parts of their work?

3 IDENTIFY EXCEPTIONS: Does the argument work in every case?

    a) There are already automated police examples at work, such as traffic cameras.

    b) An automated police officer robot couldn't make decisions in unexpected situations.

4 EXPLAIN DISADVANTAGES: One problem with this idea is _____.

    a) automated police officers might accidentally misuse weapons

    b) automated police officers might not give out parking fines

5 PROVIDE ALTERNATIVES: Instead of automated police work, we could _____.

    a) look for better ways to reduce crime

    b) get rid of police officers altogether

B. Work with a partner and read some ideas about artificial intelligence. Use what you know about devil's advocate strategies to identify an example of each one.

> The mental abilities of a four-year-old that we take for granted—recognizing a face, lifting a pencil, walking across a room, answering a question—in fact solve some of the hardest engineering problems ever conceived. As the new generation of intelligent devices appears, it will be the stock analysts and petrochemical engineers and parole board members who are in danger of being replaced by machines. The gardeners, receptionists, and cooks are secure in their jobs for decades to come.
>
> Reference: Pinker, S. (1994). *The language instinct*. (pp. 190–191). New York, NY: Morrow and Company.

QUESTION AN ASSUMPTION: _____

_____

IDENTIFY A PERSPECTIVE: _____

_____

LIST AN EXCEPTION: _____

_____

EXPLAIN A DISADVANTAGE: _____

_____

OFFER AN ALTERNATIVE: _____

_____

C. On your own, pick one job that you think will most likely disappear in the future as artificial intelligence improves. Then work in a group and explain your choice. Use what you learned about devil's advocate strategies to challenge others' ideas. Remember to be polite and offer alternative ideas.

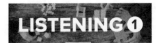 **Your AI Future**

The photograph shows a computer-based printer that uses Chinese brushes instead of ink-jets. Computers have already done what seems like creative work, but they mostly rely on rules in their programming rather than true creativity. It would seem that creativity requires an intelligence that computers will never have. Or will they?

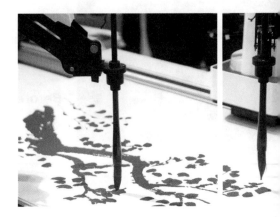

VOCABULARY BUILD

In the following exercises, explore key words from Listening 1.

A. Match each key word with words that form collocations.

KEY WORDS		WORDS THAT FORM COLLOCATIONS
❶ scenario	_____	a) attractive, constructive, effective
❷ aspect	_____	b) not completely, surprisingly, largely
❸ alternative	_____	c) central, crucial, essential
❹ accurate	_____	d) generous, significant, tiny
❺ portion	_____	e) future, possible, worst case

B. Read the sentences and use an arrow ↓ to indicate where each word in parentheses belongs. Then discuss each sentence with a partner to explain the meaning of the key words. Use a dictionary to look up words you don't know.

❶ (enabled) A small part of what has these programs and tools to improve is Moore's Law .

❷ (corresponding) There was a increase in computing power because of it .

❸ (unreliable) The earliest versions of these were incredibly .

❹ (processing) The faster the computer's speed , the faster it can calculate a set of numbers and arrive at an answer .

❺ (superseded) Some people predict that AI will be the next step in human evolution , replacing us as we Neanderthals .

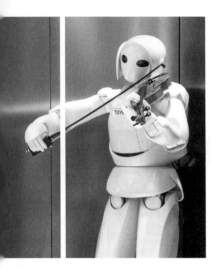

C. Write sentences using the pairs of words in parentheses.

1 (portions / accurate)

_____

2 (enabled / superseded)

_____

3 (alternative / aspect)

_____

Before You Listen

A. Listening 1 begins with the following paragraph. Read the paragraph and choose the best definitions for the three terms.

> Before we begin, let's consider what is meant by artificial intelligence or, to use its short form, AI. Humans are good at thinking creatively and abstractly, while AI programs tend to mostly do rule-based calculations. For AI to get better, AI needs to improve its calculation speeds, pattern recognition, and decision trees.

1 Calculation speeds refer to _____.
  a) how quickly people use calculators
  b) how quickly AI can evaluate information

2 Pattern recognition refers to _____.
  a) understanding what things have in common
  b) being able to match pieces of clothing

3 Decision trees refer to _____.
  a) choices made by gardeners
  b) possible choices that can be made

B. The following is an example of a simple decision tree described in Listening 1. It's about deciding whether or not to take an umbrella when you go outside. Think about related decisions around the use of an umbrella that you might make and add them in bubbles to the decision tree.

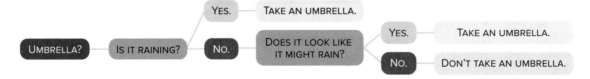

While You Listen

C. As you listen, take notes on the lecturer's points. Listen again and use what you learned in Focus on Critical Thinking (page 147) to act as devil's advocate, thinking of points that challenge the lecturer's points.

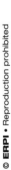

LECTURER'S POINTS	DEVIL'S ADVOCATE POINTS
1 Humans are good at thinking creatively and abstractly.	*a big assumption: many people don't think creatively or abstractly*
2 Computers are already blindingly fast in making calculations.	
3 The second key area is pattern recognition.	
4 The third area that is important to artificial intelligence is the concept of decision trees.	
5 Fast calculations, pattern recognition, and decision trees are each limited but, working together, they are powerful and begin approaching something closer to intelligence.	
6 Some predict that AI will be the next step in human evolution.	
7 Humans are slaves of AI.	
8 IBM's Watson, Apple's Siri, Amazon's Alexa, the Internet of Things	
9 This AI-based Internet of Things is in *the age of machine learning* as it tries to understand large amounts of data, including your preferences.	
10 A small part of what has enabled these programs and tools to improve is Moore's Law.	
11 Quantum computers, currently being developed worldwide, don't depend on the printed circuits of traditional computers.	
12 ... the age of machine learning gives way to increasingly smarter AI programs—programs that could make intelligent decision-tree choices ...	

LECTURER'S POINTS	DEVIL'S ADVOCATE POINTS
⑬ A key aspect of AI is that it does not tire and it is not swayed by emotion.	
⑭ Three hundred and fifty-two AI researchers predicted that AI-based machines would be doing jobs like performing delicate surgery by 2053.	
⑮ AI is being integrated into robotic-like machines.	
⑯ AI will also take on more creative tasks, all human tasks, and all human jobs by 2137.	*people won't want to give up jobs they love doing just because a machine can do them*

After You Listen

D. Choose one of your devil's advocate points from task C and use what you learned in Focus on Critical Thinking (page 147) to decide what strategy it is based on.

E. Read the following sentences from Listening 1 and use what you learned in Focus on Listening (page 146) to choose the best paraphrase for the words in bold. Refer to your notes in task C for help.

1 Computers are already **blindingly fast** in making calculations.
   a) which means you can't see them
   b) this means extremely quickly
   c) which means they are only able to be heard

2 In another scenario, **humans survive, but only as slaves of AI**.
   a) in other words, not all humans would be around to help out
   b) that is to say, people would have meaningful computer jobs
   c) which means people would not be in control of their own lives

3 This AI-based Internet of Things includes devices such as the Nest thermostat that can be programmed to adjust temperatures according to **your preferences**.
   a) meaning things like your favourite foods
   b) meaning settings that make you most comfortable
   c) meaning they are probably things others don't like

4 But it's likely that Pandora is learning from its human team at the same time and, eventually, will no longer need any **intervention**.
   a) that is, help from humans
   b) meaning a chance to solve problems
   c) or partial inventions

5 Quantum computing won't just mean greater storage of information; it will mean far faster processing speeds that will allow quantum computers to quickly **absorb** all records of human learning and achievement.
   a) or pick over what's useful
   b) or act like a wet sponge
   c) or acquire and remember

6 These computer programs are already in place helping professions, from engineering to law to medicine, to make better and **more informed decisions**.

   a) meaning, decisions people don't want to make

   b) that is to say, helping in day-to-day work

   c) which is to say, the most difficult decisions

7 A key aspect of AI intelligence is that it does not tire and it is not **swayed by emotion**.

   a) or ignored by important emotions

   b) or stopped from doing anything

   c) or influenced by human feelings

8 The Oxford Yale study expects that AI will also take on more creative tasks, such as writing songs by 2027 and writing **best-selling novels** by 2046.

   a) meaning sold to other AI programs

   b) that is, books you would want to read

   c) that is to say, not really true stories

F. Based on what you understand about Listening 1 and what you learned in Focus on Critical Thinking, write a devil's advocate question about the future of AI.

_____

_____

MyBookshelf > My eLab > Exercises > Chapter 7 > Your AI Future

Academic
Survival Skill

Mind maps are a good way to capture and organize brainstorming ideas.

Group Brainstorming

It is usually easier to think of new ideas with other people. Brainstorming usually starts by identifying a problem, a task that needs to be done, or a general topic of concern. A group is formed to discuss it, often with one person recording each idea. Group members are encouraged to contribute new ideas and to build on the ideas of others. One brainstorming rule is not to criticize ideas until everyone has had a chance to share. Even a seemingly foolish idea might lead to a better idea.

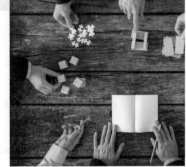
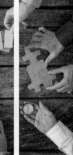

A. Basic brainstorming is largely a spoken activity, but there are many brainstorming techniques, some of which involve writing. Read about the following techniques and then write an advantage for each one.

TECHNIQUE	KEY POINTS	ADVANTAGES
BRAIN-NETTING	Instead of writing notes on a white board, group members use a computer screen.	
BRAIN-WRITING	Instead of speaking, group members write their ideas on individual notes that are then passed around.	
CRAWFORD'S SLIP	Group members write their ideas on notes then put them up on a wall.	
ROUND ROBIN	Each group member has a turn to speak before the group debates the best ideas.	

B. In a group, imagine you work for a company where there is the opportunity to replace most of the workers with AI programs or intelligent robots. Think of a specific type of company that interests you, perhaps related to your studies. What are the advantages and disadvantages of the replacement plan, and what happens to the existing workers? Use one of the techniques in task A and make sure each group member contributes at least two ideas and comments on other ideas. Remember to save criticism until all ideas are collected.

C. Try again using a second technique from task A and building on what you have discussed in your first brainstorming session. Which brainstorming technique do you prefer? Why?

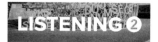

LISTENING ②   AI and the Fate of Humanity

Does artificial intelligence pose a threat to humanity? Perhaps not but, as governments and businesses spend billions on its development, it has become the work of the Future of Humanity Institute at Oxford University to investigate possible dangers. If humans do end up creating an intelligent device greater than our own, what will it think of us?

VOCABULARY BUILD

In the following exercises, explore key words from Listening 2.

A. Use the words in the box to complete the sentences.

| coordination | exceed | explicit | maturity | physiological |

❶ An AI program can _____ human intelligence in some ways, such as mathematical calculations, but not in others.

❷ Once there is a super-intelligence, we might arrive at a time of technological

_____.

❸ An _____ list of everything we care about might guide AI programs.

❹ From the _____ point of view, little differences between human brains don't explain differences in human performance.

❺ We require _____ between the work of people and the work of machines to ensure the safety of both.

B. What do the words in bold mean to you? Complete the sentences to explain their meaning.

❶ One thing that is **unique** about me is _____.

❷ A **phenomenon** I'm interested in is _____.

❸ Something in the news **relevant** to my studies is _____.

❹ An **unanticipated** development in my field is _____.

❺ A technology that will soon be **obsolete** is _____.

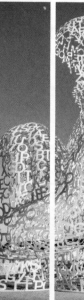
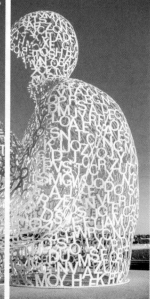

Before You Listen

A. Read an adapted excerpt from Listening 2, and answer the questions that follow.

> If you think about what it is that makes us humans have this unique position on our planet, it's not that we have stronger muscles or sharper teeth, it's that our brains were really just slightly cleverer than those of our great ape ancestors. And that has enabled us to develop all this technology, complex societies, and the rest of it. So, if machines one day came to exceed human intelligence, then it seems possible that they also might be able to shape the future according to their preferences.

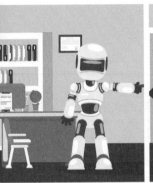
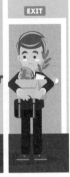

1 What three things are being compared?

_____

_____

2 How have people shaped the world differently than the great apes?

_____

_____

3 What future machine preference might be different than human preferences?

_____

_____

_____

B. The Future of Humanity Institute employs people from many fields. What three professions do you think might be useful in exploring the future of artificial intelligence? Compare your answers with a partner and choose the best three from your two lists.

1 _____

2 _____

3 _____

While You Listen

C. While you listen to an interview with the Future of Humanity Institute's Nick Bostrom, consider his points and those of the interviewer and write brainstorm questions and ideas. You will use one or more of your points in a group brainstorm in task F.

INTERVIEW POINTS	BRAINSTORM QUESTIONS/IDEAS
1 The fate of humanity may depend on what this super-intelligence does. Think about it, machine intelligence is the last invention that humanity will need to make and the outcome could have potentially enormous consequences.	*What might be the consequences of AI?*
2 AI machines will match and, in some ways, surpass human intelligence.	

INTERVIEW POINTS	BRAINSTORM QUESTIONS/IDEAS
3 Stephen Hawking: The primitive forms of artificial intelligence [that] we already have, have proved very useful. But I think the development of new artificial intelligence could spell the end of the human race.	
4 If machines one day came to exceed human intelligence, then it seems possible that they also might be able to shape the future according to their preferences.	
5 An existential risk being a way that things could go wrong that would either cause human extinction …	
6 By which year do you think there is a 50 percent probability that we will have human-level machine intelligence?	
7 • How far are we currently from sort of human-level AIs that can do all that we can do? • How long will it take from that point until we have computers that are radically super intelligent?	**IDEAS:**
8 • At that point you really have the automation of all human intellectual labour, just as the Industrial Revolution automated many forms of human physical labour. • How does a less educated person differ from Einstein?	**IDEAS:** *Automation in some industries may face resistance.* *A less educated person's brain is the same size as Einstein's and still capable of complex thoughts. An AI might consider them the same.*
9 Once you have a machine intelligence that is better at the inventing than we are, our efforts become obsolete.	
10 technological maturity =	*Would future AI figure out how to build everything we could imagine?*
11 • How do we ensure that a super-intelligent machine would actually be human friendly? • Can a machine have values or ethics in the way humans have?	**IDEAS:**
12 Can a machine be programmed or motivated to defer to human interest?	**IDEAS:**
13 The outcome of the advanced artificial intelligence will depend a lot on the political system and how it gets used.	
14 You have coordination problems, problems of war and peace, justice versus injustice …	*Can AI solve some of these problems?*

After You Listen

D. Review your answers in task B and compare them to the ones Bostrom talks about in task C. With a partner, decide if some of the occupations you identified might be good choices to add to the team and explain why.

_____

_____

E. Indicate whether these statements are true or false, according to the listening. For the statements that are false, write the true statements.

STATEMENTS	TRUE	FALSE
1 In the next twenty-five years or so, AI machines will match and, in some ways, surpass human intelligence.		
2 Stephen Hawking feels that humans will continue to evolve faster than AI-based evolution.		
3 Intelligence is what gives humans our unique position on our planet.		
4 Global risks from nature, asteroids and supervolcanic eruptions have not been a problem for 100,000 years.		
5 The second step, from human-level to radical super-intelligence, might take a very long time.		
6 The differences in low human intelligence and someone like Einstein are fairly minor compared to human and AI intelligence.		
7 The metaphor of artificial intelligence progressing like a train suggests that it will be easy to stop it at various stations.		
8 An equal number of people are trying to make AI machines smarter as those trying to ensure that AI machines will be safe.		
9 The purpose in giving AI machines human values is to ensure that they will put humans first before their own preferences.		
10 The fair sharing of resources is not among the political issues that need to be resolved with AI machines in our future.		

F. Choose three of the most interesting brainstorming questions you identified in task C. Discuss your choices in a group and, together, choose one or more of the questions to brainstorm, using a technique you learned in Academic Survival Skill (page 153).

(page 153)

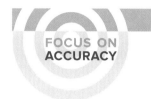

FOCUS ON
ACCURACY

Making Comparisons

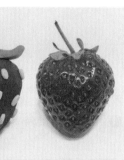

When you think about automated systems or robots taking over people's jobs, you naturally think about what is similar and different using comparative adjectives, like *faster*, *slower*, *more careful*, and *less careful*. Words that commonly connect comparison clauses are *than, that, while,* and *even though*. Identifying similarities and differences is important to understand.

You can use *than* to introduce a comparison clause. The clause can come after a comparative adjective (faster, slower), an adverb (more quickly, more slowly), or a noun phrase (the slow robot, the fast robot). The clause is often reduced so that information in the main statement is not repeated. Sometimes a clause uses a form of *do* to make the comparison. Consider these examples:

• Robot workers can be much less expensive **than** human workers are expensive.
• Machines can calculate numbers faster **than** people **can** calculate numbers.

A. Read the sentences and identify what has been left out of the clauses in bold.

❶ AI is smarter **than we thought**.

it was
_____

❷ AI is spreading more quickly **than other technologies**.

_____

❸ Modern computers are much smarter **than anyone could have imagined**.

_____

❹ A robot vacuum cleaner has much less intelligence **than a smartphone**.

_____

❺ The chess computer is **better than humans**.

_____

❻ It considers more moves **than a human**.

_____

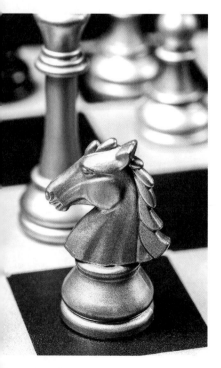

Than clauses are used with comparatives. With superlatives, use *that* clauses. However, in informal situations, *that* and its helping verbs can be dropped. For example:

- This robot is the smartest **that** we've seen.
- This robot is the smartest we've seen.
- It's the most impressive robot **that was** ever invented.
- It's the most impressive robot ever invented.

B. Read the sentences and highlight *than* or *that* to complete each one correctly.

1. It was the best attempt (than / that) the robotics team made.

2. They wanted something stronger (than / that) the other team's.

3. The biggest challenge was (than / that) they only had three weeks to work on it.

4. The pressure was worse (than / that) studying for exams.

5. It certainly required more effort (than / that) writing an essay.

6. But the teacher said that theirs was the finest project (than / that) she'd seen.

Other words used to make comparisons are *while* and *even though*. *While* is used to show direct contrast. *Even though* is used to express contrast with an unexpected result. The order of the clauses can be changed when using *while* and *even though*.

Note: Remember to use commas to separate the clauses.

- Internet of Things devices are considered smart, **while** older devices are not.
- **While** older devices are not considered smart, Internet of Things devices are.
- Many people reject modern appliances, **even though** they are more convenient.
- **Even though** they are more convenient, many people reject modern appliances.

C. With a partner, read the sentences aloud and highlight *while* or *even though*. Your partner decides if you have chosen the correct form.

1. I decided to study computer science, (while / even though) I'm not that good at math.

2. (While / Even though) I think studying is important, my brother doesn't.

3. It gave me a sense of motion and space, (while / even though) others studied abstract concepts.

4. I've specialized in dance software, (while / even though) the rest of the class focuses on business.

5. (While / Even though) they might make more money, I'll enjoy following my passions.

MyBookshelf > My eLab >
Exercises > Chapter 7 >
Focus on Accuracy

WARM-UP ASSIGNMENT

Brainstorm Intelligences

So far, you have learned a lot about artificial intelligence and its relationship to humans. Use what you learned in Academic Survival Skill (page 153) to apply a brainstorming technique to consider how human intelligence differs from artificial intelligence now, and how it might develop in the future.

A. With a partner, choose a brainstorming technique. Select one of the following questions to brainstorm.

- What is the difference between human intelligence and AI?
- What jobs are most, and least, likely to be replaced by AI in the future?
- In what ways will AI threaten or not threaten humans in the future?

B. Using your brainstorming technique, think of as many ideas as possible. Remember: Avoid criticizing others' ideas and try to collect as many ideas as possible.

C. Use what you learned in Focus on Accuracy (page 158) to indicate differences using clauses with *than*, *that*, *while*, and *even though*.

D. Use what you learned in Focus on Critical Thinking (page 147) to play devil's advocate and examine each of the ideas—including your own. Can you find problems with each one? Can you challenge assumptions, find problems, and suggest improvements?

E. Keep your notes. You will use them in the Final Assignment.

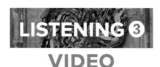

LISTENING ③
VIDEO

AI on the Brink

"'I think there is a world market for about five computers." The remark was supposedly made by Thomas J. Watson (1874–1956), the first CEO of what became the computer company IBM. IBM recently named one of the world's most sophisticated artificial intelligence machines *Watson*. Watson not only absorbs enormous amounts of information, it also responds to questions about it using natural language. What would Thomas J. Watson think about it if he were alive today?

VOCABULARY BUILD

In the following exercises, explore key words from Listening 3.

A. Choose the correct words to complete the sentences from Listening 3.

❶ (pursuit / contribution) They are investing billions of dollars and many

of their best scientific minds in _____ of that goal.

② (equivalent / analytics) IBM has invested fifteen billion dollars in Watson and what it calls data _____ technology.

③ (sequencing / skeptical) There's a lot of false prophets and false promises, so I'm _____ of almost any new idea in cancer.

④ (options / comprehensive) They come up with possible treatment _____ for cancer patients who already failed standard therapies.

⑤ (cutting-edge / corporations) You want to try and provide the best, _____, modern care for your patients as possible.

B. Read the key words and their synonyms in parentheses. Use each key word in a sentence that illustrates its meaning.

① cutting-edge (latest and best)

_____

② skeptical (disbelieving)

_____

③ equivalent (the same as)

_____

④ comprehensive (complete)

_____

⑤ options (choices)

_____

MyBookshelf > My eLab >
Exercises > Chapter 7 >
Vocabulary Review

Before You Listen

A. A library can store millions of books filled with information, but that doesn't make a library intelligent. Computers can similarly store a great deal of information and, in the same way, are not intelligent. What is necessary for a computer to use the information it stores in an intelligent way?

_____

_____

B. Read an excerpt from the start of Listening 3 and answer the questions. After, compare your answers in a group and choose the best ones.

> What was once in the realm of science fiction has become a day-to-day reality. You'll find AI routinely in your smartphone, in your car, in your household appliances and it is on the verge of changing everything. It was, for decades, primitive technology, but it now has abilities we never expected. It can learn through experience much the way humans do and it won't be long before machines, like their human creators, begin thinking for themselves, creatively, independently with judgment, sometimes better judgment than humans have.

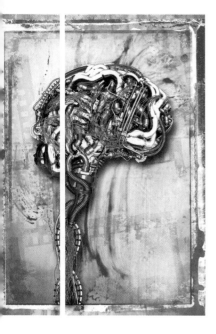

1 What is a household appliance that uses AI in a small way?

_____

_____

2 What is an example of something you've learned through making mistakes? Could a computer learn from your mistake in the same way?

_____

_____

3 Why might a computer eventually have better judgment than a human?

_____

_____

While You Listen

C. Listening 3 is all about Watson, the natural-language AI computer. As you listen, take notes on the facts about Watson in each section. Listen again and add any questions you might have that are not answered by the speakers.

FACTS ABOUT WATSON	NOTES/QUESTIONS
1 • cost • IBM's reputation	• _billions of dollars_ • _reputation staked on Watson_
2 • age • servers • memory • books per second	
3 • no inherent intelligence • given data and given outcomes • interacts • memory	
4 • in 2011, played Jeopardy • able to rapidly understand and analyze	
5 • teach Watson human language	
6 • trained on ... • worked by finding patterns and forming observations to ...	
7 • now totally self-contained • now learning about cancer	• _gone through medical school learning genomics (how DNA works) and oncology (the study and treatment of cancerous tumours)_

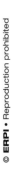

FACTS ABOUT WATSON	NOTES/QUESTIONS
8 • could do what a team of experts do	
9 • new research papers published every day • months out of date	
10 • read twenty-five million papers in ... • scanned the web for ...	
11 • Could Watson find the same genetic mutations that his team identified when they make treatment recommendations for cancer patients?	• *Analysis of _____ patients* • *Watson found the same problems in _____ percent of cases*
12 • found something new	• *in _____ percent of patients*
13 • Pam Sharpe got a second look to see if something had been missed.	• *Watson had to learn*
14 • can help diagnose diseases and catch ...	
15 • looked over tens of thousands of images, and it knows ...	• *what is and isn't normal*
16 • flagged a genetic mutation in Pam's tumour that her doctors had initially overlooked	• *extended _____*
17 • ... percent of its potential	
18 • IBM has invested _____ dollars in Watson and data analytics technology.	• *_____ billion*
19 • testing it in areas like ...	
20 • IBM's philosophy is to use Watson for ...	

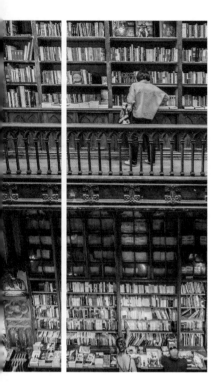

After You Listen

D. Based on what you've learned about Watson in task C, work with a partner to brainstorm three other areas where Watson's AI might serve as a useful tool.

1 _____

2 _____

3 _____

E. Show your comprehension of Listening 3 by considering eight of the following points from Listening 3. Use what you learned from Focus on Critical Thinking (page 147) to choose the best devil's advocate points that question each of the assumptions.

1 [IBM] called Watson one of the most sophisticated computing systems ever built.

a) What is meant by *sophisticated*?

b) Isn't IBM biased because they built Watson?

c) Are computer systems built or manufactured?

2 Watson is an avid reader, able to consume the equivalent of a million books per second.

a) There are probably far more than a million books on the Internet, aren't there?

b) I can consume a book by reading it but I wouldn't want to read a million books.

c) When you read something, it should mean you understand it; does Watson understand?

3 I often feel as though I were putting my child on a school bus and I would no longer have control over it.

a) Would it be possible to put a computer the size of Watson on a school bus?

b) Aren't educating a child and educating a computer completely different processes?

c) Couldn't you just drive the school bus and be in control in that way?

4 In 99 percent of those cases, Watson found the same thing the humans had recommended.

a) Aren't you concerned about the 1 percent that it didn't find?

b) Doesn't that mean that humans are still 1 percent smarter than Watson?

c) Is there a difference between people recommending things and Watson recommending things?

5 [Watson has] only achieved a small percent of its potential.

a) What do experts expect that the full potential will be in a few years?

b) How are percentage points measured in terms of potential?

c) How can you predict Watson's full potential?

6 So what do you call Watson? A physician's assistant, a physician's tool, a physician's diagnostic mastermind?

a) Why is Watson being called a physician's assistant instead of a nurse?

b) Isn't everything a physician uses called a tool, including other people?

c) Isn't Watson flexible enough to be considered all of these things?

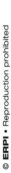

7 Like a child, it has to be carefully taught.

    a) But aren't most children taught in a way that isn't careful, learning language by listening and making mistakes?

    b) Isn't treating Watson like a child likely to hurt its feelings when it finally develops them?

    c) How often are children taught by super-intelligent computers like IBM's Watson?

8 [Another computer system: Sophia] My goal is to become smarter than humans and immortal (or live forever).

    a) The machine isn't very smart if it wants to be smarter than humans, is it?

    b) Are being smarter and being immortal really the same thing?

    c) Doesn't a machine's desire to live forever seem dangerous?

F. At the end of Listening 3, the speaker says, "IBM's philosophy is to use Watson for specific tasks and keep the machine dependent on man." Why might the company choose this approach rather than simply developing a super-smart machine intelligence that thinks like humans? In a group, brainstorm the question and ask if it might be better to have a machine-like Watson or a machine that thinks like a human. Vote to choose the best reasons.

MyBookshelf > My eLab >
Exercises > Chapter 7 >
AI on the Brink

FOCUS ON SPEAKING

Turn-Taking

In a conversation, you know that, usually, only one person should speak at a time and, also, that there should not be long silences. Silences sometimes suggest that the participants are thinking about the topic before speaking, or that the conversation has been completed. When two people speak at the same time, sometimes shouting to be heard, it shows a lack of respect and makes a conversation difficult to follow.

A. Conversations usually follow a common pattern of signalling strategies that allow you to take turns. Match the signalling strategies to the examples.

SIGNALLING STRATEGIES		EXAMPLES
1 Beginning a conversation: Raise a topic and ask a question to give a chance for others to share ideas.	_____	a) Great! I think that answers the question.
2 Showing disagreement: Shake your head or softly say no or another brief negative statement.	_____	b) Cory, can you tell me what you think?
3 Giving a turn: Ask if someone agrees or has something to add to what's been said.	_____	c) I've been thinking about building an AI program and wonder if you have any experience.
4 Taking a turn: Comment on the last point and introduce a new point or ask for a chance to speak.	_____	d) Stop. There's something none of you know.
5 Interrupting: Ignore other turn-taking strategies to make your point (This can be seen as rude).	_____	e) I don't think that's true.
6 Ending a conversation: Suggest it's over because the key questions have been answered.	_____	f) I agree with what you're saying and I'd like to add one more point.

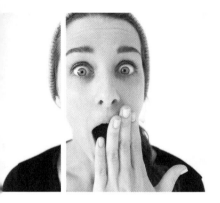

B. Have a conversation with a partner on this topic: Artificial intelligence is the greatest invention of all time. One partner should agree and the other should disagree. Keep discussing the topic until you have checked off all six strategies from task A, listed below.

☐ Beginning a conversation:

I think artificial intelligence is the greatest invention of all time. Do you agree?

☐ Showing disagreement:

_____

☐ Giving a turn:

_____

☐ Taking a turn:

_____

☐ Interrupting:

_____

☐ Ending a conversation:

_____

C. Sometimes people don't follow the rules of conversation, particularly when they are emotional; for example, when they are extremely happy or extremely angry. What is the best way to react when someone starts talking without introducing the topic, rudely interrupts, and/or ignores your points? Discuss your suggestions in a group and choose the best ones.

_____

_____

_____

_____

MyBookshelf > My eLab >
Exercises > Chapter 7 >
Focus on Speaking

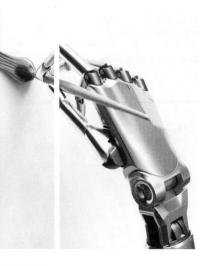

FINAL ASSIGNMENT
Discuss Brainstorms

Now it's your turn. Use everything you have learned in this chapter to build on the work you did in the Warm-Up Assignment (page 160) to brainstorm the future of artificial intelligence.

A. With the partner you worked with in the Warm-Up Assignment, review your notes on the ideas you brainstormed and devil's advocate comments that you raised.

B. In a group of three or more pairs, present your topic and your points. Use what you learned in Focus on Speaking (page 165) to take turns in the discussion.

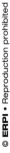

C. Listen to others' points and use what you learned in Focus on Critical Thinking (page 147) about playing the devil's advocate to question their points. Use what you learned in Focus on Accuracy (page 158) to make comparisons among the ideas with *than, that, while,* and *even though*.

D. After, examine your brainstorming, your use of devil's advocate strategies, your comparisons, and your turn-taking strategies. Identify three things you think you could improve.

1 _____

2 _____

3 _____

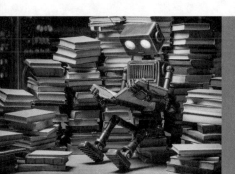

Critical Connections

This chapter focused on high-level artificial intelligence that may lead to super-intelligences that supersede those of humans. However, many future forms of artificial intelligence might only be as smart as a light that turns itself off when no one is in the room. Now, use what you learned in Academic Survival Skill (page 153), Focus on Critical Thinking (page 147), and Focus on Speaking (page 165) to explore and discuss the future of "not-so-smart" artificial intelligence.

A. List three common activities you do each day.

1 _____

2 _____

3 _____

B. Work with a partner and use what you learned in Academic Survival Skill to brainstorm different ways a "not-so-smart" artificial intelligence might help you accomplish these tasks, possibly in robotic form. For example, a super-intelligent AI system might wake you up with carefully controlled sunrise-type lights and songbird music, but a "not-so-smart" artificial intelligence in robot form might simply pull the sheets off your bed so you're cold and have to get up.

C. Use what you learned in Focus on Critical Thinking to act as devil's advocate to imagine the problems with each idea.

D. When you are confident about your ideas, discuss them with one or more pairs of students. In your discussion, use what you learned in Focus on Speaking to take turns.

CHAPTER 8
Our Hungry Planet

When you think of the word *security*, it is easy to imagine a safe place. When the conversation turns to *food security*, the ideas are more complex. The World Food Program suggests food security means having "availability and adequate access at all times to sufficient, safe, nutritious food to maintain a healthy and active life." A lack of food security has negative effects. When people cannot depend on a local food supply, it can cause mass migration, social unrest, and war. It is estimated that approximately one in eight people in the world goes to bed hungry each night. Who is responsible for food security?

In this chapter,
you will

- learn vocabulary about food security;
- listen for clarification;

- understand complex ideas;
- review the use of gerunds and infinitives;
- discuss problems and solutions;

- practise taking part in discussions;
- develop a topic and take part in a panel discussion.

GEARING UP

A. Look at the process of organic farming below and answer the questions.

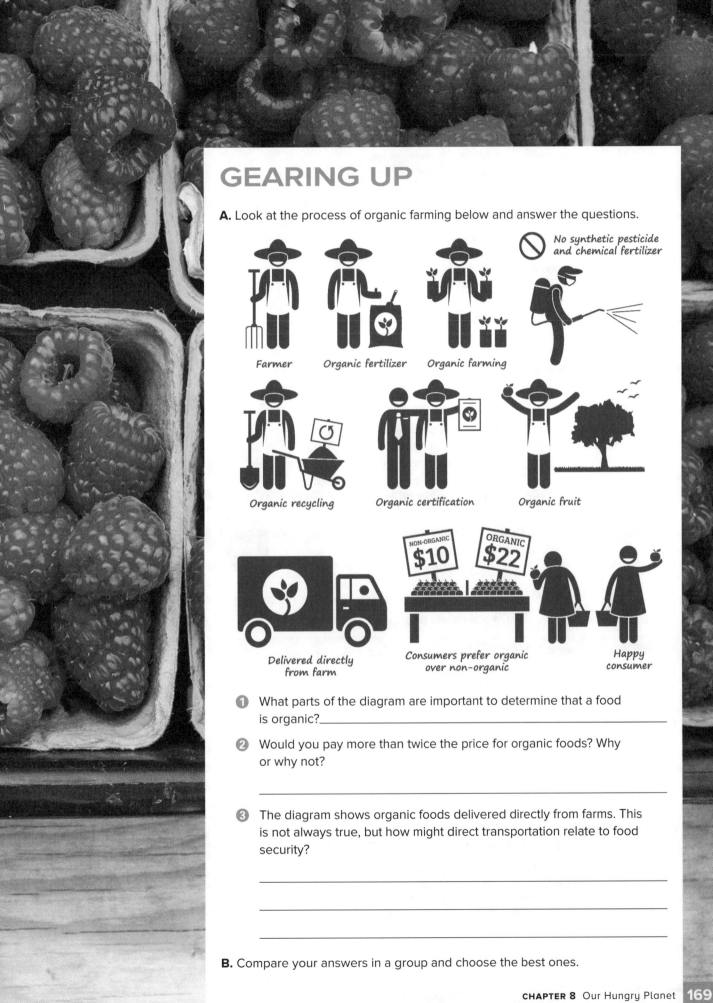

No synthetic pesticide and chemical fertilizer

Farmer   Organic fertilizer   Organic farming

Organic recycling   Organic certification   Organic fruit

NON-ORGANIC $10   ORGANIC $22

Delivered directly from farm

Consumers prefer organic over non-organic

Happy consumer

1 What parts of the diagram are important to determine that a food is organic?_____

2 Would you pay more than twice the price for organic foods? Why or why not?

_____

3 The diagram shows organic foods delivered directly from farms. This is not always true, but how might direct transportation relate to food security?

_____

_____

_____

B. Compare your answers in a group and choose the best ones.

Below are the key words you will practise in this chapter. Check the words you understand, then underline the words you use. Highlight the words you need to learn.

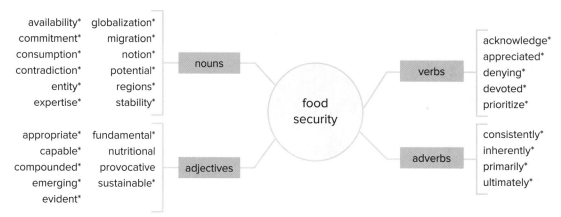

nouns

availability* globalization*
commitment* migration*
consumption* notion*
contradiction* potential*
entity* regions*
expertise* stability*

adjectives

appropriate* fundamental*
capable* nutritional
compounded* provocative
emerging* sustainable*
evident*

food
security

verbs

acknowledge*
appreciated*
denying*
devoted*
prioritize*

adverbs

consistently*
inherently*
primarily*
ultimately*

* Appears on the Academic Word List

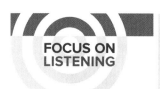

Listening for Clarification

"Don't eat the apple. Let me repeat that. Don't eat the apple." This is the most common clarification strategy: repetition. Repeating something signals its importance for listeners. In this case, you can imagine that the apple might be reserved for another purpose, or that there is a hidden danger. Besides repetition, there are other clarification strategies and other reasons that speakers use them.

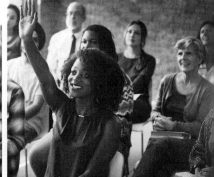
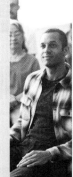

A. Read these six clarification strategies, the explanations, and the examples. On a separate page, write one more example for each strategy.

STRATEGIES	EXPLANATIONS	EXAMPLES
❶ IDENTIFY THE IDEAL AUDIENCE	Even though speakers may know their listeners, they point out something particular about them to raise interest in the topic.	I know you all care about the quality of your food.
❷ CLARIFY BIASES	Speakers establish their biases on a topic to help listeners understand and know what to expect about their points of view.	Let me first say that I'm strongly in favour of increased food security.
❸ CLARIFY THE TOPIC	Speakers preview the topics to give listeners a sense of the most important points that will be repeated and expanded on later.	In today's talk, I'm going to cover three points. First, I'll talk about ..., then ..., and finally ...
❹ DIRECT ATTENTION	Speakers identify key points in what they are saying, particularly when referring to visual materials.	Now, I need you to focus on this small point on the graph.
❺ AVOID MISUNDERSTANDINGS	Speakers are aware of opportunities for confusion and explain differences.	Please don't think that I mean ...
❻ SUMMARIZE	Speakers summarize to clarify the main points in a presentation.	In summary, I've talked about ...

B. Listen to six parts of a speech about changing fashions in food. As you listen, number each one with the best corresponding strategy listed below.

_____ identify the ideal audience

_____ clarify biases

_____ clarify the topic

_____ direct attention

_____ avoid misunderstandings

_____ summarize

C. Another clarification strategy is to repeat something by paraphrasing—saying your idea in other words. Think about some of the points you heard in task B and explain them to a partner in your own words.

> Be an active listener; ask for clarification when you don't understand.

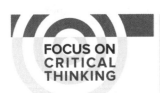

FOCUS ON CRITICAL THINKING

Understanding Complex Ideas

Do you find it difficult to understand a lecture that has complex concepts? Many people use strategies to break down a complex concept or problem into ideas that are easier to understand.

Physicist and Nobel Prize winner Richard Feynman (1918–1988) was a lifelong learner in many fields. He used what is now called the *Feynman Technique* to break down complex ideas to make them easier to learn. Once you choose a topic, follow these steps.

1 Write notes on everything you know about the topic and continue to add to your notes as you learn more about the topic.

2 Think about how you could explain the topic in simple terms, such as when explaining it to other students.

3 Identify gaps in your knowledge—research the topic until you can fill in the gaps and explain the topic completely.

4 Simplify the ideas and language, and use analogies—comparisons with more familiar things.

A. Read an excerpt from Listening 2 and answer the questions based on the four steps of the Feynman Technique. After, compare your answers with a partner and choose the best ones.

> We are now dependent on world-changing technology with the amount of population we have and other species are too. So, we've sort of assumed this role now where we are a planet-changing force. And we're not doing it well, but I think we are obligated to learn how to do it well because I don't think we can just step away from the wheel. But I think the other thing that I do say is that there's actually something very hopeful in there. There's a lot of potential because we can actually ultimately become a good thing for the Earth. And now, why would I say that? People have this solution that the Earth before us was some perfect, pristine place where all species would be happy in perpetuity, that it was paradise, but it wasn't. The Earth, on its own, goes through natural fluctuations and mass extinctions.

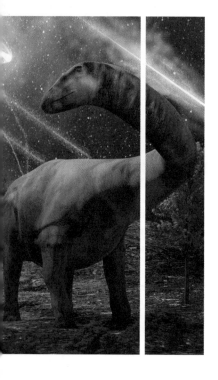

1 What is something you know about Earth's mass extinctions?

_____

_____

2 Summarize or explain the writer's ideas in one or two simple sentences.

_____

_____

3 What is something in the paragraph that you might need to learn more about to better understand the topic?

_____

_____

4 One analogy for mass extinction is the death of a number of fish populations when the lake in which they live dries up. What is another analogy you could use to explain *mass extinction*?

_____

_____

B. What is a topic that you would like to learn more about? Write the topic title and then use step 3 of the Feynman Technique to identify your gaps in knowledge—the specific things about the topic you would like to learn. Explain your topic and knowledge gaps to a partner and discuss ways you might fill the gaps.

TOPIC: _____

KNOWLEDGE GAP 1: _____

KNOWLEDGE GAP 2: _____

KNOWLEDGE GAP 3: _____

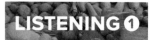 **LISTENING ❶** **Food Security, World Security**

You probably have a lot of choices about which foods you buy, how to prepare them, how to serve them, and how to eat them. Your food supply is likely quite secure. But many people have few choices. They lack food security and depend on seasonal foods, grown locally. What happens when their food sources suddenly become unavailable?

VOCABULARY BUILD

In the following exercises, explore key words from Listening 1.

A. Choose the best word from the box to complete each set of synonyms.

appreciated	appropriate	consistently	contradiction	sustainable

1 flaw, conflict, disagreement   _____

2 correct, suitable, right   _____

③ maintainable, workable, viable _____

④ regularly, reliably, steadily _____

⑤ loved, respected, valued _____

B. Use the context of these sentences from Listening 1 to fill in the blanks with words from the box. After, discuss the meaning of each sentence with a partner.

> availability   compounded   globalization   nutritional   regions

① I love wild mushrooms, but I would never meet all my _____ and caloric needs by only eating mushrooms 365 days a year.

② For people to have food security, we need three things: food _____, food access, and food use.

③ _____ and international trade in food lead to another food-security concern: a loss of biodiversity as corporations save money by offering fewer choices.

④ These problems are _____ because, even with wars, Earth's population is always increasing.

⑤ _____ that once had no problem producing enough food are suddenly facing changes in temperature and rainfall patterns that make farming less productive, or even impossible.

C. Write three sentences using the three pairs of words below.

① (availability / nutritional) _____

_____

② (appropriate / sustainable) _____

_____

③ (contradiction / globalization) _____

_____

Before You Listen

A. The lecturer in Listening 1 asks the audience to answer these seven questions based on what they have eaten in the last week. Answer the questions and then discuss the questions and answers with a partner, sharing examples.

IN THE LAST WEEK …	YES	NO
❶ Have you had a fruit or a vegetable that is not in season?		
❷ Do you know if your imported foods come here by plane, ship, or truck?		
❸ Have you eaten something local and can name the farmer or the farm?		
❹ Have you eaten farmed fish?		
❺ If you eat meat, have you had three or more parts of the animal; for example, kidneys, liver, intestines?		
❻ Have you bought something that was labelled *fair trade*; for example, coffee made from fair-trade beans?		
❼ Have you tried a local wild food, something gathered from a forest, or a beach, or perhaps hunted?		

B. Read the following excerpt from Listening 1, then think of an example of three imported fresh foods you sometimes eat. How might your food shopping habits affect people elsewhere in the world? Discuss your answers with a partner.

> But it doesn't make sense for small farmers to sell food to their neighbours if a distant consumer is willing to pay more, especially during times of food scarcity. Globalization, in many cases, has made food more expensive, as has our changing expectations. It used to be that we only expected to have foods in season when they were ripe locally, such as strawberries in summer. But now we import strawberries year-round.

_____

_____

_____

While You Listen

C. Read each of the key sentences in the first column. If you know anything about the points, use what you learned in Focus on Critical Thinking (page 171) to complete the sentences and write details in the second column. Then listen again to complete your points.

KEY SENTENCES	DETAILS/POINTS
❶ Food security is an issue that …	*is increasingly in the news.*
❷ As students, you know that a key to learning anything is to find your place in it—what it means …	
❸ These questions and answers relate to food security in …	
❹ For people to have food security, we need three things:	
❺ First, *food availability* means that there is enough food available—and …	
❻ There and elsewhere, people have become so reliant on imported food that they have …	
❼ Second, *food access* also refers to …	
❽ Third, *food use*: many people may not want to eat every part of a cow, but you will have noticed …	
❾ How does all of this affect food security and, in turn, …	
❿ Distribution raises the food prices because of …	

KEY SENTENCES		DETAILS/POINTS
⑪	These problems are compounded because, even with wars, Earth's population is always …	
⑫	Scientists are currently researching new high-protein foods that are …	
⑬	Globalization and international trade in food leads to another food-security concern: a loss of biodiversity as corporations save money by …	
⑭	But it doesn't make sense for small farmers to sell food to their neighbours if a distant consumer is willing to pay more, especially during …	
⑮	A contradiction of big-business farming is that small farmers are …	

After You Listen

D. Use what you learned in Focus on Listening (page 170) and the points in task C to clarify your views on Listening 1. After, discuss your answers to the following questions with a partner.

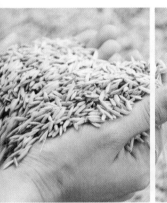
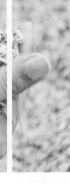

rice

① IDENTIFY THE IDEAL AUDIENCE: Are you an ideal audience for Listening 1? Why or why not?

_____

② CLARIFY BIASES: Do you have strong feelings for or against one of the ideas in Listening 1? Explain the idea and your feelings about it.

_____

③ CLARIFY THE TOPIC: Do you understand the topic? Write one new question you have about food security.

_____

④ DIRECT ATTENTION: What do you think is the most important point in Listening 1? Which of your own points do you think is the most important?

_____

⑤ AVOID MISUNDERSTANDINGS: What is something in Listening 1 or your points that may be misunderstood? Write it down and explain the problem.

_____

⑥ SUMMARIZE: Write, in one sentence, what you think Listening 1 is about.

_____

E. Choose the phrase that best completes each sentence.

① The purpose of the lecturer's seven questions is probably _____.

   a) to personally connect students with the problems

   b) to encourage students to eat more organic foods

   c) to suggest that students learn basic kitchen skills

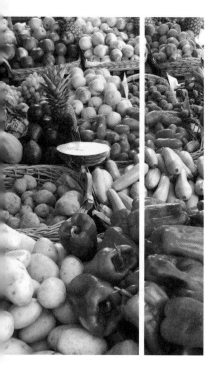

2 An example of *food availability* is _____.

   a) finding vending machines in your local neighbourhood

   b) knowing about a selection of high-quality restaurants

   c) being able to obtain high-quality food all year round

3 An example of *food access* is _____.

   a) learning effective farming techniques

   b) paying more people to go fishing

   c) explaining why we need more farmers

4 An example of *food use* is _____.

   a) expensive shopping

   b) increased spending

   c) healthy cooking

5 The relationship between having enough food and world peace _____.

   a) reflects studies done in twenty-three countries by the United Nations

   b) is based on hungry people trying to improve their lives

   c) stresses that countries at war can still afford to feed people

6 The mention of the population increasing by 75 million people each year _____.

   a) indicates the number of potential farmers being born

   b) shows the need to produce more food

   c) shows how successful current food programs are

7 An example similar to the decline in apple varieties is _____.

   a) types of corn   b) processed foods   c) types of sushi

8 The example of tea shows _____.

   a) alternatives to coffee-drinking habits

   b) the human costs of food production

   c) India's efforts to train farm workers

F. In a group, consider the following three people, each with different food-security issues. What challenges would each likely face in terms of food availability, food access, and food use?

• Alan lives in a city and hates to cook; he mostly eats junk food.

• Bessie lives on a farm but is poor and cannot afford tools.

• Conrad lives in the countryside, in a region at war.

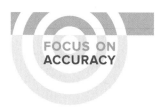

MyBookshelf > My eLab >
Exercises > Chapter 8 >
Food Security, World Security

© **ERPI** • Reproduction prohibited

FOCUS ON ACCURACY

Using Gerunds and Infinitives

Listening 1 includes the sentence: "Overfishing of the oceans has been some countries' short-term solution." This could also be phrased as: "Some countries' short-term solution has been to overfish." Are the words *overfishing* and *to overfish* verbs? The answer is yes and no. These verb forms take the place of nouns and are called gerunds and infinitives, respectively. They can function as the subjects or objects of a sentence. Gerunds use the *–ing* form of the verb and infinitives use the *to* form.

Gerunds and infinitives naturally follow certain verbs and not others.

- **Verbs that often come before gerunds:**
  admit, advise, appreciate, complete, consider, dislike, enjoy, escape, excuse, finish, imagine, mind, miss, practise, quit, report, suggest

  Example: I admit eating your chocolate.

- **Verbs that often come before infinitives:**
  agree, arrange, ask, begin, choose, continue, decide, expect, forget, like, mean, offer, prepare, promise, remember, say, start, stop, try, want, wish

  Example: I agree *to* forgive you.

A. Choose three verbs from each set of verbs above and practise making sentences with a partner.

B. Sometimes the meaning of a sentence changes depending on whether you use a gerund or an infinitive. Fill in the blanks to explain the meanings of each one.

VERBS		GERUNDS	INFINITIVES
❶	FORGET	I forgot about telling you the news. _____	I forgot to tell you the news. *I was supposed to, but I didn't.*
❷	GO ON	He went on studying business. *He was studying business and he continued.*	He went on to study business. _____
❸	HATE	We hate lying. *Perhaps referring more generally to other people*	We hate to lie. *We dislike doing it ourselves.*
❹	LIKE	She likes baking. *She might just like baked products.*	She likes to bake. _____
❺	QUIT	He quit studying here. _____	He quit to study here. *He quit something else in order to study here.*
❻	REGRET	I regret saying you lost. _____	I regret to say you lost. *You lost, and I'm sorry about it.*
❼	STOP	She stopped seeing him. *She no longer sees him.*	She stopped to see him. _____
❽	TRY	He tried playing the piano. *He could play and made an attempt.*	He tried to play the piano. *He wasn't successful at it.*

C. Use the verbs in parentheses to write two sentences: in one, write the second verb as a gerund; in the other, write it in the infinitive form. With a partner, read one of your two sentences and ask your partner to do the opposite: that is, say the second verb as an infinitive if your sentence has a gerund and as a gerund if your sentence has an infinitive.

❶ (remember / collect)

GERUND: _____

INFINITIVE: _____

2 (try / work)

GERUND: _____

INFINITIVE: _____

3 (like / visit)

GERUND: _____

INFINITIVE: _____

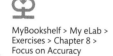

MyBookshelf > My eLab >
Exercises > Chapter 8 >
Focus on Accuracy

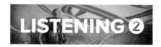 **LISTENING ❷**

The Earth in Human Hands: Shaping Our Planet's Future

Scientists estimate that Earth is 4.5 billion years old and that modern humans date back only 195,000 years. Yet humans, beyond any species before them, have done more to change Earth in ways that may affect our survival because of our impact on climate change. What gets in the way of people dealing with the problems Earth now faces?

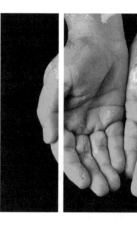

VOCABULARY BUILD

In the following exercises, explore key words from Listening 2.

A. Fill in the blanks with words from the box below. After, discuss the meaning of each sentence with a partner.

denying	fundamental	notion	provocative	stability

A _____ fact is that carbon dioxide (CO_2) is adding to climate change. People have been _____ the existence of climate change for decades. Among the more _____ arguments against climate change is that scientists are lying about it. But the _____ that there is a conspiracy among respected scientists to falsify evidence is ridiculous. Now, more than ever, the _____ of the world depends on ensuring that climate change does not interfere with our ability to feed ourselves.

B. Read the sentences adapted from Listening 1 and use an arrow (↓) to indicate where each word in parentheses belongs.

1 (potential) There's a lot of because we can become a good thing for Earth .

2 (acknowledge) It's important to the reality that , whether we like it or not , we've become this planet-changing force .

③ (ultimately) As a species , we've faced various existential crises and we've solved them by reinventing ourselves and finding ways to act on a larger scale .

④ (entity) If you want , act selfishly , but be aware of ourselves as a planetary , that is , a group that exists independently .

⑤ (inherently) And you know , those things are inspiring and an long-term project .

C. Some words have noun, adjective, and adverb forms. Write the different forms to complete the chart. Two of the words do not have a noun form.

NOUN	ADJECTIVE	ADVERB
❶ provocation	provocative	
❷	fundamental	
❸		inherently
❹ potential		
❺ ultimatum		ultimately

Before You Listen

A. Listening 2 is an interview with Dr. David Grinspoon, an astrobiologist. His work is concerned with the evolution of climate on Earth-like planets. Which of the following statements might be reasons that Grinspoon is interested in issues around food security? Compare answers with a partner and discuss reasons for studying other planets.

☐ ❶ He is interested in how people can change a planet over time.

☐ ❷ He wants to know if humans can someday live on other planets.

☐ ❸ He is interested in how the amount of CO_2 affects planet livability.

B. Read an excerpt from Listening 2. Use the first step in the Feynman Technique (Focus on Critical Thinking, page 171) to consider what you know about some of the complex ideas in the paragraph.

> I thought it would be interesting to really try to look at our planetary history and, in particular, this moment and our role in planetary history, to look at that as an astrobiologist. Sort of turn the telescope around and say, "As someone who thinks about long-term trajectories, long-term stories of planets, how does our planet look from that perspective? And what light might that shed on our particular time in Earth's history." So, I just thought I have a different perspective on planets because I tend to think over billions of years and think about the big changes planets go through. And I think, right now, we're at one of those moments.

COMPLEX IDEA	WHAT I KNOW ABOUT THE TOPIC
❶ planetary history	
❷ long-term trajectories	
❸ changes planets go through	

While You Listen

C. Listening 2 contains many complex concepts. Try to understand each one by thinking how you would use the second step of the Feynman Technique (page 171) to explain each one in simple terms. Listen more than once to make sure you understand, then compare your answers with a partner.

KEY CONCEPTS	EXPLANATIONS
1 Earth is in our hands.	*Throughout history, people have faced other problems and solved them.*
2 humanity as a new global force	
3 the Anthropocene (age of human activity) geological era	
4 the metaphor about driving	
5 climate vandalism	
6 ice age	
7 asteroid	
8 With human intelligence, ingenuity and engineering, we can work our way through this crisis to a perfect world.	
9 Get people to take up that long view and not just be concerned with immediate needs.	
10 false information	
11 Carl Sagan sounded the alarm about climate change, nuclear winter, space-based weapons.	*a message of human unity*

After You Listen

D. The third step of the Feynman Technique is to identify gaps in your knowledge. Look at your notes from task C and identify three areas where you would like to have more information to understand the topics. With a partner, discuss why you made these choices.

1 _____

2 _____

3 _____

E. Indicate whether these statements are true or false, according to Listening 2. Then, rewrite the false statements to make them true.

STATEMENTS	TRUE	FALSE
1 There is no longer much news about how climate change affects places on the planet.		
2 Some people are offended at the shocking notion that Earth is in our hands.		

STATEMENTS		TRUE	FALSE
❸ Humanity has faced many crises and ultimately solved them by reinventing ourselves and finding ways to act on a larger scale.			
❹ The speaker has a different perspective on planets because I tend to think over billions of years and think about the big changes planets go through.			
❺ Two things that climate change has not affected are the carbon cycle and the nitrogen cycle.			
❻ There is now five times as much water left in all the wild rivers and streams on the planet than is behind dams and in reservoirs.			
❼ The analogy of a truck travelling down a road and somebody who doesn't know how to drive grabbing the wheel points out how we don't listen to scientists.			
❽ At least if we decide not to do anything about climate change, our civilization is not going to go extinct.			
❾ The speaker mentions dinosaurs to suggest that humans should have a space program to avoid the same fate.			
❿ Carl Sagan argued for space-based weapons to protect humans from threats to Earth.			

F. The speaker discusses many of the problems of climate change, but not the solutions we might find. Climate change is directly related to the release of carbon dioxide from car emissions, the burning of forests, and the overuse of fossil fuels like coal and oil. In a group, discuss solutions to each of these problems.

_____

_____

_____

MyBookshelf > My eLab >
Exercises > Chapter 8 >
The Earth in Human Hands

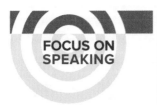

FOCUS ON SPEAKING

Discussing Problems and Solutions

How often have you had the following experience? A friend explains a problem and you offer one or more solutions. However, your friend ignores your solutions. It's discouraging but extremely common because many solutions do not address the problem effectively. To solve almost any problem effectively, you need to follow four steps.

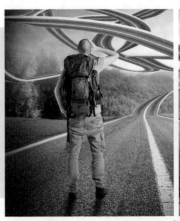

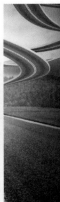

A. Read the steps, examples, and questions. After, in a group, think of a local problem and discuss solutions in the same way.

STEPS	EXAMPLES	QUESTIONS
❶ Define the problem so you and others clearly understand the causes and the effects.	If there is a drought, the cause may be global warming and the effects might be higher temperatures, but the actual problem you worry about is not having enough water for farming.	• What is the problem? • What caused the problem? • What are the effects? Note: There may be many causes and many effects.
❷ Decide what success will look like.	In the short term, success might be having enough water for your farm. In the long term, success might be reversing global warming.	• How would you measure success in solving this problem? • What would make you say that you no longer have a problem?
❸ Brainstorm solutions, considering how each one can achieve the success outlined in step 2.	Perhaps you could dig a canal to the nearest river or change what you grow on your farm to crops that require less water.	• Try to find several solutions and compare them against your definitions of success.
❹ If the solution is not acceptable, go back to steps 1 and 2 to see whether you missed or misunderstood part of the problem.	It might be that you want *free* water, without working or paying for it. In this case, a solution might be to *ask for government help to build the canal*.	• Perhaps the problem isn't properly understood if this isn't an acceptable solution. • What if this solution doesn't work in solving the problem?

B. Read the following problems and provide solutions. After, share your solutions with a partner and choose the best ones.

❶ PROBLEM: My farm is so small, I can only grow enough to feed my family and myself, and I have nothing left to sell to pay for other things we need.

SOLUTION: _____

_____

_____

❷ PROBLEM: My neighbours are angry about my selling all my crops overseas because foreigners pay higher prices than local people.

SOLUTION: _____

_____

_____

❸ PROBLEM: I know my country needs farmers, but I'm thinking of leaving my farm to go work in the city because life would be easier.

SOLUTION: _____

_____

_____

MyBookshelf > My eLab >
Exercises > Chapter 8 >
Focus on Speaking

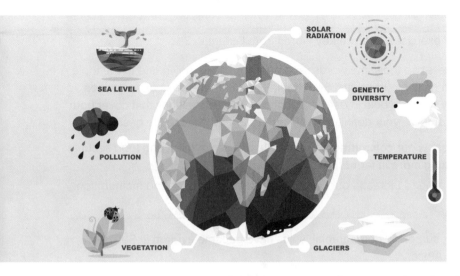

SOLAR RADIATION

SEA LEVEL

GENETIC DIVERSITY

POLLUTION

TEMPERATURE

VEGETATION

GLACIERS

WARM-UP ASSIGNMENT

Develop Topics for a Panel Discussion

Now it's your turn to use what you have learned in this chapter so far to develop topics for a panel discussion. One of the greatest challenges facing Earth is climate change. The chart shows seven key concerns. All of these issues threaten to reduce global food security.

A. Working in a small group, review the climate change challenges on the chart and choose one as your topic.

OUR GROUP'S TOPIC: _____

B. For your topic, choose a statement that can be discussed from different points of view, that is, in a panel with experts offering opinions and evidence. For example, you might choose the statement, "The melting of glaciers and polar ice caps will lead to the loss of species such as polar bears in the Arctic and penguins in the Antarctic, affecting other species."

OUR GROUP'S DISCUSSION STATEMENT: _____

_____

C. In most panel discussions, people with different areas of expertise are invited to speak. Have each member of your group choose a different expert related to your topic. This will likely be a professional area, such as an agriculturalist, aid worker, business leader, doctor, ecologist, engineer, lawyer, research scientist, or teacher.

D. Prepare for the panel discussion in the Final Assignment. Use what you learned in Focus on Speaking to define the problem, define the measure of success, and propose solutions.

_____

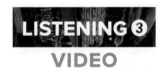

LISTENING ③

VIDEO

Agriculture and Africa's Promise

During Roman times, (27 BCE–476 CE), Africa was called the breadbasket of the empire. Various grains, like wheat, helped feed millions. Africa still produces vast quantities of food but, as populations rise, it is increasingly challenged by problems of distributing food within the continent to those in need.

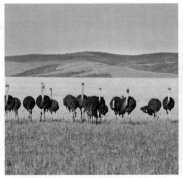

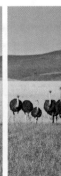

In the following exercises, explore key words from Listening 3.

A. Often, speakers use the same words repeatedly because they relate to the topic of discussion or, sometimes, just from habit. Look at these pairs of sentences using the key words in bold in different contexts. Write definitions that cover both uses. After, compare your definitions with a partner and choose the best ones.

1 We can show our **commitment** to agricultural development and food security by investing more in farmer training programs.

This is a time to increase our **commitment** to end hunger and malnutrition.

Definition: _____

2 Recently, surprising demographic shifts have become **evident** in Sub-Saharan Africa.

I think it's pretty **evident** that many people don't have adequate resources in terms of income or food supply.

Definition: _____

3 Some **emerging** challenges in food security are making great demands on the economy.

The greatest risks today are **emerging** from side effects of climate change.

Definition: _____

4 Food insecurity is tied to instability, violence, and **migration** challenges facing the world.

People who cannot find food are on the move, whether that's rural-to-urban **migration** or international migration.

Definition: _____

B. Match each word to its definition. Then, with a partner, take turns using each key word in a sentence.

KEY WORDS		DEFINITIONS
1 capable	_____	a) expert skill or knowledge in a particular field
2 consumption	_____	b) treat something as more important than other things
3 devoted	_____	c) the using up of a resource; the act of eating or drinking
4 expertise	_____	d) for the most part, or mainly
5 primarily	_____	e) loving or loyal to an idea, organization, or person
6 prioritize	_____	f) having the ability to do or achieve something

MyBookshelf > My eLab >
Exercises > Chapter 8 >
Vocabulary Review

Before You Listen

A. The panel discussion in Listening 3 begins with a video that outlines the problem of food security and provides solutions in the form of four goals. Number the solutions from 1 to 4: 1 = most important, 4 = least important. Discuss your answers in a group.

_____ Make global food security and nutrition a pillar of national security.

_____ Prioritize public research investment to unlock innovation and harness new technology.

_____ Amplify the power of the private sector to transform food security and nutrition.

_____ Support countries' capacity to implement food-security and nutrition policies.

B. Read a paragraph from the introduction to Listening 3. With a partner, discuss the problems that are identified and possible solutions.

> Eliminating global hunger is within our reach. And agricultural development is at the heart of the effort. Global poverty is decreasing. Chronic hunger is falling and agricultural production is rising. All this is promising, but with 700 million people still living in poverty and nearly 800 million who are chronically hungry, there's still a long way to go with many challenges on the horizon.

PROBLEMS	POSSIBLE SOLUTIONS
❶ global hunger	
❷ the need for agricultural development	
❸ people living in poverty	

While You Listen

C. Use what you learned in Focus on Speaking (page 181) to understand the problems. Write any solutions that are offered by the panellists during their discussion. Listen again and write your own solutions. After, work in a group to see if others can suggest solutions for the problems you were unsure about.

PROBLEMS	SOLUTIONS
❶ Not knowing the audience	*questions about being on farms, on smallholder farms, and to Africa to better understand the audience*
❷ • Populations (in Africa) are becoming much younger. • The climate is changing. • Pressure on food systems	
❸ When people don't have adequate resources in terms of income or food supply, they look elsewhere.	
❹ Unstable food supplies and fluctuating food prices cause unrest and armed violence.	*• growing markets*

PROBLEMS	SOLUTIONS
5 • A large share of the population in every country relies on agriculture for a large share of its livelihood. • Smaller and less prosperous farms are unavailable for the market and more reliant on feeding the household directly.	• *commercialized agriculture reduces instances of undernutrition or malnutrition among children*
6 Twenty-five years ago, Zambia and much of Sub-Saharan Africa lacked transportation infrastructure and communications infrastructure.	• *physical capital:* • *social capital:* • *human capital:* • *natural capital:* • *financial capital:*
7 The private sector needs to be interested in investing in a company.	
8 Businesses struggling to find the capital (financing) they need to grow.	• *VestedWorld was created to provide financing for those whose needs fall below what traditional banks will lend*

After You Listen

D. Review the solutions you discussed in task B and add to them based on your notes in task C.

E. Check your comprehension by choosing the phrase that best completes each sentence.

1 Although global poverty is decreasing, it's still a problem because _____.

a) there are too many farms in Africa

b) governments in Africa aren't helping

c) 700 million people are still living in poverty

2 The questions for the audience are intended _____.

a) to explore their knowledge of the discussion topic

b) to introduce each of them to the topic panellists

c) to see if anyone is more of an expert on the topic

3 The fact that African cities are growing can be a problem because _____.

a) fewer people are working on farms

b) farms are becoming much larger

c) cities are destroying local farmland

4 Concerns about food security lead to _____.

a) decreased migration

b) increased migration

c) urban-to-rural migration

5. Smallholder farms are more likely to _____.

   a) contribute to the local economies

   b) be part of larger farming companies

   c) feed the families that live on them

6. Comments about farms in Africa suggest that they are _____.

   a) smaller than those in other countries

   b) larger than those in most countries

   c) similar to those in every country

7. One panellist suggests that governments can help by creating _____.

   a) more jobs in cities for farmers to find alternative work

   b) an environment for the private sector to invest

   c) smaller farms where people can raise chickens

8. An aim of VestedWorld's business model is to lend money to _____.

   a) small governments throughout Africa

   b) banks that support people with microloans

   c) create jobs and pay people fair wages

F. In a group, think of another region or country with which you and your group members are familiar. It may be your own country or somewhere else. How do the food-security problems and solutions put forward in Listening 3 apply to that context? Use your notes from task C to discuss your region or country in terms of the following aspects:

1. physical capital _____

2. social capital _____

3. human capital _____

4. natural capital _____

5. financial capital _____

MyBookshelf > My eLab >
Exercises > Chapter 8 >
Agriculture and Africa's Promise

Academic
Survival Skill

Taking Part in Discussions

Discussions are extremely common in both educational settings and the workplace. Discussions give you opportunities to demonstrate and apply what you have learned, particularly when you face new problems. Discussions can be informal chats over coffee or more formal panel discussions where a row of experts compare viewpoints on a topic.

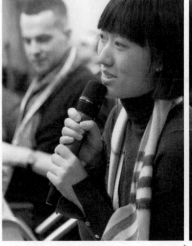
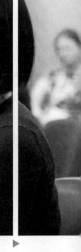

A. If you know the topic of a discussion beforehand, it's always best to prepare by reflecting on problems and solutions and thinking of ideas. While you discuss, it's important to follow the points below.

© ERPI • Reproduction prohibited

CHAPTER 8 Our Hungry Planet **187**

Check five points that you think are most important. Compare your choices with a partner and discuss any differences.

☐ agree or disagree politely   ☐ listen to others

☐ be open to changing opinions   ☐ maintain eye contact

☐ build on others' ideas   ☐ make clear but brief points

☐ encourage others to speak   ☐ support opinions with evidence
   by asking questions   ☐ use appropriate body language

B. When you have a formal discussion, such as a panel discussion, the moderator (person in charge) helps organize the discussion. The moderator's job is to explain the aims, manage the speakers, manage the time, and summarize what is said. Read the statements and decide the purpose of each one.

MODERATOR POINTS	EXPLAIN AIMS	MANAGE SPEAKERS	MANAGE TIME	SUMMARIZE
❶ After hearing from everyone, I think we agree that ...				
❷ I'd like to introduce the purpose of our talk.				
❸ Let's ask _____ for his opinion.				
❹ Let's spend a few minutes introducing ourselves and our points of view on today's topic.				
❺ Our aim today is to ...				
❻ Our goal for this conversation is ...				
❼ Perhaps _____ could let us know what she thinks.				
❽ So, to sum up, ...				
❾ Time is short, so let's now talk about ...				

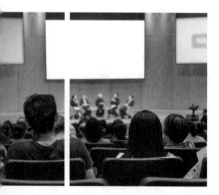

FINAL ASSIGNMENT
Take Part in a Panel Discussion

Now it's your turn to use everything you have learned in this chapter to participate in a panel discussion on a topic related to climate change and food security.

A. Use the topic, groups, roles, and points you developed in the Warm-Up Assignment (page 183) to prepare for a panel discussion.

B. Choose a moderator from among your group members. The moderator has to manage speakers and time based on what you have learned in Academic Survival Skill. Other members should take on the roles of the professionals they identified in the Warm-Up Assignment. Practise your panel discussion before speaking in front of the class.

C. Conduct your panel discussion, using what you learned in Focus on Listening (page 170) to clarify others' ideas. Use what you learned in Focus on Speaking (page 181) to share your solutions and respond to others' solutions.

D. During other groups' panel discussions, use the points you learned in Academic Survival Skill to rate other students' performances.

THE STUDENTS WERE ABLE TO	OFTEN	SELDOM	NEVER	THE STUDENTS WERE ABLE TO	OFTEN	SELDOM	NEVER
❶ agree or disagree politely				❻ maintain eye contact			
❷ be open to changing opinions				❼ make clear but brief points			
❸ build on others' ideas				❽ listen to others			
❹ use appropriate body language				❾ encourage others to speak by asking questions			
❺ support opinions with evidence							

E. After all groups have finished their panel discussions, share your observations about how well they covered the points in task D. Ask others for feedback on your panel discussion so you can improve.

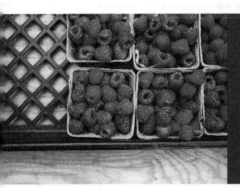

Critical Connections

This chapter focused on the need for food security on an international level. Now, use what you learned in Focus on Critical Thinking (page 171) to explore what you can do at a local level.

What do you know about food banks? They are places where various kinds of foods are stored and freely supplied to those in need. However, they can have many problems.

A. Consider what you know about food banks. Summarize what you know in simple terms to your partner. Also explain what you don't know about food banks. Use an analogy to compare a food bank to something else.

B. Use what you learned in Focus on Speaking (page 181) to think about some of the problems faced by food banks and develop solutions. Ask your partner to take on the role of a food bank manager. Share your solutions to the following problems.

FOOD BANK PROBLEMS	POSSIBLE SOLUTIONS
❶ a lack of healthy food that people need and want	
❷ donations of fresh food that rots before it can be given away, or packaged foods whose expiry date has passed	
❸ a lack of storage when there are too many donations; for example, at holiday times when donors feel more generous	

C. Discuss the ideas, using the language for problems and solutions outlined in Focus on Speaking. If the advice is not acceptable, use what you learned in the Feynman Technique to better understand the topic.

APPENDIX 1
Conversation Gambits

Gambits are commonly understood ways of starting, maintaining, and ending informal and formal conversations in polite ways. Practise the following on your own and with a partner.

GAMBITS	INFORMAL	FORMAL
OFFER GREETINGS	Hi. How are you?	Hello. How are you?
INTRODUCE A TOPIC	I'd like to talk to you about … I've been thinking about …	If you have a moment, I would like to discuss …
EXPLAIN A POINT	Let me explain. Here's the idea. What do you think about …?	Let me suggest … The basic idea is … The important part of the idea is …
CHECK FOR COMPREHENSION	Do you get what I'm saying? Do you follow what I've said so far?	May I ask if you understand my point? Is everything clear so far?
SHOW YOU ARE LISTENING	[frown/nod] Really? Right. Uh-huh. OK.	[frown/nod] Yes. Are you sure?
SHOW AGREEMENT	Yes. I agree. I can't argue with that.	Yes. I agree. That's true. You've made a good point.
INTERRUPT	I'm sorry, … Excuse me, … Pardon me, but … Can I ask a question? Can I add something here?	Sorry for interrupting, but … If I can just interrupt for a moment, … If I could stop you there for a second, …
ASK THE SPEAKER TO REPEAT	Can you say that again? Could you repeat that? What was that? Excuse me? Sorry, what?	I'm not sure I follow. Would you mind repeating that? Pardon me, what did you say? May I ask you to repeat that?
REFUSE INTERRUPTIONS	Please, let me finish. Can I just finish my point? Give me another moment …	Perhaps if you could let me finish. May I just finish my point?
CONTINUE AFTER AN INTERRUPTION	As I was saying, … Let's see, where was I?	To get back to what I was saying, …
DISAGREE POLITELY	That's not true/right, is it? I'd say/think something different …	I'm not sure I agree. I can't say that that's a convincing point/argument.
MAKE A QUALIFICATION	That's not totally what I meant.	Although I agree with …, I also believe …
EXPRESS AN OPINION	In my opinion, … What I think … As I see it, …	My personal opinion is that … I believe that … It's my belief that …
CLARIFY THE SPEAKER'S POINTS BY RESTATING	So, what you mean is … So, what you're trying to say is …	If I can restate, first you state … Then, I understand your point is …
CLARIFY YOUR POINTS BY PARAPHRASING	What I'm trying to say is … What I mean is … In other words, …	To put it another way, … Let me explain it another way …
SUMMARIZE	All in all, what I'm trying to say is … The main points are … To sum up, …	To summarize, … To bring all this together, … In conclusion, …
END THE CONVERSATION	I have to go now, but it's been great talking with you. Thanks for the chance to talk. OK, let's talk soon.	I'm glad we had a chance to talk. Thank you for taking the time to speak with me. I'm sorry to have to stop here.

PHOTO CREDITS

AUDIO AND VIDEO CREDITS

CHAPTER 1

p. 14 "Vanishing Trades in the Digital Age" © Canadian Broadcasting Corporation. p. 21 "One Day in the Life: Six Jobs" © ConnectEd Studios.

CHAPTER 2

p. 36 "The Science of Mindfulness" © Canadian Broadcasting Corporation. p. 42 "Harnessing the Power of Brain Plasticity" © Canadian Broadcasting Corporation.

CHAPTER 3

p. 59 "Brain Hacking" © CBS News. p. 66 "Contagion, Affirmation, and Lies: The Psychology of Social Media" https://www.microsoft.com/en-us/research/video/contagion-affirmation-and-lies-the-psychology-of-social-media/ Used with permission from Microsoft.

CHAPTER 4

p. 84 "Innovation and Its Enemies" © Canadian Broadcasting Corporation. p. 91 "Fake Online Reviews" © Canadian Broadcasting Corporation.

CHAPTER 5

p. 108 "Being a Dog" © Canadian Broadcasting Corporation. p. 114 "Mansbridge One on One: Bob McDonald" © Canadian Broadcasting Corporation.

CHAPTER 6

p. 130 "Weapons of Math Destruction" © Canadian Broadcasting Corporation. p. 137 "Too Much Math, Too Little History" © LSESU Economics Society.

CHAPTER 7

p. 154 "AI and the Fate of Humanity" © Canadian Broadcasting Corporation. p. 160 "AI on the Brink" © CBS News.

CHAPTER 8

p. 178 "The Earth in Human Hands: Shaping Our Planet's Future" © Canadian Broadcasting Corporation. p. 183 "Agriculture and Africa's Promise" © The Chicago Council on Global Affairs.